Lecture Notes: Oncology

Lecture Notes
Oncology

Mark Bower
Professor of Oncology
Chelsea & Westminster Hospital and
Imperial College School of Medicine
London, UK

Jonathan Waxman
Professor of Oncology
Hammersmith Hospital
Imperial College School of Medicine
London, UK

Second Edition

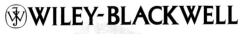

WILEY-BLACKWELL

A John Wiley & Sons, Ltd., Publication

This edition first published 2010, © 2010 by Mark Bower and Jonathan Waxman
Previous editions: 2006

Blackwell Publishing was acquired by John Wiley & Sons in February 2007. Blackwell's publishing program has been merged with Wiley's global Scientific, Technical and Medical business to form Wiley-Blackwell.

Registered office: John Wiley & Sons Ltd, The Atrium, Southern Gate, Chichester, West Sussex, PO19 8SQ, UK

Editorial offices: 9600 Garsington Road, Oxford, OX4 2DQ, UK
              The Atrium, Southern Gate, Chichester, West Sussex, PO19 8SQ, UK
              111 River Street, Hoboken, NJ 07030-5774, USA

For details of our global editorial offices, for customer services and for information about how to apply for permission to reuse the copyright material in this book please see our website at www.wiley.com/wiley-blackwell

Library of Congress Cataloging-in-Publication Data

Bower, Mark.
  Lecture notes: Oncology / Mark Bower, Jonathan Waxman. – 2nd ed.
    p. cm.
  Other title: Oncology
  Includes index.
  ISBN 978-1-4051-9513-3 (pbk.)
1. Cancer–Outlines, syllabi, etc. 2. Oncology–Outlines, syllabi, etc. I. Waxman, Jonathan. II. Title.
III. Title: Oncology.
  [DNLM: 1. Neoplasms. QZ 200 B786L 2010]
  RC254.5.B69 2010
  616.99′4–dc22

                                  2010005587

A catalogue record for this book is available from the British Library.

Set in 8 on 12 pt Stone Serif by Toppan Best-set Premedia Limited
Printed in Singapore by Ho Printing Singapore Pte Ltd.

1   2010

Contents

Colour plate section faces p. 146

v

Preface to the second edition

We are delighted that *Lecture Notes: Oncology* has progressed to a second edition, returning by popular demand with an updated format, enormous revisions and a few poor jokes.

The last decade has seen tremendous changes in oncology, with marvellous developments in targeted therapies, based on an understanding of the molecular biology of cancer. We are at a stage in oncology where death rates have fallen in many cancers, and where the survival for patients with metastatic disease has, in many instances, doubled. Cancer doctors used to proudly talk about curing a small minority of tumours such as lymphoma, leukaemia, choriocarcinoma and testicular cancer, but currently this shortlist of survivable cancers has increased, providing optimism in oncologists and delight in patients.

Oncology involves an understanding of the processes that lead to the development of malignant disease, and this understanding has led Medicine by its nose to the frontiers of science. These are exhilarating times to be an oncologist and we hope that the reader of this book enjoys our efforts to convey our excitement in oncology.

Mark Bower
Jonathan Waxman

Part 1

Introduction to Oncology

Chapter 1

What is cancer?

Cancer is not a single illness but a collection of many diseases that share common features. Cancer is widely viewed as a disease of genetic origin. It is caused by mutations of DNA and epigenetic changes that alter gene expression, which make a cell multiply uncontrollably. However, the description and definitions of cancer vary depending on the perspective as described below.

Epidemiological perspective

Cancer is a major cause of morbidity in the United Kingdom with around 289 000 new cases diagnosed in 2005. There are more than 200 different types of cancer, but four of them (breast, lung, colorectal and prostate) account for over half of all new cases. Overall it is estimated that one in three people will develop some form of cancer during their lifetime. In the 30-year period 1976–2005 the overall age-standardized incidence rates for cancer increased by 35% in men and 16% in women but have remained fairly constant over the last decade (1996–2005). The cancers whose incidence is rising fastest in men are malignant melanoma, mesothelioma, prostate cancer and hepatocellular cancer, while in women they are mesothelioma, melanoma, endometrial cancer and oral cancer.

Cancer incidence refers to the number of new cancer cases arising in a specified period of time. Prevalence refers to the number of people who have received a diagnosis of cancer who are alive at any given time, some of whom will be cured and others will not. Therefore prevalence reflects both the incidence of cancer and its associated survival pattern. In 2008 approximately 3% of the population of the UK (around two million people) are alive having received a diagnosis of cancer. The single cancer that contributes most to the prevalence is breast cancer, with an estimated 550 000 women alive who have had a diagnosis of breast cancer.

Sociological perspective

Patients with cancer adopt a medically sanctioned form of deviant behaviour described in the 1950s by Talcott Parsons as 'the sick role'. In order to be excused their usual duties and to not be considered responsible for their illness, patients are expected to seek professional advice and to adhere to treatments in order to get well. Medical practitioners are empowered to sanction their temporary absence from the workforce and family duties as well as to absolve them of blame. This behavioural model minimizes the impact of illness on society and reduces the secondary gain that the patient benefits from as a consequence of their illness. However, as Ivan Illich pointed out it also sets up physicians as agents of social control by

Lecture Notes: Oncology, 2nd edition. By M. Bower and J. Waxman. Published 2010 by Blackwell Publishing Ltd.

Table 1.1 The top cancer books (in the authors' opinion).

	Title	Author
1	Cancer Ward	Alexander Solzhenitsyn
2	A Very Easy Death	Simone de Beauvoir
3	Age of Iron	J. M. Coetzee
4	Cancer Vixen	Marisa Acocella Marchetto
5	One in Three	Adam Wishart
6	C: Because Cowards get Cancer, Too	John Diamond
7	Before I Say Goodbye	Ruth Picardie
8	Illness as Metaphor	Susan Sontag
9	The Black swan	Thomas Mann
10	Mom's Cancer	Brian Fies
11	Coda	Simon Gray
12	Cancer Tales	Nell Dunn

medicalizing health and contributing to iatrogenic illness – 'a medical nemesis'. Of all the common medical diagnoses, cancer probably carries the greatest stigma and is associated with the most fear. The many different ways in which cancer affects people has been explored in literature (Table 1.1).

Experimental perspective

In the laboratory, a number of characteristics define a cancer cell growing in culture. The four features listed below are used by scientists experimentally to confirm the malignant phenotype of cancer cells:

1. Cancer cells are clonal, having all derived from a single parent cell.
2. Cancer cells grow on soft agar, in the absence of growth factors.
3. Cancer cells cross artificial membranes in culture systems.
4. Cancer cells form tumours if injected into immunodeficient strains of mice (Box 1.1).

Histopathological perspective

Cancer is usually defined by various histopathological features, most notably invasion and metastasis, that are observed by gross pathological and microscopic examinations. Laminin staining of

---

Box 1.1: Onco-mice

Mice have been used as a laboratory model in cancer research for a century. In the 1930s, Sir Ernest Kennaway showed that polycyclic aromatic hydrocarbons were carcinogenic by inducing skin cancers in mice. In 1969 the first inbred mice were developed that were essentially genetically identical except for gender. These strains allowed the transfer of cells and tissues between mice without rejection as they are syngeneic (genetically identical). This has allowed the effects of experimental treatments on murine cancers to be evaluated in laboratory mice. Some inbred strains also spontaneously develop cancers (e.g. BALB/c mice frequently develop lung tumours) so that the effects of cancer prevention strategies can be studied. The development of immunodeficient mice allowed the transfer and study of human cancer cells in mice without the mice rejecting the xenograft (graft between different species). The first immunodeficient mice were 'nude mice', an inbred strain that lacks a thymus gland and T lymphocytes; they are hairless because of a mutation in a linked genetic locus. Subsequently, in 1983, even more immunodeficient SCID (severe combined immunodeficiency) mice were developed that lack both T and B cells. Genetically modified transgenic mice have been manufactured by knocking out specific genes ('knockout mice') or adding extra trans-genes, usually from different species ('transgenic mice'), to embryonic stem cells. These mice are used to elucidate the influence of individual genes on the phenotype. Finally, mice were the original source of monoclonal antibodies produced by immunizing inbred mice with the desired antigen and fusing spleen cells from the mouse with myeloma cells to yield hybridoma cells that produce monoclonal antibodies.

---

the basement membrane may assist the histopathologist in identifying local invasion by tumours that breach the basement membrane. In addition a number of microscopic features point to the diagnosis of cancer:

- Cancer cells differ morphologically from normal cells
- Tumour architecture is less organized than that of the parent tissue
- Cancer cells have increased nuclear DNA and nuclear:cytoplasmic ratio
- Cancer cells have hyperchromatic nuclei with coarsening of chromatin and wrinkled nuclear edges

• Cancer cells may be multinucleated or have macronucleoli

• Cancer cells may have numerous and bizarre mitotic figures

Cancers may be heterogenous with cells of varying sizes and orientation with respect to one another despite their clonal origin.

Molecular perspective

The molecular features that identify a cancer are described in 'Six steps to becoming a cancer' in Chapter 2. These six properties are:

1. Grow without a trigger (self-sufficiency in growth stimuli).

2. Don't stop growing (insensitivity to inhibitory stimuli).

3. Don't die (evasion of apoptosis).

4. Don't age (immortalization).

5. Feed themselves (neoangiogenesis).

6. Spread (invasion and metastasis).

How to read a histology report

The diagnosis of cancer is most commonly established following a histopathological report of a biopsy or tumour resection. A histopathological report should include both gross pathological features (tumour size and number and size of lymph nodes examined) and microscopic findings (tumour grade, architecture, mitotic rate, margin involvement and lymphovascular invasion). The grade and stage of a cancer are important prognostic factors that may influence therapy options (Box 1.2).

Box 1.2: Histopathology definitions

Quantitative changes: too small

Atrophy
Acquired shrinkage due to a decrease in the *size or number* of cells of a tissue, e.g. decrease in size of the ovaries after the menopause.

Quantitative changes: too big

Hypertrophy
Increase in the size of an organ or tissue due to an increase in the *size* of individual cells, e.g. pregnant uterus.

Hyperplasia
Increase in the *size* of an organ due to an increase in the *number* of cells, e.g. lactating breast.

Qualitative changes

Metaplasia
Replacement of one cell type in an organ by another. This implies changes in the differentiation programme and is usually a response to persistent injury. It is reversible so that removal of the source of injury results in reversion to the original cell type, e.g. sqamous metaplasia of laryngeal respiratory epithelium in a smoker. Chronic irritation from smoking causes the normal columnar respiratory epithelium to be replaced by the more resilient squamous epithelium.

Dysplasia
Dysplastic changes are changes in cell type, as for metaplasia, that do not revert to normal once the injury is removed, e.g. cervical dysplasia initiated by human papillomavirus infection persists after eradication of the virus. Dysplasia is usually considered to be part of the spectrum of changes leading to neoplasia.

Invasion
The capacity to infiltrate the surrounding tissues and organs is a characteristic of cancer.

Metastasis
The ability to proliferate in distant parts of the body after tumour cells have been transported by lymph or blood or along body spaces.

Table 1.2 Histological features of benign and malignant tumours.

Features of malignancy	Features of benign tumours
Macroscopic features	
Invade and metastasize	Do not invade or metastasize
Rapid growth	Slow growing
Not clearly demarcated	Clearly demarcated from surrounding tissue
Surface often ulcerated and necrotic	Surface smooth
Cut surface heterogenous	Cut surface homogenous
Microscopic features	
Often high mitotic rate	Low mitotic rate
Nuclei pleomorphic and hyperchromatic	Nuclear morphology often normal
Abnormal mitoses	Mitotic figures normal

A histopathological definition of cancer: is it malignant or benign?

Malignancy is usually characterized by various behavioural features, most notably invasion and metastasis. However, the histopathologist may have to identify a cancer without this information. Cancers are composed of clonal cells (all are the progeny of a single cell) and have lost control of their tissue organization and architecture. In addition to the natural history, a number of physical properties help to distinguish between benign and malignant tumours (Table 1.2). However, there is no single histological feature that defines a cancer nor indeed that separates benign from malignant tumours. In general, benign tumours are rarely life-threatening but may cause health problems on account of their location (by pressure or obstruction of adjacent organs) or by overproduction of hormones. In contrast malignant tumours usually follow a progressive course and unless successfully treated are frequently fatal.

Is it *in situ* or invasive?

Invasive cancers extend into the surrounding stroma (see Plate 1.1). However tumours that exhibit all the microscopic features of cancers but do not breach the original basement membrane are termed *in situ* (non-invasive) cancers. Examples include *in situ* breast cancer confined to the mammary ducts (ductal carcinoma *in situ* or DCIS) or lobules (lobular carcinoma *in situ* or LCIS) (see Plate 1.2). Similar pre-invasive *in situ* cancers have been found in many organs (e.g. cervix, anus, prostate, bronchus) and are believed to represent a stage in the progression from dysplasia to cancer (see Plate 1.3).

Histopathologist's nomenclature: name that cancer

The histopathologists' lexicon often can be a tool for obfuscation, but follow a few simple rules and you can translate their lingo. The suffix -oma usually denotes a benign tumour (although it simply means 'swelling' and some -omas are not tumours, e.g. xanthoma). If a tumour is malignant the suffix -carcinoma (Greek for crab) is used for epithleial cancers or -sarcoma (Greek for flesh) for connective tissue cancers. The prefix is determined by the cells of origin of the tumour (e.g. adeno- for glandular epithelium), qualified by the tissue of origin (e.g. prostatic adenocarcinoma). There are numerous exceptions to this systematic nomenclature; for example leukaemias and lymphomas are malignant tumours of bone marrow and lymphoid tissue, respectively. As a general rule neoplasms are classified according to the type of normal tissue they most closely resemble. The four major categories are: epithelial, connective tissue, lymphoid and haemopoietic tissue, and germ cells (Tables 1.3–1.6). The latter arise in totipotential cells, and can develop into any cell type. Germ cell tumours contain a variety of different mature and/or immature tissues from different embryonic germ layers, and these are given names with the root terato- (Greek for monster). In addition, as with most fields of medicine where physicians try to leave their mark, there are a number of eponymous names (e.g. Hodgkin's disease). (Thomas Hodgkin (of Guy's Hospital) described seven cases in 1832 of the tumour that bears his name but re-examination in 1926 revealed that the diagnosis was inaccurate in four of the seven cases.)

Table 1.3 Nomenclature of epithelial tumours.

Epithelium	Benign tumour	Malignant tumour
Squamous	Squamous papilloma	Squamous carcinoma
Glandular	Adenoma	Adenocarcinoma
Transitional	Transitional papilloma	Transitional carcinoma
Liver	Hepatic adenoma	Hepatocellular carcinoma
Skin	Papilloma	Squamous cell carcinoma
		Basal cell carcinoma
Skin melanocyte	Naevus	Malignant melanoma

Table 1.4 Nomenclature of connective tissue tumours.

Tissue	Benign tumour	Malignant tumour
Bone	Osteoma	Osteosarcoma
Cartilage	Chondroma	Chondrosarcoma
Fat	Lipoma	Liposarcoma
Smooth muscle	Leiomyoma	Leiomyosarcoma
Striated muscle	Rhabdomyoma	Rhabdomyosarcoma
Blood vessel	Angioma	Angiosarcoma
Fibrous tissue	Fibroma	Fibrosarcoma

Table 1.5 Nomenclature of haematological tumours.

Tissue	Malignant tumour
Node lymphocyte	Lymphoma
Marrow lymphocyte	Lymphocytic leukaemia
Granulocyte	Myeloid leukaemia
Plasma cell	Myeloma

Table 1.6 Nomenclature of germ cell tumours.

Tissue	Benign tumour	Malignant tumour (male)	Malignant tumour (female)
Germ cell	Mature teratoma/dermoid cyst	Non-seminomatous germ cell tumour/malignant teratoma	Immature teratoma/embryonal carcinoma
	–	Seminoma	Dysgerminoma

Tumour grading

Tumours are graded according to the degree of tissue differentiation. Cancers that closely resemble their tissue of origin are graded as well differentiated cancers. Cancers that look nothing like the original tissue and have histological features of aggressive growth with high mitotic rates are graded as poorly differentiated cancers. The grade of a tumour is of prognostic significance.

In the case of breast cancer, the Scarff–Bloom–Richardson system is usually used to grade cancers based upon three features: the frequency of cell mitosis, tubule formation, and nuclear pleomorphism. Each of these features is assigned a score ranging from 1 to 3 (1 indicating slower cell growth and 3 indicating faster cell growth). The scores of each of the cells' features are then added together for a final sum that will range between 3 and 9. A tumour with a final sum of 3, 4 or 5 is considered a grade 1 tumour (well differentiated). A sum of 6 or 7 is considered a grade 2 tumour (moderately differentiated), and a sum of 8 or 9 is a grade 3 tumour (poorly differentiated). The five-year overall survival for grades 1, 2 and 3 are 95%, 75% and 50%, respectively.

In addition, pathologists may identify other features that relate to the natural behaviour of a tumour, such as lymphovascular invasion, which usually denotes a worse prognosis. The molecular properties of a cancer can also influence the biology, prognosis and treatment of a tumour. For example, the gene expression prolife of a breast cancer may be determined by gene expression microarray chip technology and the results assist clinicians in optimizing adjuvant therapy (see Plate 1.4).

Unknown primary identification (standard histological techniques)

Occasionally patients present with metastatic cancer without an obvious primary tumour site and, in addition to a careful clinical and radiological examination, the pathologist may provide a clue to the origins of the cancer. Most unknown primary cancers are adenocarcinoma (60%), and the remainder are poorly differentiated carcinomas (30%) and squamous cell carcinomas (5%). Light microscopy may provide pointers, for example the presence of melanin pigment favours melanoma, whilst mucin production is common in gastrointestinal, breast and lung cancers but less common in ovarian cancers and is rare in renal cell and thyroid cancers. Immunocytochemical staining of tissue samples can aid the pathologist in tissue identification. For example, the presence of oestrogen and progesterone receptors favours a diagnosis of breast cancer, whilst prostate-specific antigen and prostatic acid phosphatase staining points to prostatic adenocarcinoma. Similarly, cytokeratin expression patterns may provide helpful hints about the origin of metastatic cancers (Box 1.3 and see Plate 1.5). Cell surface immunophenotyping is a sophistication of immunocy-

---

Box 1.3: Cytokeratins

Cytokeratins are intermediate filament proteins expressed in pairs comprising a type I (cytokeratins 9–20) and a type II (cytokeratins 1–8) cytokeratin. Different tissues express different pairs and immunocytochemical staining for cytokeratins can help identify the likely tissue origins of cancers cells. For example in disseminated peritoneal metastases, CK7 expression favours an ovarian origin, whilst lack of CK7 is more common in colorectal cancer (Figure 1.3).

---

tochemistry that is frequently applied to haematological malignancies. The pattern of immunoglobulin, T-cell receptor and cluster designation (CD) antigen expression on the surface of lymphomas is helpful in their diagnosis and classification. Immunophenotyping can be achieved by immunohistochemical staining, immunofluorescent staining or flow cytometry.

Unknown primary identification (special histological techniques)

The study of intracellular organelles by electron microscopy may identify the cellular origin of a tumour; for example, the presence of melanosomes in melanomas and dense core neurosecretory granules in neuroendodermal tumours. Further laboratory techniques to aid diagnosis include molecular studies of DNA rearrangements that characterize malignancies. Monoclonal immunoglobulin gene rearrangements are present in B-cell malignancies and rearrangements of T-cell receptors occur in T-cell tumours. In addition, a number of chromosomal translocations involving the immunoglobulin genes (heavy chain on chromosome 14q32, light chains on 2p12 and 22q11) and T-cell receptor genes (TCRα on 14q11, TCRβ on 7q35, TCRγ on 7p15, TCRδ on 14q11) occur in malignancies arising from these cell types. For instance, low-grade follicular lymphomas rearrange the Bcl-2 gene on 18q21 (e.g. t(14;18)(q32;q21)), most Burkitt lymphomas rearrange the Myc gene on 8q24 (e.g. t(8;14)(q24;q32)) and most mantle cell lymphomas rearrange Bcl-1 on 11q13 (e.g. t(11;14)(q13;q32)). These rearrangements may be detected by karyotype analysis of mitotic chromosome preparations or by molecular techniques including Southern blotting and polymerase chain reaction (Box 1.4 and Table 1.7). Less commonly these same methods may assist the diagnosis of solid tumours that are associated with specific chromosomal abnormalities such as the i(12p) isochromosome found in germ cell tumours and the t(11;22)(q24;q12) translocation seen in Ewing's sarcoma and peripheral neuroectodermal tumours. In addition to translocations, gene amplification may be detected and may have prognostic

Box 1.4: The language of chromosomes – karyotype nomenclature

Each arm of a chromosome is divided into one to four major regions, depending on chromosomal length; each band, positively or negatively stained, is given a number, which rises as the distance from the centromere increases. The normal male is designated as 46,XY and the normal female as 46,XX.

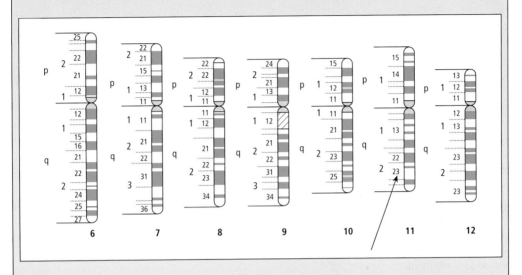

For example, 11q23 designates the chromosome (11), the long arm (q), the second region distal to the centromere (2) and the third band (3) in that region.

Polyploid
Cell with more than one complete chromosome set or with multiples of the basic number of chromosomes characteristic of the species; in humans this would be 69,92, etc.

Aneuploid
Individual with one or more chromosomes in addition or missing from the complete chromosome set; for example trisomy 21 (47,XX +21).

Deletion
The loss of a chromosome segment from a normal chromosome.

Duplication
An extra piece of chromosome segment which may be attached to the same homologous chromosome or transposed to another chromosome in the genome.

Inversion
A change in linear sequence of the genes in a chromosome that results in the reverse order of genes in a chromosome segment. Inversions may be pericentric (two breaks on either side of the centromere) or paracentric (both breaks on the same arm).

Isochromosome
breaks in one arm of a chromosome followed by duplication of the other arm of the chromosome to produce a chromosome with two arms that are both short (p) or both long (q) arms.

Translocations
Translocations are the result of the reciprocal exchange of terminal segments of non-homologous chromosomes.

Table 1.7 Examples of chromosomal abnormalities in cancers.

Chromosome defect	Karyotype	Tumour	Candidate gene
Monosomy	45,XY −22	Meningioma	NF2
Trisomy	47,XX +7	Papillary renal carcinoma	MET
Deletion	46,XY del(11)(p13)	Wilms' tumour	WT1
Duplication	46,XX dup(2)(p23-24)	Neuroblastoma	n-Myc
Inversion	46,XY inv(16)(p13q22)	Acute myeloid leukaemia (M4Eo)	MYH11/core-binding factor b
Isochromosome	47,XX i(12p)	Testicular germ cell tumour	
Translocation	46,XX t(9;22)(q34;q11)	Chronic myeloid leukaemia	bcr/abl

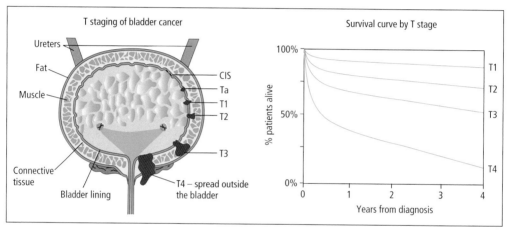

Figure 1.1 T-stage classification for bladder cancer and influence on survival. CIS, carcinoma *in situ*.

significance, e.g. the amplification of the n-Myc oncogene in neuroblastoma is an adverse prognostic variable.

How to stage a tumour

In addition to the histological grade of a tumour, an important criterion in treatment decisions and the major determinant of outcome is the extent of spread or stage of a cancer (Figure 1.1). Staging a tumour is essentially an anatomical exercise that uses a combination of clinical examination and radiology. A uniform staging system is employed for most tumour sites that is based upon the size of the primary **T**umour, the presence of regional lymph **N**odes and of distant **M**etastases. The details of this **TNM** classification vary between different tumour sites. As always there are exceptions, including the staging system for lymphomas that was originally set out following a conference at the University of Michigan in Ann Arbour. It is known as the Ann Arbour Staging System and most radiologists assume that it is named after a person rather than a town, so this is a chance to score points at the X-ray meetings.

Radiology techniques

Staging depends to a large extent upon radiology and this is the most commonly used tool to evaluate the response of cancers to therapies. Anatomical imaging by plain films, computed tomography (CT), ultrasound and magnetic resonance imaging (MRI) are the standard methods. Using the correct terms impresses other clinicians and may make a trip to the radiology department less daunting for junior doctors requesting an investigation. X-rays measure radiodensity (radiolucency and radio-opacity) and ultrasound measures echogenicity and echoreflectivity, whilst CT scans report attenuation values measured in Hounsfield units and MRI reports signal intensity.

Computed tomography

CT scanning is the production of three-dimensional images using X-rays that have been directed through tissues and the images produced depend on the density of the tissues. CT was developed in the 1970s by Sir Godfrey Hounsfield and Allan McLeod Cormack who shared the Nobel Prize in 1979. The first CT scanner built at EMI Central Research Laboratories is said to have been funded by the success of the Beatles who were signed to the EMI label. CT measures the attenuation of different tissues to ionizing radiation and calculates a mean value for a volume of tissue known as a voxel. This is displayed on a two-dimensional image as a single pixel. The attenuation is calculated relative to water which has a Hounsfield unit (HU) value of 0, so high attenutation tissues have a positive HU value (e.g. bone +400 HU) and low attenuation tissues a negative HU value (e.g. fat −120 HU). Different window settings are used to look at different ranges of the Hounsfield greyscale. For example, in the bone windows setting the lungs will look uniformly black whilst in the lung windows the bones look uniformly white. Intravenous iodinated contrast agents improve the sensitivity and specificity of CT but are contraindicated in patients with asthma or allergies to contrast.

Magnetic resonance imaging

Unlike CT, MRI does not use ionizing radiation but instead a powerful magnetic field aligns the spin of protons, especially hydrogen atom protons, in water and fat. A radiofrequency pulse then energizes the protons and the gradual release of this energy from the protons as they relax back to their original magnetic alignment may be detected as radiofrequency signals. The signal intensity relates to the concentration of mobile hydrogen nuclei in tissues. T1 (longitudinal relaxation or spin-lattice) and T2 (transverse relaxation or spin-spin) relaxation time constants depend on the physical properties of the tissues. If you want to impress the neuroradiologists (not always a useful ploy in the authors' experience), water such as cerebrospinal fluid (CSF) is black (low signal intensity) on T1 images and white (high signal intensity) on T2 images (Figure 1.2). Whilst CT is a good tool to examine tissues composed of high atomic weight elements such as bone, MRI is better suited to non-calcified tissues. For similar reasons CT contrast agents usually are composed of high atomic number atoms such as iodine or barium, whilst MRI contrast agents such as gadolinium are paramagnets that have magnetic properties only in the presence of an externally applied magnetic field. MRI is generally superior for imaging the brain, whilst CT is better for solid tumours of the chest and abdomen as it is faster and generates fewer motion artifacts. MRI is also better suited to patients who may require many examinations because it does not carry the risks of ionizing radiation. MRI is, however, contraindicated in patients with metallic objects such as pacemakers *in situ* and it is also quite claustrophobic and noisy in the scanner.

Positron emission tomography

Positron emission tomography (PET) is a functional imaging modality that detects γ-rays emitted by positrons (positively charged electrons) emitting radionuclide tracers. Positrons have a short half-life and are generated by cyclotrons. Common positron-labelled radionuclides include fluorine (^{18}F), carbon (^{11}C), oxygen (^{15}O) and nitrogen (^{13}N). In oncology the most frequently used tracer is ^{18}F-fluorodeoxyglucose (FDG), a short half-life glucose analogue that is taken up into actively metabolizing cells including cancer cells and following intracellular phosphorylation is trapped in these cells. Hence the distribution in the body of

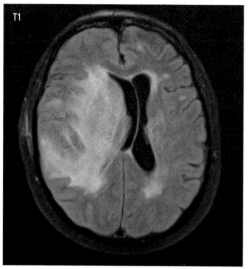 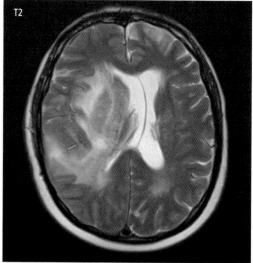

Figure 1.2 T1 and T2 MRI scan images of a primary cerebral lymphoma mass, showing a large right basal ganglia lesion with midline shift, compression of the right lateral ventricle and peritumoral oedema. In the T1 image the CSF is black (low attenuation) and the bone is white (high attenuation), whilst in the T2 image the CSF is white (high attenuation) and the bone is black (low attenuation).

FDG reflects glucose uptake within the body. This means that PET scanning may differentiate between residual masses and active disease in lymphoma. As a consequence FDG-PET scanning is used in both staging and monitoring cancer treatment (Figure 1.3 and see Plate 1.6).

Radio-isotope scanning

In addition to PET scanning other functional images may be used in the diagnosis and staging of specific cancers, using isotope-labelled radionuclide tracer elements (Table 1.8 and Figure 1.4). The isotope-labelled tracers that are used diagnostically may also be used therapeutically. Bone scintigraphy uses bisphosphonates labelled with ^{99}Tc and is more sensitive than X-rays for detecting metastases.

Performance status

In addition to the histological grade and the stage of a cancer, the general health of patients will determine how long they survive and may influence treatment decisions. Scales that measure the performance status or functional capacity of patients include the ECOG (Eastern Co-operative Oncology Group) grading system and the Karnovsky scale (Table 1.9). The performance status, however estimated, is an important prognostic indicator for almost all tumour types.

Prognosis: it's not cancer is it doc?

Although a very significant stigma is attached to the diagnosis of cancer, for most of the general population the fear outweighs the reality and comparison with other more palatable illnesses yield results that are not always expected (Table 1.10).

Cancer epidemiology

Epidemiology in UK

Cancer is now the commonest cause of death in the UK (if cardiovascular and cerebrovascular diseases are classed separately).

- One in three people in the UK will develop a cancer (289 000/year)
- One in four die of cancer (150 000/year).

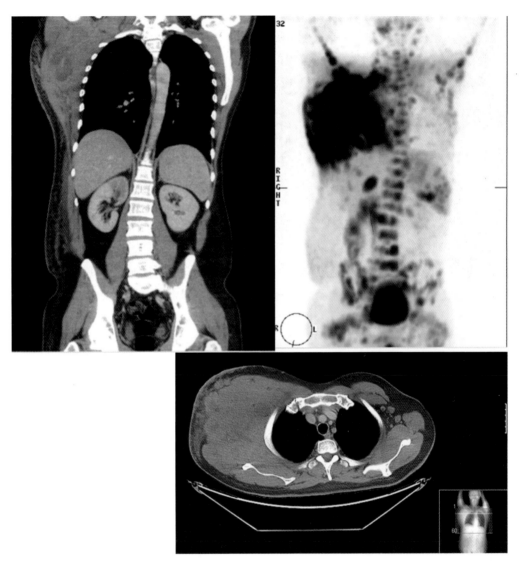

Figure 1.3 Coronal CT (top left), transverse CT (below) and FDG-PET (top right) scans demonstrating a huge right axillary and anterior chest wall mass due to Burkitt lymphoma. The FDG-PET also demonstrates extensive involvement of the other nodal groups, bones and right kidney upper pole (stage 4B).

Table 1.8 Commonly used isotopes in nuclear imaging in oncology.

Isotope	Half-life	Tracer	Oncological use
^{99}Tc (technetium)	6 hours	Methylene diphosphonate (MDP)	Bone scan
^{111}In (indium)	67 hours	Octreotide	Neuroendocrine tumours
^{131}I (iodine)	8 days	Sodium iodide	Thyroid cancer
^{131}I (iodine)	8 days	Meta-iodobenzylguanidine (MIBG)	Phaeochromocytoma neuroblastoma
^{67}Ga (gallium)	68 hours	Gallium citrate	Lymphoma

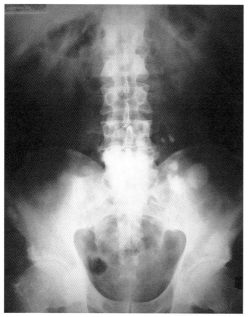

LT

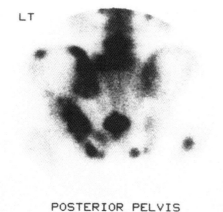

POSTERIOR PELVIS

Figure 1.4 Plain pelvic radiograph (above) and corresponding area of technetium pyrophosphate bone scan (below) of a patient with sclerotic bone metastases from prostate cancer.

The top ten cancers diagnosed in the UK excluding non-melanomatous skin cancers are shown in Table 1.11.

Global epidemiology

The incidence of different types of cancer varies geographically according to the risk factors and demographics of the local population (Figure 1.5). However, there is a general correlation between

Table 1.9 Functional capacity grading (ECOG) and Karnovsky performance scales.

ECOG functional capacity grading

0	Asymptomatic
1	Symptomatic but fully ambulant
2	Symptomatic, ambulant >50% waking hours
3	Symptomatic, confined to bed >50% waking hours
4	Symptomatic, bedfast

Karnovsky performance status score (%)

100	Normal; no complaints; no evidence of disease
90	Able to carry on normal activity; minor signs or symptoms
80	Normal activity with effort; some signs or symptoms
70	Care for self; unable to carry on normal activity or do active work
60	Requires occasional assistance, but able to care for most of needs
50	Requires considerable assistance and frequent medical care
40	Disabled; requires special care and assistance
30	Severely disabled; hospitalization indicated but death not imminent
20	Very sick; hospitalization necessary; active supportive treatment necessary
10	Moribund; fatal processes progressing rapidly

Table 1.10 Survival rates for various diseases.

	Myocardial infarction	Hodgkin's disease	Heart failure (NYHA III/IV)	Metastatic breast cancer
1-year survival rate	75%	90%	50%	60%
5-year survival rate	45%	85%	15%	20%

NYHA, New York Heart Association grading scale.

increasing wealth and increasing cancer incidence. This is attributable to tobacco use, diet and increased longevity in wealthy populations. There are intriguing exceptions, for example the Gulf states of Kuwait, Qatar, Bahrain, United Arab Emirates and Saudi Arabia have lower cancer incidences

Table 1.11 The 12 most common cancers diagnosed in UK.

Tumour	As percentage of all cancers diagnosed
Breast	15%
Lung	13%
Colorectal	13%
Prostate	12%
Non-Hodgkin's lymphoma	3.6%
Bladder	3.5%
Melanoma	3.3%
Stomach	2.7%
Oesophageal	2.7%
Pancreas	2.6%
Kidney	2.5%
Leukaemia	2.5%

than would be predicted from their per capita gross national product.

Cancer charities

Cancer charities

The UK has 640 cancer charities to counter the disease. Their expenditure increases awareness of cancer, improves diagnosis and treatment capability, and provides care for patients with the disease. The total income generated by the top 20 UK cancer charities in 2004 was £758m, and the average charitable efficiency was 64% providing £488m for spending on patients' care and research. The two largest UK cancer charities, the Imperial Cancer Research Fund (ICRF) and the Cancer Research Campaign (CRC) merged to form Cancer Research UK (CRUK) in 2002. CRUK is the largest volunteer-supported cancer research organization in the world, with 3000 scientists and an annual scientific spend of more than £339 million – raised almost entirely through public donations.

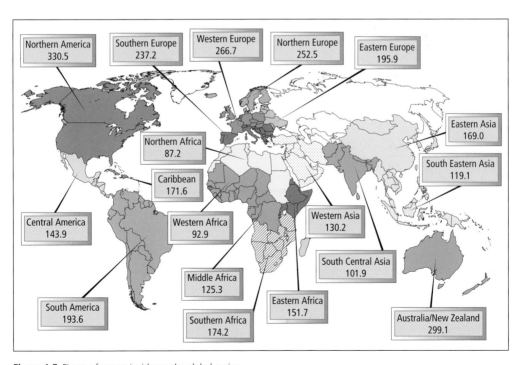

Figure 1.5 Figure of cancer incidences by global region.

Table 1.12 Rock star cancer deaths.

	Year of death	Age	Cause of death
Richard Wright (Pink Floyd)	2008	65	Cancer (type undisclosed)
Eartha Kitt	2008	81	Colon cancer
Johnny Ramone	2004	55	Prostate cancer
Little Eva	2003	60	Cervical cancer
George Harrison	2001	58	Non-small cell lung cancer
Joey Ramone	2001	49	Non-Hodgkin's lymphoma
Ian Dury	2000	58	Colorectal cancer
Dusty Springfield	1999	60	Breast cancer
Carl Wilson (Beach Boys)	1998	52	Lung cancer
Eva Cassidy	1996	33	Melanoma
Frank Zappa	1993	53	Prostate cancer
Freddy Mercury	1991	45	Kaposi's sarcoma
Mel Appleby (Mel & Kim)	1990	24	Spinal tumour
Bob Marley	1981	36	Melanoma

Cancer hospitals

Philanthropists and social reformers during the 19th century tried to provide free medical care for the poor. William Marsden, a young surgeon opened a dispensary for advice and medicines in 1828. His grandly named London General Institution for the Gratuitous Cure of Malignant Diseases – a simple four-storey house in one of the poorest parts of the city – was conceived as a hospital to which the only passport should be poverty and disease and where treatment was provided free of charge. The demand for Marsden's free services was overwhelming and by 1844 his dispensary, now called the Royal Free Hospital, was treating 30 000 patients a year. In 1846 when his wife died of cancer, Marsden opened a small house in Cannon Row, Westminster, for patients suffering from cancer. Within 10 years the institution moved to Fulham Road and became known as the Cancer Hospital, of which Marsden was the senior surgeon. The hospital was incorporated into the National Health Service in 1948 and renamed the Royal Marsden Hospital in 1954. Although other cancer hospitals have been established in Manchester (the Christie Hospital) and Glasgow (the Beatson Hospital), the Royal Marsden Hospital remains the most renown. With the recent emphasis on multi-disciplinary approaches to cancer, single specialty hospitals are less in vogue and the majority of cancer departments are within large teaching hospitals.

Cancer celebrities

Celebrities influence public perceptions and behaviour inordinately and this is as true in oncology as elsewhere. Celebrities with cancer have contributed in three main ways: personal accounts bring patients' experiences into the limelight, reports of celebrity patients increase public awareness and may encourage health-seeking behaviour such as stopping smoking, and celebrity patients may support cancer charities and encourage donations. Prominent examples of patient's perspectives include John Diamond's account in *C: Because Cowards get Cancer, Too* and Ruth Picardie's *Before I Say Goodbye*, both moving accounts by accomplished journalists. Celebrity patients can influence the treatment choices that the public make. Following Nancy Reagan's mastectomy for localized breast cancer in 1987, there was a 25% fall in American women choosing breast-conserving surgery over mastectomy. Her husband's successful surgery for Dukes' B colon cancer whilst president in 1984 increased awareness and propelled the warning signs of colon cancer into the media. Similarly, the diagnosis and death from cervical cancer in 2009 of Jade Goody, a *Big Brother* celebrity, led to an increased uptake of cervical cancer screening especially amongst young women in the UK. Successful cancer treatment is often most widely publicized and no article describing Lance Armstrong's seven consecutive Tour de France cycling victories is complete without a mention of his treatment for metastatic non-seminomatous germ cell tumour and his two children conceived with stored sperm banked prior to chemotherapy.

Other celebrity patients have used their wealth and fame to establish and support charitable projects to support cancer research and treatment including Bob Champion, the steeple chase jockey treated for testicular cancer in the 1979, and Roy Castle, a life-long non-smoker who was diagnosed with lung cancer in 1992. Of course, no one is immune to cancer; even rock stars whose deaths are more traditionally associated with suicide and substance abuse (Table 1.12).

Chapter 2

The scientific basis of cancer

Six steps to becoming a cancer

At a molecular level cancer cells are characterized by six acquired biological properties:

1. Self-sufficiency in growth stimuli (keep on doubling).
2. Insensitivity to inhibitory stimuli (don't stop doubling).
3. Evasion of apoptosis (don't die).
4. Immortalization (don't age).
5. Neoangiogenesis (feed themselves).
6. Invasion and metastasis (spread).

It is not certain, but probable, that all six features are necessary to a greater or lesser extent for a cell to posses malignant behaviour (Figure 2.1). Some single molecular changes in cancer cells may produce more than one of the six attributes (e.g. mutations of p53 may cause both avoidance of apoptosis and insensitivity to inhibitory stimuli). A number of mechanisms may contribute to the acquisition of these six properties, including genomic instability as a consequence of deficient DNA repair or loss of cell cycle arrest/death in response to DNA damage as well as epigenetic dysregulation of gene expression.

Lecture Notes: Oncology, 2nd edition. By M. Bower and J. Waxman. Published 2010 by Blackwell Publishing Ltd.

1. Autonomous growth signals

The instruction to a cell to grow and start dividing is communicated by extracellular growth factor ligands that bind to cell surface receptors. This usually results in the reversible phosphorylation of tyrosine, threonine or serine amino acid residues of the receptor. The transfer of these molecular switches from activated phosphorylated receptors to downstream signalling enzyme effectors and then to non-enzymatic second messengers in the cytoplasm and finally to nuclear transcription activators, is known as signal transduction (Figure 2.2). This cascade results in amplification of the initial stimulus. Cancers achieve self-sufficiency in growth factors and do not depend on these extracellular ligands for continued growth. The majority of dominant oncogenes act on this signal transduction mechanism by one of the following mechanisms:

- Overproducing growth factors, e.g. glioblastomas produce platelet-derived growth factor (PDGF)
- Overproducing growth factor receptors, e.g. epidermal growth factor receptor (EGFR/erbB) overexpression in breast cancers
- Mutations of the receptor or components of the signalling cascade that are constitutively active, e.g. mutations of Ras in lung and colonic cancers.

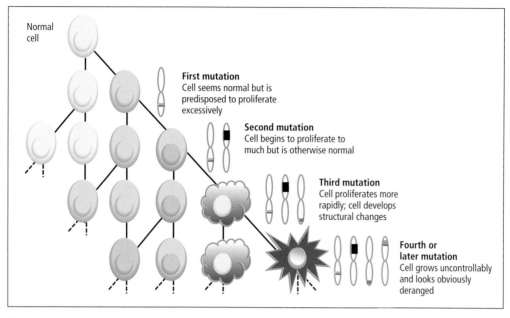

Figure 2.1 Stepwise accumulation of genetic mutations contributing to oncogenic phenotype.

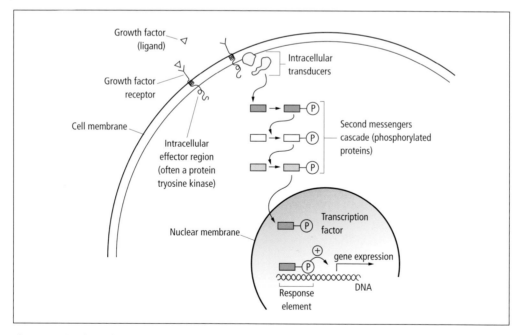

Figure 2.2 Signal transduction pathway.

2. Insensitivity to cell cycle checkpoints

Many normal cells grow throughout their lifespan and the co-ordination of their growth, differentiation, senescence and death is controlled by the cell cycle. Antiproliferative signals may be received by cells as soluble growth inhibitors or fixed inhibitors in the extracellular matrix. They act on the cell cycle clock (Box 2.1), most frequently arresting transit through G1 into S phase. Cancer cells ignore these stop signals.

The co-ordination of the cell cycle and its arrest at checkpoints in response to DNA damage is achieved by sequential activation of kinase enzymes that ultimately phosphorylate and dephosphorylate the retinoblastoma protein (Rb). Periodic activation of these cyclin–cyclin-dependent kinase (CDK) complexes drives the cell cycle

---

Box 2.1: The cell cycle

There are five cell cycle phases:
- **Quiescent phase (G0)**: Normal cells grown in culture will stop proliferating once they become confluent or are deprived of growth factors, and enter a quiescent state called G0. Most cells in normal tissue of adults are in a G0 state.
- **First gap phase (G1)** (duration 10–14 hours): This occurs prior to DNA synthesis. Cells in G0 and G1 are receptive to growth signals but once they have passed a restriction point (R), are committed to DNA synthesis (S phase).
- **Synthesis phase (S)** (duration 3–6 hours): During this phase DNA replication occurs and the cell becomes diploid.
- **Second gap phase (G2)** (duration 2–4 hours): This occurs after DNA synthesis and before mitosis (M) and completion of the cell cycle.
- **Mitosis (M)** (duration 1 hour).
  Cell division completes the cell cycle.

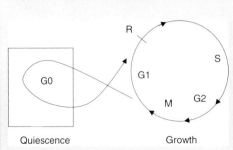

Quiescence   Growth

---

forward (Figure 2.3). Phosphorylation of Rb releases E2F, a transcription factor which is then able to promote the expression of a number of target genes resulting in cell proliferation. The brakes that balance this system are CDK inhibitors (CKIs). Interference in elements of the cell cycle regulatory process is a common theme in malignancy (see Table 2.2).

G1/S checkpoint

An important checkpoint or restriction point in the cell cycle occurs in G1 to ensure that errors in DNA are not replicated but instead are either repaired or that the cell dies by apoptosis. This is initiated by damaged DNA and is co-ordinated by p53, the gene that is probably most commonly mutated in cancers overall. Additional checkpoints are present in the S and G2 phases to allow cells to repair errors that occur during DNA duplication and thus prevent the propagation of these errors to daughter cells.

3. Evasion of apoptosis

Apoptosis is a pre-programmed sequence of cell suicide that occurs over 30–120 minutes. Apoptosis commences with condensation of cellular organelles and swelling of the endoplasmic reticulum. The plasma membrane remains intact but the cell breaks up into several membrane-bound apoptotic bodies, which are phagocytosed. Confining the process within the cell membrane reduces activation of both inflammatory and immune responses, so that programmed cell death does not cause autoimmune disease or inflammation. Amongst the molecules that control apoptosis are the Bcl-2 family that confusingly includes both pro-apoptosis members (e.g. Bax) and anti-apoptosis members (e.g. Bcl-2).

In mammalian cells two pathways initiate apoptosis (Figure 2.4):

1. **Intracellular triggers:** DNA damage leads via p53 to activation of pro-apoptotic members of the Bcl-2 family. This causes release of cytochrome c from mitochondria, which in turn activates the caspase (**c**leaves after **asp**artate prote**ase**) cascade.

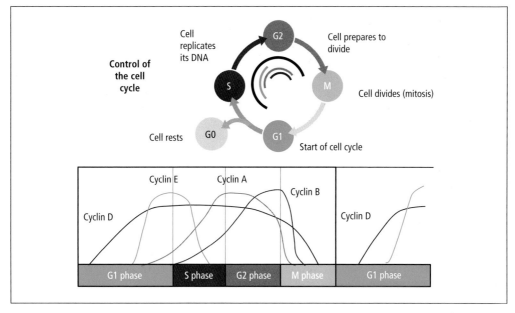

Figure 2.3 Oscillating levels of cyclins through the phases of the cell cycle.

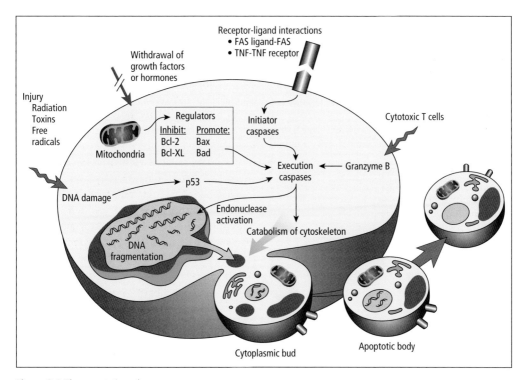

Figure 2.4 The apoptotic pathway.

2. **Extracellular triggers:** Binding of extracellular ligands to the cell surface death receptor superfamily (including CD95/Fas and tumour necrosis factor receptors) leads to a death-inducing cytoplasmic signalling complex that activates the caspase cascade.

Ultimately both pathways activate the caspase cascade, a series of protease enzymes that result in cell apoptosis. Evasion of this pathway is a prerequisite for malignant cell proliferation and a number of strategies to this end have been identified (see Table 2.2).

4. Immortalization

In culture, cells can divide a limited number of times, up to the 'Hayflick limit' (60–70 doublings in the case of human cells in culture), before the cell population enters crisis and dies off. This senescence is attributed to progressive telomere loss, which acts as a mitotic clock (Figure 2.5). Telomeres are the end segments of chromosomes and are made up of thousands of copies of a short 6 base pair sequence (TTAGGG). DNA replication always follows a 5′ to 3′ direction so that manufacturing the 3′ ends of the chromosomes cannot be achieved by DNA polymerases and each time a cell replicates its DNA ready for cell division, 50–100 base pairs are lost from the ends of chromosomes. Eventually the protective ends of chromosomes are eroded and end-to-end chromosomal fusions occur with karyotypic abnormalities and death of the affected cell.

Normal germ cells and cancer cells avoid this senescence, acquiring immortality in culture usually by upregulating the expression of human telomerase reverse transcriptase (hTERT) enzyme, which uses an RNA template and RNA-dependent DNA polymerase to add the 6 base pair sequence back onto the ends of chromosomes to compensate for the bases lost during DNA replication (see Table 2.2). Dyskeratosis congenita is an inherited condition, characterized by many abnormalities, including premature ageing and an increased risk of skin and gut cancers. It is due to mutations of components of the telomerase complex including the telomerase RNA and dyskerin.

5. Angiogenesis

All tissues including cancers require a supply of oxygen and nutrients. For cancers to grow larger

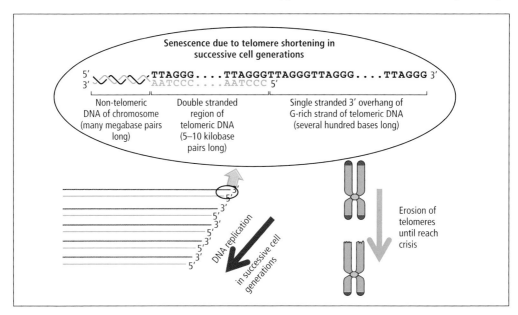

Figure 2.5 With every round of cell replication the chromosomes become shorter due to loss of the telomere repeats. Eventually this encroaches on the non-telomeric DNA of the chromosome and the cell enters crisis and dies.

Table 2.1 The angiogenic switch of angiogenic factors and inhibitors.

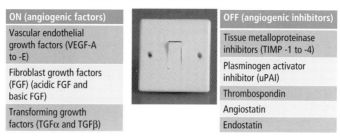

ON (angiogenic factors)	OFF (angiogenic inhibitors)
Vascular endothelial growth factors (VEGF-A to -E)	Tissue metalloproteinase inhibitors (TIMP -1 to -4)
Fibroblast growth factors (FGF) (acidic FGF and basic FGF)	Plasminogen activator inhibitor (uPAI)
	Thrombospondin
Transforming growth factors (TGFα and TGFβ)	Angiostatin
	Endostatin

than about 0.4 mm in diameter, a new blood supply is needed to deliver these. The growth of new blood vessels from pre-existing vasculature is termed angiogenesis. The 'angiogenic switch' denotes the ability of tumours to recruit new blood vessels by producing growth factors and is necessary for tumour growth and metastasis. Angiogenesis is determined by the relative balance of angiogenesis promoters and inhibitors (Table 2.1).

Vascular endothelial growth factors (VEGF-A to -E) are a family of growth factor homodimers that act via one of three plasma membrane receptors (VEGFR-1 to -3) on endothelial cells. Overproduction of VEGF and/or FGF (fibrobast growth factor) is a common theme in many tumours (see Table 2.2). Angiogenesis may be measured microscopically as microvessel density in an area of tumour, or by assays of angiogenic factors. These measures are of prognostic significance in several human tumours. Angiogenesis is becoming a major focus of anticancer drug development. It is an attractive target for several reasons. Angiogenesis is a normal process in growth and development but is quiescent in adult life except during wound healing and menstruation, so side effects are predicted to be minimal. As the target will be normal endothelial cells without any genetic instability, there should be little capacity to acquire resistance. Each capillary supplies a large number of tumour cells, so the effects should be magnified in terms of tumour cell kill. Anti-angiogenic agents should have easy access to their target through the blood stream. In combination, these elements make anti-angiogenic therapies attractive and several pharmaceutical companies have invested heavily in attempts to develop these agents. Bevacizumab is a

monoclonal antibody that binds VEGF; it was originally licensed for use in colon cancer and is also a valuable treatment for age-related macular degeneration, which is caused by retinal vessel proliferation.

6. Invasion and metastasis

The properties of tissue invasion and metastatic spread are the histopathological hallmarks of malignant cancers that discriminate them from benign (see Plate 2.1). A number of sequential steps have been identified in the process of metastatic spread of cancers:

1. Motility and invasion from the primary site.
2. Embolism and circulation in lymph or blood.
3. Arrest in a distant vascular or lymphatic capillary and adherence to the endothelium.
4. Extravasation into the target organ parenchyma.

Central to many of these steps is the role of cell–cell adhesion that controls the contact between cells, and cell–extracellular matrix connections that influence the relationship between a cell and its environment. These interactions are regulated by cell adhesion molecules. Members of the cadherin and immunoglobulin superfamilies modulate cell–cell interactions whilst integrins control cell–extracellular matrix interactions. Alterations of cadherin, adhesion molecule and integrin expression are a common feature of metastatic cancer cells (see Table 2.2).

Tumours may migrate as single cells or as collections of cells. The former strategy is used by lymphoma and small cell lung cancer cells. It requires changes in integrins that mediate the

Box 2.2: How cancers metastasize: routes and destinations

Routes of metastasis

Breast cancer cells that leave a primary tumour in blood vessels will be carried in the blood first through the heart and then to the capillary beds of the lungs. Some cancer cells might form metastases in the lung (Figure 2.6) whilst others pass through the lung to enter the systemic arterial system, where they are transported to remote organs, such as bone. By contrast, colon cancer cells will be taken by the hepatoportal circulatory system first to the liver. There is no direct flow from the lymphatic system to other organs, so cancer cells within it – for example, melanoma cells – must enter the venous system to be transported to distant organs. Rarely, routes other than blood and lymphatic vessels are used in metastasis. Transcoelomic spread across the abdominal cavity occurs for gastric tumours that metastasize to the ovaries (known as Krukenberg tumours). Spread within the cerebrospinal fluid is thought to be responsible for the metastasis of medulloblastoma up and down the spinal column.

Where cancers metastasise

Certain cancers tend to metastasize to particular organs and this cannot be accounted for by blood flow alone. The basis for this tissue tropism has been found to relate to chemokine and chemokine receptor expression. Breast cancer cells express high levels of the CXCR4 chemokine receptor. Lung tissue expresses high levels of a soluble ligand for the CXCR4 receptor. Therefore, breast cancer cells that are taken to the lung find a strong chemokine receptor 'match', which may lead to chemokine-mediated signal activation. By contrast, in other organs where breast cancers less commonly metastasize, there are low levels of the ligand.

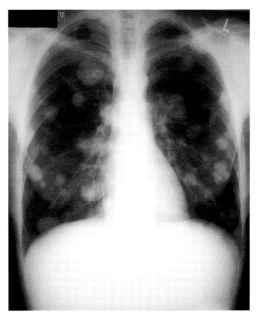

Figure 2.6 Plain chest radiograph showing multiple rounded metastases of varying sizes in a man with a metastatic testicular non-seminomatous germ cell tumour. Other tumours that commonly metastasize to the lungs include lung, breast, renal and thyroid cancers and sarcomas.

Figure 2.7). A number of mechanisms are in place to prevent cells acquiring all six properties, including efficient mechanisms to correct errors in DNA and to eradicate cells with extensive DNA damage. In fact, DNA mutation is facilitated in cancer cells by error-prone DNA replication (mutator phenotype), including deficient DNA repair leading to genetic instability, and uncoupling of the DNA damage cell cycle arrest/apoptosis response.

Genome instability

DNA damage or mutation will normally result in cell cycle arrest followed by DNA repair or apoptosis. Interference in this process may occur either by deficient DNA damage recognition and repair, or abnormal gatekeeping of the cell cycle arrest/apoptosis response. This will result in the uncorrected accumulation of a large number of genetic abnormalities, which is referred to as 'genomic instability'. It is thought that this allows cells to acquire

cell–extracellular matrix interaction and matrix-degrading proteases. Metastatic migration as clumps of cancer cells is common for most epithelial tumours. In addition, this needs changes in cell–cell adhesion through cadherins and other adhesion receptors, as well as cell–cell communication via gap junctions.

How to acquire the six capabilities

Cancer is a somatic genetic disease caused by DNA mutations and epigenetic changes (Table 2.2 and

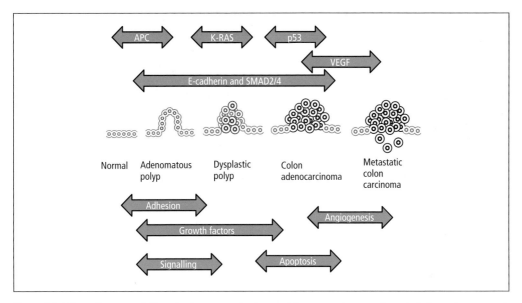

Figure 2.7 Schematic representation of colon cancer development from normal mucosa to metastatic carcinoma associ-ated with stepwise acquisition of oncogenic mutations. APC, adenomatous polyposis coli gene; K-RAS, Kirsten-rat sarcoma viral oncogene homologue; p53, tumour protein 53 (TP53); SMAD, *Homo sapiens* homologue of *Drosophila* protein MAD (mothers against decapentaplegic); VEGF, vascular endothelial growth factor.

Table 2.2 Examples of the six features and their molecular basis in cancers.

Feature	Colorectal cancer	Glioma	Head and neck squamous cancer
1. Growth factor independence	K-Ras mutation	EGFR amplification or mutation NF1 loss	EGFR mutation
2. Over-riding inhibitory signals	SMAD2/SMAD4 mutation	CDK4/p16 mutation	Cyclin D amplification p16 and p21 mutation
3. Evasion of apoptosis	p53 mutation	p53 mutation/MDM2 overexpression	p53 mutation
4. Immortalization	hTERT re-expression	hTERT re-expression	hTERT re-expression
5. Angiogenesis	VEGF expression	PDGF/PDGFR overexpression	Nitric oxide pathway activation of VEGF
6. Invasion and metastasis	APC, inactivate E-cadherin	Cathepsin D, MMP-2 and -9 and UPA overexpression	Cathepsin D, MMP-1, -2 and -9 overexpression

APC, adenomatous polyposis coli gene; EGFR, endothelial growth factor receptor; hTERT, human telomerase reverse transcriptase; MMP, matrix metalloproteinase; PDGF, platelet-derived growth factor; PDGFR, platelet-derived growth factor receptor; VEGF, vascular endothelial growth factor; UPA, urokinase-type plasminogen activator.

the six capabilities that characterize the cancer cell phenotype and physiology.

DNA repair

Environmental damage to DNA occurs commonly and eukoryotes have developed several techniques for repairing both double strand and single strand errors in DNA.

1. Repair of double strand breaks in DNA:
   - homologous recombination using the sister chromatid as a template
   - non-homologous end joining (NHEJ).
2. Repair of single strand mutations in DNA:
   - nucleotide excision repair (NER) for bulky lesions
   - mismatch repair (MMR) for single mispaired bases and short deletions
   - base excision repair (BER) for alkylated bases.

Hereditary mutations of the enzymes involved in DNA repair will predispose to malignancy as they confer genome instability (Table 2.3).

DNA damage recognition

Another group of enzymes are required to recognize damaged DNA, leading to cell cycle arrest to allow DNA repair to be completed before the damage is replicated and passed on to the progeny cells. A number of cancer-predisposing syndromes are associated with inherited mutations of these enzymes. Examples include p53, whose inactiva-tion is an early step in the development of many cancers. Patients with the Li–Fraumeni syndrome carry one mutant germline p53 allele and are at high risk for the development of sarcomas, leukae-mia and cancers of the breast, brain, and adrenal glands.

Epigenetic changes

Most of the discussion above about the molecular mechanisms of malignancy has described somatic and occasional germline mutations of DNA that lead to aberrant proteins that in turn contribute to oncogenesis. This argument follows the central dogma of molecular biology introduced by Francis Crick in the late 1950s that stated that information flows in a unidirectional course from DNA sequence via RNA sequence to protein sequence. Although there are recognized exceptions to the central dogma, such as retroviruses and prions, it remains broadly true. However, some inheritable changes in phenotype or gene expression arise by mechanisms other than changes in the sequence of DNA bases. These inheritable changes passed on from a cell to her daughters are called epigenetic changes and perhaps the most obvious of these is cell differentiation.

The term epigenetics was introduced by the British developmental biologist Conrad Hal Wad-dington in 1942 as a metaphor for cell differentia-tion and development from a progenitor stem cell. Waddington likened differentiation to a marble

Table 2.3 Table of hereditary DNA repair syndromes.

DNA repair mechanism	Example of defect of DNA repair	Examples of cancers associated with defects
Homologous (sister chromatid) repair	BRCA1 (herediatry breast and ovarian cancer)	Breast and ovarian cancers
Non-homologous end joining (NHEJ)	XRCC4 (X-ray repair complementing defect gene) (lethal)	None (lethal defect)
Nucleotide excision repair (NER)	XP (xeroderma pigmentosa)	Skin cancers, leukaemia and melanoma
Mismatch repair (MMR)	MSH and MLH (hereditary non-polyposis colon cancer)	Colon, endometrium, ovarian, pancreatic and gastric cancers
Base excision repair (BER)	MYH (hereditary non-polyposis colon cancer)	Colon cancers

rolling down a landscape of hills and valleys to reach a final destination. The destination (cell fate) was determined by the landscape (epigenetics) and the marble could not travel back to the top (terminal differentiation). Today the term refers to modification of DNA and chromatin that influences gene transcription, alteration of post-transcriptional RNA and finally to protein degradation.

DNA methylation

Perhaps the most recognized epigenetic modification of DNA is nucleotide base methylation, typically the addition of a methyl group to the cytosine pyrimidine ring. In vertebrates, DNA methylation usually occurs in a CpG dinucleotide. Unmethylated CpGs are grouped in clusters called 'CpG islands' that occur in the 5′ regulatory regions of many genes. DNA methylation of CpG islands inhibits gene transcription by impeding the binding of transcriptional proteins and by binding methyl-CpG-binding domain (MBDs) proteins. MBD proteins recruit additional proteins, such as histone deacetylases, that modify histones to form compact, inactive chromatin termed silent chromatin. Since epigenetic changes such as DNA methylation are inherited during cell replication, maintenance of the pattern of DNA methylation is required following each cycle of DNA replication and this is achieved by DNA methyltransferases using the conserved DNA strand as the template (Figure 2.8). DNA methylation of tumour suppressor genes has been found to be a common mechanism of epigenetic gene silencing in cancers.

Chromatin modification

Chromatin is composed of DNA and proteins, chiefly the histone proteins around which the DNA is wound. There are six classes of histones organized into core histones (H2A, H2B, H3 and H4) and linker histones (H1 and H5). The core histones, which are highly conserved through nature, share N-terminal amino acid sequences that are the sites for post-transcriptional modification, for example acetylation and methylation. These histone modifications alter the binding of the DNA to the nucleosome, and modify RNA polymerase activity and hence gene expression. In general, tightly bound DNA is less expressed. Numerous enzymes have been identified that are involved with the modification of histone protein leading to alterations of chromatin structure and regulation of gene expression. These include histone methyltransferase (HMT) and histone acetlytransferse (HAT); other enzymes catalyze the removal of these modifications including histone deacetylase (HDAC) (Figure 2.9). Acetylation of histone tails reduces their binding affinity for DNA, allowing access for RNA polymerase and enhancing gene transcription. HDAC, therefore, by reversing histone tail residue acetylation suppresses gene expression, including tumour suppressor gene expression contributing to oncogenesis. A number

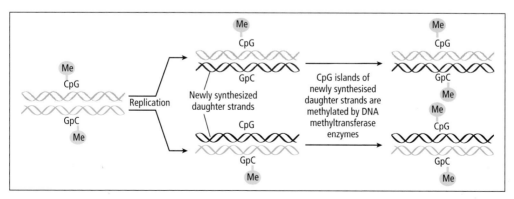

Figure 2.8 DNA methylation is passed on during cell replication to progeny cells by DNA methyltransferase enzymes that methylate CpG islands. CpG refers to the DNA dinucleotide sequence C G joined by the phosphate backbone of DNA.

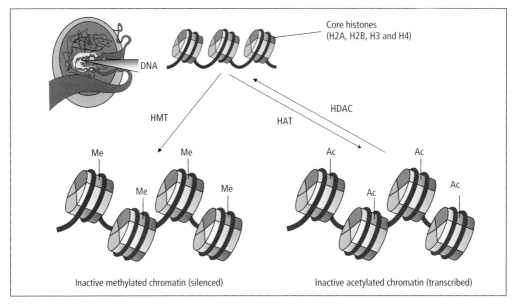

Core histones
(H2A, H2B, H3 and H4)

DNA

HMT

HDAC

HAT

Me

Me

Me

Me

Ac

Ac

Ac

Ac

Inactive methylated chromatin (silenced)

Inactive acetylated chromatin (transcribed)

Figure 2.9 Mechanism of chromatin modification. Ac, acetyl; HAT, histone acetyltransferase; HDAC, histone deacetylase; HMT, histone methyltransferase; Me, methyl.

of HDAC inhibitors have been studied including valproate and more recently vorinostat or suberoylanilide hydroxamic acid (SAHA), which is licensed for the management of cutaneous T-cell non-Hodgkin's lymphoma.

RNA interference

Post-translational interference of messenger RNA (mRNA) transcripts can also modify the expression of genes without altering the DNA sequence. Two types of small RNA molecules, microRNA (miRNA) and small interfering RNA (siRNA), can bind to specific complementary sequences of RNA or DNA and either increase or decrease their activity, for example by preventing an mRNA from producing a protein (Figure 2.10). RNA interference was originally identified in petunia plants. Botantists attempting to produce darker and darker petunia flowers inserted additional genes of an enzyme that catalyzes pigment synthesis. However, the transgenic plants produced white or variegated white flowers and this was subsequently found to be due to post-transcriptional inhibition of gene expression brought about by rapid mRNA degrada-

tion. The eventual explanation of this gene silencing phenomenon was identified in *Caenorhabditis elegans* by Craig Mello and Andrew Fire in 1998 who demonstrated that double stranded RNA caused the gene silencing. They called this RNAi (RNA interference) and won the Nobel Prize in 2006 for this work. Both the role of RNAi in the epigenetic generation of cancers and the potential of RNAi as a therapeutic approach are the focus of fevered research.

Protein degradation

A further form of epigenetic modification that contributes to the cellular phenotype is the destruction of proteins chiefly by proteosomes. Proteins are tagged for degradation by a small protein called ubiquitin and this reaction is catalyzed by enzymes including the product of the gene disrupted in Von Hippel–Lindau syndrome and Fanconi's anaemia. At least four ubiquitin molecules attach to the condemned protein, in a process called polyubiquitination, and the protein then moves to a proteasome, where the proteolysis occurs (Figure 2.11). Epigenetic regulation of protein degradation

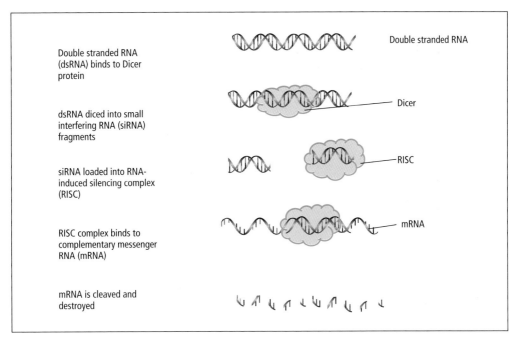

Figure 2.10 Mechanism of RNA interference.

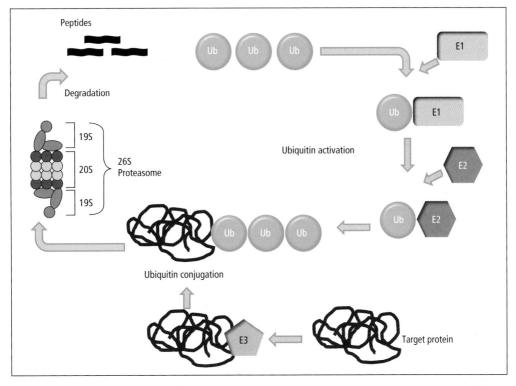

Figure 2.11 Proteosome pathway of protein ubiquitination and degradation. E, ubiquitination enzymes; Ub, ubiquitin.

could contribute to oncogenesis in a variety of ways. Gankyrin, a component of the proteosome is overexpressed in hepatocellular cancers. Bortezomib, a new treatment for myeloma, acts by inhibiting proteosome function.

Genetic causes of cancer

The causes of cancer may be usefully divided into genetic and environmental factors. The genetic factors are either germline mutations that are present in every cell of the body or somatic alterations only found in the tumour cells. Germline mutations may be either inherited, in which case they follow a familial pattern, or may be new sporadic mutations that neither parent has. Some of the germline mutations have been outlined as mutator phenotypes (DNA repair and damage recognition genes) above. Other germline cancer-predisposing mutations occur in tumour suppressor genes and oncogenes.

Oncogenes

The first clue to the identification of specific genes involved in the development of cancer came from the study of tumour viruses. Although cancer is generally not an infectious disease, some animal leukaemias, lymphomas and solid tumours, particularly sarcomas, can be caused by viruses. Oncogenes were identified following the discovery by Peyton Rous in 1911 that sarcomas could be induced in healthy chickens by injecting them with a cell-free extract of the tumour of a sick chicken. This was due to transmission of Rous sarcoma virus (RSV), an oncogenic retrovirus with just four genes:

- *gag* (group-specific antigen), which encodes the capsid protein
- *pol* (polymerase), which encodes the reverse transcriptase
- *env* (envelope), which encodes the envelope protein
- *src*, which encodes a tyrosine kinase.

It is the *src* gene that is necessary for cell transformation and is therefore an oncogene – literally a gene capable of causing cancer. In the late 1970s

Harold Varmus and Michael Bishop discovered that a homologous proto-oncogene (c-SRC) is present in the normal mammalian genome (the human *src* locus is on chromosome 20q12-q13) and has been hijacked by the retrovirus. The prefix v- denotes a viral sequence and the prefix c- a cellular sequence. In 1956, 55 years after his discovery of RSV and at the age of 87, Peyton Rous was (finally) awarded a Nobel Prize, whilst Bishop and Varmus only waited 10 years from their discovery to the award of their Nobel Prize in 1989. Around 50 oncogenes have been identified by their presence in transforming retroviruses (e.g. erbB, H-RAS, JUN) and further oncogenes have been discovered by positional cloning of chromosomal translocations (e.g. Bcl-2, BCR-ABL) and by transfection studies (e.g. N-RAS, RET). Most oncogenes contribute to cancer's autonomy in growth factors, either as plasma membrane receptors (e.g. RET, PTCH), signal transduction pathways (e.g. PTEN, NF1 and 2, VHL) or transcription factors (e.g. c-MYC, WT1) (Table 2.4).

Tumour suppressor genes

In contrast to oncogenes, tumour suppressor genes act as cell cycle brakes, slowing the proliferation of cells, and mutations in these genes also contribute to cancer. Germline mutations of tumour suppressor genes behave as autosomal-dominant familial cancer predispositions. Tumour suppressor genes require the loss of both functional alleles to support a cancer (unlike oncogenes where one mutant allele suffices). In 1971 Alfred Knudson proposed the two hit model of tumour suppression to account for the differences between familial and sporadic retinoblastoma in children. In familial cases, tumours arose at a younger age and were more frequently bilateral. Knudson hypothesized that these children had inherited one defective retinoblastoma gene allele, followed by loss of the function of the second allele in the cancer cells through a somatic mutation (see Plate 2.3). Tumour suppressor genes, like oncogenes, also involve a variety of functional categories, including cell cycle regulation (e.g. p53, Rb), DNA repair and maintenance (e.g. BRCA1 and 2, MLH1, MSH2), as

Table 2.4 Table of hereditary cancer predisposition syndromes.

Syndrome	Malignancies	Inheritance	Gene	Function
Breast/ovarian	Breast, ovarian, colon, prostate	AD	BRCA1	Genome integrity
		AD	BRCA2	
Cowden	Breast, thyroid, gastrointestinal, pancreas	AD	PTEN	Signal transduction (tyrosine phosphatase)
Li–Fraumeni	Sarcoma, breast, osteosarcoma, leukaemia, glioma, adrenocortical	AD	p53	Genome integrity
Familial polyposis coli	Colon, upper gastrointestinal	AD	APC	Cell adhesion
Hereditary non-polyposis colon cancer (Lynch type II)	Colon, endometrium, ovarian, pancreatic, gastric	AD	MSH2	DNA mismatch repair
		AD	MLH1	
		AD	PMS1	
		AD	PMS2	
MEN 1 (multiple endocrine neoplasia 1)	Pancreatic islet cell, pituitary adenoma	AD	MEN1	Transcription repressor
MEN 2 (multiple endocrine neoplasia 2)	Medullary thyroid, phaeochromocytoma	AD	RET	Signal transduction (receptor tyrosine kinase)
Neurofibromatosis 1 (see Plate 2.2)	Neurofibrosarcoma, phaeochromocytoma, optic glioma	AD	NF1	Signal transduction (regulates GTPases)
Neurofibromatosis 2	Vestibular schwannoma	AD	NF2	Cell adhesion
von Hippel–Lindau	Haemangioblastoma of retina and central nervous system, renal cell, phaeochromocytoma	AD	VHL	Ubiquination
Retinoblastoma	Retinoblastoma, osteosarcoma	AD	RB1	Cell cycle regulation
Xeroderma pigmentosa	Skin, leukaemia, melanoma	AR	XPA	DNA nucleotide excision repair
		AR	XPC	
		AR	XPD	
		AR	XPF	
Gorlin	Basal cell skin, brain	AD	PTCH	Signal transduction (repressor of hedgehog signalling)

AD, autosomal dominant; AR, autosomal recessive; GTPase, guanosine triphosphatase.

well as signal transduction (e.g. NF1, PTEN) and cell adhesion (e.g. APC) (Table 2.3).

Environmental causes of cancer

The multitude of environmental factors that are associated with the development of malignancy may be usefully divided into:

- Physical (radiation)
- Chemical (chemical carcinogens)
- Biological (infections).

Radiation

The major physical carcinogen is radiation. Radiation is ubiquitous and may either be ionizing (e.g. γ-rays from cosmic radiation and isotope decay, α-particles from radon, X-rays from medical imaging) or non-ionizing (e.g. ultraviolet (UV) light from the sun, microwave and radiofrequency radiation from mobile phones, electromagnetic fields from electricity generators and pylons, ultrasound radiation from imaging). Ionizing radiation ejects electrons from atoms yielding an ion pair and requires 10–15 eV (electronvolts). Ionizing radiation may be either electromagnetic (X-rays, γ-rays) or particulate (α-particles, neutrons). Non-ionizing radiation does not yield an ion pair but can still excite electrons resulting in chemical change.

Ultraviolet radiation

UV radiation is subdivided into three wavelength bands:

- UVA (313–400 nm)
- UVB (290–315 nm)
- UVC (220–290 nm).

UVC has the most potent effects on DNA, which absorbs most strongly at 254 nm. However, UVC is quickly absorbed in air and hence UVB is considered to be the greater environmental hazard. Most UV radiation is absorbed by atmospheric ozone in the stratosphere and this ozone layer is being depleted in part due to chlorine in chlorofluorocarbons (CFCs), resulting in increasing UV exposure levels. One of the major lesions induced in DNA by UV radiation is the thymidine dimer, a covalent bonding of adjacent thymidine residues on the same DNA strand. This causes local distortion of the double helix which is repaired by the nucleotide excision repair (NER) pathway. The seven identified xeroderma pigmentosa genes encode essential components that undertake NER and hence xeroderma pigmentosa predisposes to UV-induced skin malignancies. Melanin pigment in the skin normally absorbs UV radiation, thus protecting the skin. Basal cell and squamous cell skin cancers increase with cumulative UV exposure, whilst the relationship is less straightforward for melanoma. The evidence for an association with cancer for other forms of non-ionizing radiation (microwave, radiofrequency, ultrasound and electromagnetic radiation) is weak and inconsistent.

Ionizing radiation

Natural sources

Exposure to natural sources of ionizing radiation varies in different populations. Higher altitude and further latitude from the equator are both associated with higher cosmic radiation exposure. In addition, various regions have higher natural background levels from radon. Radon is a colourless, odourless gas formed from decay as part of the uranium-238 series. The radon-222 isotope, along with a number of its progeny, is an α-particle emitter. Radon gas levels are normally quoted in Bq/m³ (1 becquerel (Bq) is one decay per second) and the average indoor levels in the UK are about 20 Bq/m³. Local geology (igneous granite) with high levels of uranium produces high levels of radon in soil gas, but for it to escape to the surface the soil must be highly porous. In the UK, radon levels are particularly high in Devon and Cornwall, Derbyshire and Northamptonshire. From the results of eight case–control studies, it is believed that radon exposure accounts for a small fraction of lung cancers with a 14% increased risk for a person living for 30 years in a house with levels of 150 Bq/m³.

Nuclear warfare

Most of the information on the induction of cancers by ionizing radiation comes from exposed populations, including Japanese people exposed to atomic bombs at Hiroshima (Little Boy was a uranium-235-enriched bomb) and Nagasaki (Fat Man was a plutonium-239 bomb). The estimated populations of the two cities at the time of bombing was 560 000 and approximately 200 000 people died within the first few months of the acute effects of blast, burns and radiation exposure (Table 2.5).

Table 2.5 How atomic bombs kill.

Timing	Effect
1–2 hours	Radiation sickness (acute nausea and vomiting)
2–10 days	Denuded intestinal epithelium (intractable diarrhoea, gastrointestinal haemorrhage, septicaemia)
7–21 days	Pancytopenia (neutropenic sepsis, haemorrhage)
3–10 years	Acute myeloid leukaemia
10–50 years	Solid tumours (breast, bone, thyroid, lung, gastrointestinal, ovary, skin)

Table 2.6 Cancer deaths in the hibakusha (survivors of Hiroshima and Nagasaki atomic bombs).

	Total number of deaths	Estimated number of deaths due to radiation	Percentage of deaths attributable to radiation
Leukaemia	176	89	51%
Solid tumours	4687	339	7%
Total	4863	428	9%

Box 2.3: Chernobyl

On 26 April 1986, nuclear reactor number 4 at Chernobyl exploded in the world's worst nuclear accident. Over 10^{19} Bq of radioactive isotopes were released, including 5.2×10^{18} Bq of β-emitting isotopes of iodine that concentrate in the thyroid gland. An increase in thyroid cancer in children was first reported in 1990 but an excess of other tumours has not (yet?) been reported. Fallout from Chernobyl affected millions of people living within a few hundred kilometres of the reactor and caused a 30–100-fold increase in the incidence of thyroid cancer, especially in children. The younger the child at exposure, the greater the risk is. The increase so far is almost entirely papillary carcinoma of the thyroid and the dominant subtype has solid papillary morphology. At a molecular level, these tumours show rearrangement of the RET oncogene by inversion or translocation with partner genes to yield constitutively active c-RET tyrosine kinases.

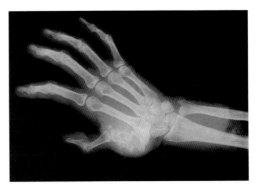

Figure 2.12 Osteosarcoma of the first metacarpal 15 years after radiotherapy for arthritis (no longer used). This radiograph shows cortical destruction, a soft tissue mass with internal calcification and periosteal reaction.

The Radiation Effects Research Foundation has followed 86 000 survivors or hibakusha, and, up to 1990, 7827 had died of cancer. The excess risk of leukaemia was seen especially in those exposed as children and was highest during the first 10 years after the bombing. However, the excess risk of solid tumours occurred later and still persists (Table 2.6).

Medical radiation

The hazards of medical ionizing radiation may be difficult to determine as ionizing radiation-induced tumours are not identifiable by a particular signature DNA mutation (unlike the thymidine dimers induced by UV radiation). Some tissues, such as breast, thyroid and bone marrow, are more susceptible to the carcinogenic effects of ionizing radiation, although tumours have been described in every organ site following radiation exposure

(Figure 2.12). Well-described examples of iatrogenic tumours include acute leukaemias induced by radiation treatment for ankylosing spondylitis prescribed in the late 1930s in the UK. Similarly, 20 000 Israelis received radiation for *Tinea capitis* (ringworm) in the 1950s, and by the 1980s there was a significantly increased risk of meningioma. Similar increases in tumours have been observed in patients treated with radiotherapy, including men treated for prostate cancer, women treated for cervical cancers and Hodgkin's disease survivors. Diagnostic imaging radiation doses are shown in Table 2.7.

Occupational radiation

The first victims of occupational exposure to radiation included Marie Curie and her daughter Irène Joliot-Curie (also a Nobel laureate), who both died of leukaemia. In the 1920s, watch dials were hand painted with radium-based luminous paint. The female radium dial painters often licked their paint brushes to give them a sharp point and

Table 2.7 Diagnostic imaging radiation doses.

Imaging procedure	Radiation dose	Equivalent to natural background radiation for:
Chest X-ray	0.02 mSv	3 days
Chest CT scan	8 mSv	3.6 years
Abdominal CT scan	10 mSv	4.5 years
Intravenous urogram	2.5 mSv	14 months
Brain CT scan	2.3 mSv	1 year
Mammogram	0.7 mSv	3 months

Box 2.4: Units of radiotherapy

The becquerel (Bq) is the SI unit of radioactivity and 1 Bq is equivalent to one nuclear decay per second. It is named after Henri Becquerel who shared the Nobel Prize with Marie and Pierre Curie for the discovery of radioactivity. The Hiroshima bomb produced 8×10^{24} Bq.

The gray (Gy) is the SI unit of absorbed radiation dose for ionizing radiation. One gray is the absorption of 1 joule (J) of ionizing radiation by 1 kg of matter, usually human tissue. It is named after Hal Gray, a British pioneer of radiation biology and physics who also established the Gray Laboratories at Mount Vernon Hospital.

The sievert (Sv) is the SI unit of radioactive dose equivalence and reflects the biological effects in tissue of radiation rather than its physical attributes. The equivalent dose will depend on the absorbed dose (measured in grays) as well as the type of radiation, as well as the time and volume and part of body irradiated. It is named after Rolf Sievert, a Swedish medical physicist. A dose of 3 Sv will lead to a lethal dose (LD) 50/30, or death in 50% of cases within 30 days, and over 6 Sv survival is very unusual.

---

ingested the radium. Up to 3% of these women subsequently developed osteosarcomas after a latency of 5–10 years. These 'radium girls' successfully sued their employer and this litigation resulted in the introduction of industrial safety standards and health and safety regulations at work. Similarly, pitchblende (uranium oxide) and uranium miners in Czechoslovakia, Sweden, Newfoundland and Colorado who have been exposed to radon are at increased risk of lung cancers.

Chemical carcinogenesis

Cancer is essentially a genetic disease arising from mutations of genes that affect the control of normal cell function (proto-oncogenes and tumour suppressor genes) or from polymorphic genes that govern enzyme systems that activate or detoxify environmental carcinogens (phase I and phase II enzyme reactions). Carcinogenic mutations can arise in several ways: genotoxic environmental factors (e.g. radiation and many chemical carcinogens), spontaneous DNA aberrations occurring during normal cell replication, or hereditary germline mutations. Chemical carcinogenesis was shown to be a multistep process following studies in the 1940s using PAHs (polycyclic aromatic hydrocarbons) and a murine skin cancer model system. This identified three steps – initiation, promotion and progression – that involve separate biological processes. Chemical carcinogens may operate at any or all three stages. The minority of chemical carcinogens act directly on DNA (e.g. alkylating agents), whilst the majority are procarcinogens that require metabolic activation to the ultimate carcinogen forms. Many ultimate carcinogens are potent electrophiles, capable of accepting electrons (e.g. epoxides derived from polycyclic hydrocarbons, vinyl chloride and aflatoxins, the N-hydroxylated metabolites of azo dyes, and the alkyldiazonium ions derived from nitrosamines).

Initiation

The key feature of initiation is the need for cell replication without repair of the chemically induced DNA damage. Initiation is irreversible, usually involves simple DNA mutations that are 'fixed' by cell division, and results in no morphological changes to the cells. Single exposure to a carcinogen may be sufficient for initiation. For example, aflatoxin B1 is one of a family of mycotoxin contaminants of food crops such as grain and groundnuts (peanuts). It is produced by *Aspergillus flavus*, which favours hot and humid conditions and is therefore most likely to contaminate food in Africa and Asia. Aflatoxin B1 is oxidized by hepatic P450 microsomal enzymes into aflatoxin B1 2,3-epoxide, which binds to DNA bases forming mutagenic adducts that preferentially induce GC to TA transversions. These transversions have been identified frequently in codon 249 of the p53 gene in hepatocellular carcinomas in patients from southern Africa and China who are exposed to high levels of aflatoxin B1 and may also have hepatitis B virus infection.

Promotion

Promotion is a reversible process requiring multiple exposures to the carcinogen, usually with a dose–response threshold. Promotion does not usually involve DNA mutations (non-genotoxic carcinogenesis) but provides a chemically mediated selective growth advantage. Thus, promotion results in the clonal expansion of cells. In the 1940s it was noted that 5% of mice treated with penzpyrene developed tumours but this figure rose to 80% when croton oil was added. Croton oil alone, however, produced no tumours. Subsequently, it was found that tetradecanoylphorbol acetate (TPA), a natural component of croton oil (from the seeds of *Croton tiglium*, a tree cultivated in India that resemble castor seeds), interacts with the protein kinase c signal pathway, stimulating growth and thus acting as a promoter. TPA is the most widely used tumour promoter in cellular experimental models of oncogenesis. Similarly, oestrogens are believed to act as carcinogenic promoters. Indeed, transplacental diethylstilboestrol (DES) was shown to induce vaginal clear cell adenocarcinomas in young women whose mothers had been treated with DES during pregnancy.

Progression

Progression is an irreversible step that results in morphologically identifiable cellular changes and frequently involves multiple complex DNA changes, such as chromosomal alterations. Progression and the accumulation of multiple genetic abnormalities that characterize cancer cells may occur spontaneously or may be driven by chemical carcinogens. Since individual cells may acquire these genetic changes, progression leads to heterogeneity of the cell population. Ultimately some cells will acquire a mutator phenotype and the six genetic attributes that characterize a cancer cell.

Diet and cancer

A role for dietary constituents has been described for a number of cancers and the evidence for some of these relationships is more robust than for others. Alcohol intake has been convincingly associated with an increased risk of oral, oesophageal and hepatic cancers. In contrast, dietary fat was believed to play an important role in breast cancer development based on animal studies, migrant studies and a few case–control trials. This led to great enthusiasm for reduced dietary fat intake to reduce the incidence of breast cancer. However, results from large prospective studies have failed to confirm a strong relationship between dietary fat intake and breast cancer. Two paths may contribute to dietary carcinogenesis. Firstly, foodstuffs may include dietary genotoxins formed by contaminating moulds, products of storage or fermentation of food, products of cooking and food additives (e.g. aflatoxin contamination of food). Secondly, endogenous genotoxins, such as reactive oxygen species, may be formed and higher calorific intake may yield more genotoxins.

Carcinogenic infections

The association between infection and cancer is usually attributed to Peyton Rous, who described the acellular transmission of sarcoma between chickens in 1911. However, six years earlier, Goebel had reported a link between bladder tumours and bilharzia (schistosomiasis). It is estimated that 15% of cancers globally are attributable to infections (11% viruses, 4% bacteria and 0.1% helminths) (Table 2.8).

Oncogenic human DNA viruses

Human papillomavirus (HPV)
The papillomaviruses are non-enveloped, icosahedral, double stranded DNA viruses. Around 100

Box 2.5: A brief epidemiological history of smoking and cancer

Tobacco was one of the 'gifts' from the New World to the Old along with syphilis and potatoes. Nicotine is named after Jean Nicot, a 15th century French ambassador to Lisbon, who was a great advocate of smoking and who in 1559 sent tobacco to Catherine de Medici, the then Queen of France. Tobacco was subsequently introduced to England by Sir Walter Raleigh in 1586. Smoking was actively encouraged amongst soldiers in the Thirty Years War, Napoleonic campaigns, Crimean War and, most notably, the First World War. Smoking reduces fear and anxiety and suppresses appetite and these were deemed beneficial to soldiers.

Early epidemiological links with non-lung cancers

In 1761, John Hill, a London doctor, wrote up several cases of nasal cancer amongst heavy tobacco snuff users and, in 1795, Thomas van Soemmering suggested a link between pipe smoking and lip cancer. The American Civil War Yankee general and later USA president, Ulysses S. Grant died in 1885 of throat cancer and this was attributed to his cigars. In an early cohort study in the 1920s, Dr R. Abbe observed that, of 90 patients with oral cancer, 89 were smokers.

Epidemiological links with lung cancer

In 1939, Dr Franz Muller of the University of Cologne performed what is generally recognized as the earliest case–control study of smoking, which showed that a very high proportion of lung cancer patients were heavy smokers. However, the results were dismissed as unreliable because Hitler was a fanatical antismoker. Shortly after the Second World War, Austin Bradford Hill, Edward Kennaway, Percy Stock and Richard Doll set out to investigate links between smoking and lung cancer, at a time when 90% of adult males in the UK smoked, using a case–control dose–response strategy. Their case–control study was performed in 1948 in 20 London hospitals, interviewing two controls with gastric or colonic cancer as controls for each lung cancer patient. In all analyses, there was a dose–response relationship between the number of cigarettes smoked and the risk of lung cancer. This was published in 1950 in the *British Medical Journal*.

In 1951, Doll and Hill set up a prospective cohort study of 60 000 doctors on the medical register who were recruited via a letter in the *BMJ*; 40 000 replies were received and, in the following 2.5 years, there were 789 deaths, including 36 from lung cancer. There was a significant increase in the risk of lung cancer with increased tobacco consumption (see table below). However, they noted that the only two doctors who definitely died of smoking had died after setting fire to their beds whilst smoking in bed! This relationship was maintained in a 1993 update of the original cohort, which now includes 20 000 deaths (883 from lung cancer), and the relative risk for smoking >25 g tobacco a day was 20-fold.

	N	Tobacco 1 g/day	Tobacco 15 g/day	Tobacco >25 g/day
Lung cancer deaths	36	0.4/10 000	0.6/10 000	1.1/10 000
All deaths	789	13/10 000	13/10 000	16/10 000

Similar findings were reported in the early 1950s in the USA by Ernst Wynder, a medical student, and Evarts Graham, a thoracic surgeon, who, in 1950, published 'Tobacco smoking as a possible etiologic factor in bronchiogenic carcinoma: a study of 684 proven cases' in the *Journal of the American Medical Association*. Evarts, a chain smoker, did not take enough heed of his own findings and himself died of lung cancer.

---

genotypes have been identified and >30 of these infect the female genital tract. Some genotypes are associated with benign lesions, such as warts (e.g. HPV-6 and -11), whilst others are known as high-risk genotypes and are associated with invasive cancer (e.g. HPV-16, -18, -31, -33, -45, -51, -52, -58 and -59) (Table 2.9). The prevalence of infection varies between populations but is 20–30% in women aged 20–25 years and declines to 5–10% in women over 40 years old. HPV is sexually transmitted and the main determinant of infection is the number of sexual partners. Most infections are cleared spontaneously but a small proportion persist and are believed to be the origin of cervical dysplasia and invasive cancers. Latent infection is associated with cervical intraepithelial neoplasia

Table 2.8 Cancers attributed to infection.

Infection	Cancer	Number of cancer cases worldwide per year
RNA viruses		
Human T-cell leukaemia virus	Leukaemia	3 000
HIV (and Epstein–Barr virus)	Non-Hodgkin's lymphoma	9 000
HIV (and human herpesvirus 8)	Kaposi's sarcoma	45 000
Hepatitis C virus	Hepatocellular cancer	110 000
DNA viruses		
Human papillomavirus	Cervical cancer	360 000
Hepatitis B virus	Hepatocellular cancer	230 000
Epstein–Barr virus	Burkitt lymphoma, Hodgkin's disease, nasopharyngeal cancer	100 000
Bacteria		
Helicobacter pylori	Gastric cancer, gastric lymphoma	350 000
Helminths		
Schistosoma haematobium	Bladder cancer	10 000
Liver flukes	Cholangiocarcinoma	1 000

HIV, human immunodeficiency virus.

Table 2.9 Human papillomavirus genotypes and associated conditions.

Human disease	HPV genotype
Skin warts	HPV-1, -2, -3, -7 and -10
Epidemodysplasia verruciformis	HPV-5, -8, -17 and -20
Anogenital warts: exophytic condylomas	HPV-6 and -11
Anogenital warts: flat condylomas	HPV-16, -18, -31, -33, -42 and -43
Respiratory tract papillomas	HPV-6 and -11
Conjunctival papillomatosis	HPV-6 and -11
Focal epithelial hyperplasia	HPV-13 and -32

(CIN), which is graded 1 to 3 according to the severity of cytological changes. The histological equivalents of these lesions are called squamous intraepithelial lesions, which may be low or high grade. Over 99% of invasive cervical cancers have detectable HPV DNA present and HPV can transform cells in culture. The molecular basis of papillomavirus-induced neoplasia is attributed to two viral oncogenes, E6 and E7. HPV E6 inactivates p53 and E7 degrades Rb protein. High-risk HPV geno-types have also been associated with anal, penile, vaginal and vulval cancers. In addition HPV is thought to play a role in the development of a number of other malignancies, including head and neck cancers, conjunctival squamous cancers, oesophageal cancers and possibly cutaneous squamous cell cancers.

Studies have suggested that the detection of HPV in the cervix may be more sensitive for detecting CIN than conventional cytological screening. Prophylactic HPV vaccines that induce neutralizing antibodies may prevent infection and the associated malignancies. Most of the vaccines have used virus-like particles constructed of major capsid proteins without viral DNA or enzymes present. A nationwide HPV vaccination programme for teenage girls was started in UK in 2008.

Hepatitis B virus (HBV)

Hepatitis B virus is a double stranded DNA virus that includes a single stranded DNA region of variable length. The virus possesses a DNA-dependent DNA polymerase as well as a reverse transcriptase and replicates via an RNA intermediate. HBV has three main antigens: the 'Australian antigen' is

Table 2.10 Serological markers of hepatitis B virus infection.

	HBsAg	HBeAg	Anti-HBe	Anti-HBs	Anti-HBc	Anti-HBc IgM
Acute infection	+	+/−	+/−	−	+	+++
Highly infectious carrier	+++	+	−	−	+	−
Low infectious carrier	+	−	+	−	+	−
Past infection	−	−	+	+	+	−
Past immunization	−	−	−	+	−	−

associated with the surface (HBsAg), the 'core antigen' (HBcAg) is internal, and the 'e antigen' (HBeAg) is part of the same capsid polypeptide as HBcAg. All of these antigens elicit specific antibodies and are used diagnostically (Table 2.10).

Hepatitis B is one of the most common infections worldwide with two billion people having been infected and 300–350 million chronic carriers. Hepatitis B is the ninth most common cause of death worldwide. Acute hepatitis B infection may be associated with extrahepatic immune-mediated manifestations and 1–4% of patients develop a fulminant form. Following acute infection, up to 10% will develop chronic hepatitis, either chronic persistent hepatitis, which is asymptomatic with modest elevation of transaminases and little fibrosis, or chronic active hepatitis, which causes jaundice and cirrhosis and is associated with a 100× increased risk of hepatocellular cancer 15–60 years after infection. It is uncertain how hepatitis B leads to cancer, although the X protein of hepatitis B may interact with p53 causing disruption of the cell cycle control, or the virus may act indirectly by causing increased hepatic cell turnover associated with cirrhosis.

Although treatment with α-interferon and antiviral agents (e.g. lamivudine, tenofovir, telbivudine, entecavir, adefovir) may lead to clearance of hepatitis B in chronic infection, recombinant subunit vaccines have been available since the early 1980s. The introduction of a mass immunization programme in Taiwan has been associated with a dramatic reduction in liver cancer in children.

Epstein–Barr virus (EPV)

Epstein–Barr virus (or HHV-4, human herpesvirus 4) is a ubiquitous double stranded DNA gamma-

Table 2.11 Diseases associated with Epstein–Barr virus infection.

Non-malignant
Infectious mononucleosis
X-linked lymphoproliferative syndrome (Duncan's syndrome)
Oral hairy leukoplakia

Malignant
Burkitt lymphoma
Nasopharyngeal cancer
Post-transplant lymphoproliferative disorder
Hodgkin's disease
Primary cerebral lymphoma
Primary effusion lymphoma (with HHV8)
Leiomyosarcoma in children with HIV
Nasal T/NK non-Hodgkin's lymphoma

herpesvirus. It was first identified by Epstein and his colleagues by electron microscopy of a cell line derived from a patient with Burkitt lymphoma in 1964. Burkitt lymphoma had been described only a few years earlier in 1956 by Dennis Burkitt, a surgeon working in Uganda. The subsequent finding that EBV was the cause of infectious mononucleosis arose serendipitously when a laboratory technician in Philadelphia developed mononucleosis and was found to have acquired antibodies to EBV. EBV infects over 90% of the world's population, is transmitted orally and, in normal adults, from 1 to 50 B lymphocytes per million are infected by latent EBV. A carcinogenic role for EBV has been confirmed for several types of lymphoma (Burkitt lymphoma, Hodgkin's disease and immunosuppression-associated non-Hodgkin's lymphoma) and nasopharyngeal cancer (Table 2.11). EBV is estimated to be responsible for 100 000 cancers per year in the world.

Primary infection of epithelial cells by EBV is associated with the infection of some resting B lymphocytes. The majority of infected B cells have latent virus with a small percentage undergoing spontaneous activation to lytic infection. During lytic infection EBV replicates in the cell and when the progeny virions are released the host cell is destroyed. In contrast, during latent infection there is neither virus replication nor host cell destruction. Most infected B lymphocytes have latent virus expressing at most ten of the >80 genes of EBV. The roles of these latent genes include maintenance of the episomal virus DNA, growth and transformation of B cells and evasion of the host immune system. A number of these latent genes are thought to contribute to the oncogenicity of EBV. For example LMP-1 (latent membrane protein 1) mimics a constitutively activated receptor for tumour necrosis factor (TNF), and BHRF1 and BALF1 are viral homologues of the anti-apoptotic protein bcl-2 that leads to evasion of programmed cell death. Thus, in contrast to retroviruses, which generally possess a single oncogene, EBV uses a number of genes that contribute to the steps towards cancer.

Human herpesvirus 8 (HHV-8/KSHV)

Kaposi's sarcoma (KS) was originally described over a century ago and four forms have subsequently been recognized. The first is classic KS and is usually found on the lower legs of elderly men of Mediterranean or Jewish descent without any immunosuppression. A second form, endemic or African KS, is found in all age groups in sub-Saharan Africa, where even before the HIV epidemic it was as common as colorectal cancer is in Europe. A third form associated with iatrogenic immunosuppression was recognized in patients who had received an allogeneic organ transplant. The fourth and most common form of the disease is associated with AIDS (acquired immune deficiency syndrome). All forms of KS are associated with HHV-8 (also known as Kaposi sarcoma herpesvirus, KSHV), which was identified in 1994. In addition, this virus is most prevalent in the populations at risk of KS. HHV-8 is also implicated in the pathogenesis of two rare lymphoproliferative diseases, primary effusion lymphoma and multicentric Castleman's disease (see Plate 2.4). Like EBV, HHV-8 includes a number of cellular gene homologues that are thought to contribute to its oncogenic potential.

Oncogenic human RNA viruses

Hepatitis C virus (HCV)

Hepatitis C virus was identified in 1989 as the cause of transfusion-acquired non-A non-B hepatitis by Houghton, Choo and Kuo. HCV is a single stranded RNA virus belonging to the flavivirus genus along with yellow fever and dengue. The prevalence of HCV varies geographically from 1–1.5% in Europe and the USA to 3.5% in Africa, and transmission is chiefly parenteral, particularly by blood transfusion prior to the introduction of blood product screening. In contrast to HBV, 85% develop persistent HCV and 65% progress to chronic liver disease including hepatocellular cancer for which the relative risk is 20-fold (Table 2.12). The oncogenic mechanism for HCV remains unclear. Unlike retroviruses, there is no evidence of genome integration but cancer is preceded by cirrhosis and it is hypothesized that the virus induces

Table 2.12 Comparison of HIV and hepatitis B and C viruses.

	HCV	HBV	HIV
Global prevalence	3%	35%	0.5%
Global prevalence	170 million	1.2 billion	36.1 million
Chronic infection rate	2.30%	6%	0.5%
Chronic infection	129 million	350 million	36.1 million
Deaths per year	476 000	1.2 million	2.8 million
Annual death rate	0.40%	0.49%	7.80%

a cycle of inflammation, repair and regeneration and thus indirectly contributes to the formation of cancer. There are at least six genotypes of HCV and the diagnosis is usually made by enzyme immunoassay for anti-HCV antibodies and confirmed by polymerase chain reaction (PCR) for HCV RNA. Treatment with pegylated interferon and ribavarin leads to clearance of the virus in 40–60% depending in part upon the HCV genotype. Promising specific protease and polymerase inhibitors are in late phase trials for HCV.

Human T-cell leukaemia virus type 1 (HTLV-1)

HTLV-1 is the main cause of adult T-cell leukaemia/lymphoma, a malignancy characterized by hypercalcaemia, lymphadenopathy, hepatosplenomegaly and myelosuppression. It is associated with a particularly poor prognosis and occurs almost exclusively in areas where HTLV-1 is endemic, such as the Caribbean, Japan and West Africa or in immigrants from these regions and their offspring. HTLV-1 is also associated with tropical spastic paraparesis and uveitis. HTLV-1 is an enveloped retrovirus that integrates into the host cellular genome. The virus is able to immortalize human T lymphocytes and this property is attributable to a specific viral oncogene, *tax*. Tax is a trans-activating transcription factor that can also lead to repression of transcription. Adult T-cell leukaemia/lymphoma develops in 2–5% of HTLV-1 infected people and is commoner in those infected at a younger age.

Oncogenic bacteria

Helicobacter pylori

Helicobacter pylori is a spiral, flagellated, Gram-negative bacteria that colonizes the human gastrointestinal tract. It causes gastritis leading to peptic ulceration, although many infections are asymptomatic. The discovery of *H. pylori* and the recognition of its place in the pathogenesis of peptic ulcer disease are chiefly due to Barry Marshall, who, in order to prove his point, swallowed a solution of the organism and developed acute gastritis 1 week later. It is believed that half of the world population is chronically infected with *H. pylori*. Prospective sero-epidemiological data suggest that *H. pylori* infection is associated with a two to four-fold increase in the risk of gastric cancer as well as an increase in gastric low-grade mucosa-associated lymphoid tissue (MALT) lymphoma. As with the hepatitis viruses, the mechanism of oncogenesis is obscure but is believed to be an indirect result of chronic inflammation and consequential epithelial cell proliferation. The combination of two antibiotics with either a bismuth preparation or a proton pump inhibitor for 14 days eradicates *H. pylori* in 80% patients. However, re-infection is common, *H. pylori* is very prevalent and the time interval between *H. pylori* infection and gastric cancer is thought to be several decades. For these reasons, it may prove very difficult to assess the value of eradication interventions in reducing cancer risk.

Oncogenic helminths

Schistosomes

Schistosomes are parasitic blood flukes or flatworms (platyhelminths) belonging to the trematode class whose intermediate hosts are snails. Three species infect humans: *Schistosoma haematobium*, *Schistosoma mansoni* and *Schistosoma japonica*. Humans are infected by contact with fresh water where the parasite cercaria form penetrates the skin. It is estimated that 200 million people are infected with schistosomes (Table 2.13). Acute infection may produce swimmer's itch dermatitis and tropical pulmonary eosinophilia, although most people remain asymptomatic. The development of adult worms, days to weeks after infection, may cause Katayama fever, a systemic illness of fevers, rigors, myalgia, lymphadenopathy and hepatosplenomegaly. Chronic infection leads to granuloma formation at sites of egg deposition, in the bladder for *S. haematobium* and in the bowel and liver for *S. mansoni* and *S. japonica*. The late sequelae include squamous cell carcinoma of the bladder in the case of *S. haematobium* and probably hepatocellular cancer with *S. japonica*. A single oral dose of praziquantel resolves the infection.

Table 2.13 Global distribution of schistosomiasis.

Species	Geographical distribution	Number of humans infected
Schistosoma haematobium	North Africa, Middle East, sub-Saharan Africa	114 million
Schistosoma mansoni	Sub-Saharan Africa, Middle East, Brazil	83 million
Schistosoma japonica	China, the Philippines, Indonesia	1.5 million

Table 2.14 Global distribution of liver fluke infection.

Species	Geographical distribution	Number of humans infected
Opisthorchis viverrini	Northern Thailand, Laos	9 million
Opisthorchis felineus	Kazakhastan, Ukraine	1.5 million
Clonorchis sinensis	China, Korea, Taiwan, Vietnam	7 million

Liver flukes

Three species of food-borne liver flukes of the trematode class cause illness in humans. Infection is acquired by eating raw or undercooked freshwater fish and the flukes migrate to the biliary tree and mature in the intrahepatic bile ducts. There are two intermediate hosts in the life cycle – snails and fish. As many as 17 million people are estimated to be infected (Table 2.14). Cholangiocarcinoma has been recognized as a complication of chronic infection and case–control studies have found a five-fold increased risk with liver fluke infection. The oncogenic mechanism is again unclear although chronic inflammation is believed to play a role. The antihelminth drug praziquantel is the treatment of choice.

Worldwide contributions to cancer

The current world population is six billion and the global burden of cancer is estimated to be 10 million new cases and six million deaths annually. Projections for 2020, when the global population is estimated to have risen to eight billion, are 20 million new cases and 12 million deaths annually. Tobacco contributes to three million cases of cancer (chiefly lung, head and neck, bladder), diet to an estimated three million cases (upper gastrointestinal, colorectal) and infection to a further 1.5 million cases (cervical, stomach, liver, bladder and lymphomas) globally. Prevention by tobacco control, dietary advice and affordable food, and infection control and immunization could have a major impact in reducing the global burden of cancer. The differences in outcome for tumours between the developed and the developing worlds are most marked for the rare but curable cancers where access to therapy dramatically improves survival (e.g. acute leukaemias, Hodgkin's disease and testicular cancers). Small differences are recorded where screening programmes aimed at early detection are effective (e.g. cervical and breast cancers), whilst there are little differences in outcome in the common tumours where prevention has a major role (e.g. lung, stomach and liver cancers). These observations have led to a World Health

Table 2.15 WHO cancer priority ladder.

1. Tobacco control
2. Infection control
3. Curable cancer programme
4. Early detection programme
5. Effective pain control
6. Sample cancer registry
7. Healthy eating programme
8. Referral guidelines
9. Clinical care guidelines
10. Nurse education
11. National cancer network
12. Clinical evaluation unit
13. Platform technology focus for region
14. Clinical research programme
15. Basic research programme
16. International aid programme

Organization (WHO) list of priorities to reduce global cancer, that starts not with scientific research or expensive chemotherapy, but with tobacco and infection control (Table 2.15). In an optimistic scenario the implementation of these priorities could reduce the estimated cancer incidence of 20 million in 2020 to 15 million and could reduce the expected mortality of 12 million to 6 million.

Chapter 3

The principles of cancer treatment

Appropriate care

The care of people with cancer requires careful deliberation and consultation with the patient. The appropriate care will depend upon the prognosis, the effectiveness and toxicity of any therapy, and finally, most importantly, on the patient's wishes. To empower patients to participate in this decision-making process requires them to be fully informed and the clear delivery of this information is essential. A number of resources are available to supplement the information divulged by clinicians to their patients. These include a number of web-based resources as well as patient information leaflets published by charities including Macmillan Cancerbackup and individual tumour-type patient groups such as Breast Cancer Breakthrough. It is increasingly appreciated that the management of patients with cancer requires a multidisciplinary approach involving a team of professionals including surgeons, clinical and medical oncologists, palliative care physicians, radiologists, histopathologists, specialist oncology and palliative care nurses, clinical psychologists, counsellors, dieticians, occupational therapists, physiotherapists, social workers and clinical geneticists.

The aims of therapy should be clearly identified before embarking on a course of treatment. Treatment may either be curative, aiming to prolong the quantity of life, or palliative, aiming to improve the quality of life. When considering the management of individual tumour types, the maxim that prevention is better than cure should be recalled. Cancer prevention and screening are essential if the global burden of malignancy is to be minimized.

During the last quarter of the 20th century, the role of chemotherapy, radiotherapy and endocrine therapy after primary surgery for localized breast cancer was recognized. These additional treatments are defined as adjuvant therapies. Thus adjuvant therapy is treatment after the primary tumour has been removed surgically and in the absence of detectable residual disease. Whilst large clinical trials demonstrated the advantages of adjuvant therapy to a population of women with breast cancer, the benefits for an individual woman are not measurable. In part for this reason and with a view to facilitating surgery, oncologists developed neoadjuvant treatments. Neoadjuvant therapy, usually chemotherapy or endocrine therapy, is delivered prior to surgery or radiotherapy to downsize the tumour, thus demonstrating the sensitivity of the tumour and potentially reducing the extent of the surgical resection or radiation field.

Surgical oncology

Surgery has six major roles in the management of people with cancer:

Lecture Notes: Oncology, 2nd edition. By M. Bower and J. Waxman. Published 2010 by Blackwell Publishing Ltd.

1. Cancer prevention.
2. Cancer diagnosis and staging.
3. Treating cancer.
4. Management of oncological emergencies.
5. Palliation of cancer symptoms.
6. Surgical reconstruction following cancer therapy.

Surgical oncology is the oldest discipline for the management of cancer and originates with attempts at curative resections. Surgical oncology enjoyed a golden era at the end of the 19th century and early 20th century prior to the First World War (Table 3.1). Subsequent advances in surgical oncology included the development of endocrine surgery for metastatic disease. Surgical hormone ablation was pioneered by George Beatson, a Glaswegian surgeon who gave his name to Scotland's largest cancer centre for the management of breast cancer over 100 years ago (Table 3.2).

Table 3.1 Landmarks in radical surgical oncology.

Year	Surgeon	Operation
1881	Albert Billroth	Subtotal gastrectomy
1890	William Halsted	Radical mastectomy
1897	Carl Schlatter	Total gastrectomy
1898	Johann von Mikulicz	Oesophagogastrectomy
1900	Ernest Wertheim	Radical hysterectomy
1906	W. Ernest Miles	Abdominoperineal excision of rectum
1913	Franz Torek	Oesophagectomy
1913	Wilfred Trotter	Partial pharyngectomy
1933	Evarts Graham	Pneumonectomy
1935	A. O. Whipple	Pancreaticoduodenectomy

Table 3.2 Landmarks in endocrine surgery for advanced cancer.

Year	Surgeon	Operation
1896	George Beatson	Oophrectomy for breast cancer
1941	Charles Huggins and Clarence Hodges	Orchidectomy for prostate cancer
1951	Rolf Luft and Herbert Olivecrona	Hypophysectomy for breast cancer
1952	Charles Huggins and D. M. Bergenstal	Adrenalectomy for breast cancer

Surgical cancer prophylaxis

The prevention of cancer by surgery has expanded greatly in recent years with the identification of individuals at high risk of developing malignancies because they have inherited germline genetic mutations associated with cancer predisposition. However, perhaps the most widespread example of surgical cancer prevention is the role of orchiopexy in the management of undescended testes. Undescended testes are the most common birth defect of the male genitalia, affecting up to 3% of live births. Although in many cases the testes will descend to the scrotum during the first year of life, undescended testes are associated with a 4–40-fold increased risk of malignancy, especially testicular seminoma. Orchiopexy, surgey to move the undescended testis into the scrotum, has been shown to reduce infertility although it remains controversial whether it also reduces the risk of malignancy. Nevertheless, it certainly makes the detection of testicular tumours easier to recognize and diagnose at an earlier stage. Familial adenomatous polyposis (FAP) is an autosomal dominant disorder characterized by the development of multiple polyps in the colon which may undergo transformation to malignant tumours. Most patients with FAP will develop a colonic cancer by the age of 40 years old, so prophylactic colectomy is generally recommended before the age of 25 years. Similarly, risk-reducing prophylactic mastectomy may be advocated for women with inherited mutations of BRCA genes (Table 3.3).

Table 3.3 Prophylactic surgery.

Indication	Prophylactic operation
Cryptorchidism	Orchiopexy
Polyposis coli/chronic ulcerative colitis	Colectomy
Familial medullary thyroid cancer (MEN 2 and 3)	Thyroidectomy
Familial breast cancer (BRCA 1 and 2)	Mastectomy
Familial ovarian cancer (BRCA 1 and 2)	Oophrectomy

BRCA, breast cancer; MEN, multiple endocrine neoplasia.

Surgical diagnosis and staging of cancer

Oncological diagnosis hinges on histopathology, and surgeons play a major role along with interventional radiologists in obtaining tissue specimens. Whilst aspiration cytology and fine-needle biopsies can be undertaken radiologically or endoscopically, more extensive incision or excision biopsies require surgical involvement. Careful specimen orientation and inking prior to histological sectioning may be required to assess the status of tumour margins. The optimal surgical approach and biopsy technique for tumour sampling must take into account concerns about contaminating new tissue planes with cancer cells that could jeopardize subsequent therapy. For example, thoracoscopic pleural biopsy of mesothelioma may result in needle-track metastases along the path of surgical instrumentation. The risk of this surgical spread of the cancer is reduced in mesothelioma by postoperative radiotherapy to the biopsy track. Surgery had a major role in the staging of tumours prior to the development of improved radiological techniques and a staging laparotomy was routine care in the management of Hodgkin's disease until the late 1980s. Surgical staging retains a role in the management of ovarian epithelial cancer and the surgical placement of radio-opaque titanium clips (that are non-ferrous and thus safe in the magnetic resonance imaging (MRI) scanner) may guide postoperative radiotherapy in some tumours.

Surgical treatment of cancer

The surgical treatment of cancer includes definitive curative surgery (with or without adjuvant treatments), debulking operations, metastasectomy and endocrine ablation surgery for advanced disease, although the later is largely historical as pharmacological hormone manipulations have taken over most of this role. It is really important to avoid unnecessary surgery in patients with extensive unresectable cancer whilst ensuring that patients with potentially curative tumours are not denied surgery. The treatment of cancer by multidisciplinary teams including radiologists, pathologists, physicians and surgeons is designed to ensure the right patients have the right operations at the right time. For example, this approach aims to guarantee that patients who are candidates for neoadjuvant down-staging therapy prior to surgery are not wheeled straight into the operating theatre. Most early curative surgery aimed to remove tumours *en bloc*, that is with the draining lymph nodes. In recent times surgeons have developed the use of more conservative function-preserving operations. Examples of the latter include wide local excision rather than mastectomy and partial nephron-sparing nephrectomy rather than radical nephrectomy for small renal tumours. A further development in surgery for skin tumours was introduced by Dr Frederic Mohs when he was still a medical student at the University of Wisconsin-Madison. Mohs' surgery for skin tumours involves the sectioning and mapping of surgical margins during the operation to ensure completeness of tumour resection. Instead of using a breadknife and the pathologist looking at each slice, the Mohs' technique is like a vegetable peeler with the pathologist examining each peeling for involvement during the surgery. Whilst this is a more laborious technique, it is especially valuable for tumours at specific anatomical sites such as the eyelids and in recurrent disease.

Debulking operations that do not result in complete surgical removal of the tumour are not always futile. They can provide important clinical benefits in selected tumour types including ovarian cancer and primary brain tumours and are usually followed by either chemotherapy or radiotherapy. Debulking surgery forms part of the treatment algorithm in several uncommon tumours such as thymomas and pseudomyxoma peritonei. Mucin secretion into the abdominal cavity by mucinous adenocarcinomas most commonly arising in the appendix is the usual cause of pseudomyxoma peritonei. The term 'myxoma' is derived from the Greek for mucin but the etymology of the medical terms myxoma and pseudomyxoma seem to have got mixed up. Myxomas are benign, pedunculated connective tissue tumours usually arising in the atria of the heart and are not mucinous, whilst pseudomyxoma peritonei fills the abdominal cavity with true jelly-like mucin.

The surgical resection of secondary deposits may seem perverse since the presence of metastases implies systemic dissemination of the cancer. Nevertheless, surgical oncologists have embraced this approach enthusiastically, mainly on the basis of relatively weak evidence from uncontrolled retrospective series that have been interpreted as demonstrating a survival benefit. The resection of lung, liver and brain metastases has become a part of the routine treatment strategy for a number of types of cancer. The most common indication for surgical metastasectomy is for hepatic secondaries from colorectal cancer. The rationale for this approach is based upon reported five-year survivals of around 30% in patients undergoing surgery compared to around 10% in those who received chemotherapy. However, there are no randomixed controlled studies that support hepatic metastasectomy and the case series are inevitably confounded by selection and reporting bias. Similarly, pulmonary metastasectomy has been widely adopted for osteogenic sarcomas, soft tissue sarcomas, renal cell tumours and melanomas and cerebral metastasectomy has also been advocated in a similar spectrum of malignancies. In contrast to metastasectomy, the surgical resection of residual masses following the completion of chemotherapy forms part of the multidisciplinary treatment of advanced non-seminomatous germ cell tumours to remove residual differentiated teratoma that could relapse at a later date. Finally, surgical endocrine ablation is nowadays rarely indicated for metastatic cancer although surgical castration is occasionally performed for advanced prostate cancer.

Surgery for oncological emergencies

Surgery has an important role in the optimal management of oncological emergencies, in particular metastatic spinal cord compression where rapid surgical decompression reduces neurological disability (see Cord compression in Chapter 46). Surgical decompression and spinal column stabilization should be offered to patients with a good prognosis and needs to be undertaken as swiftly as possible, preferably before patients lose the ability to walk. The optimal neurosurgical approach will depend upon the anatomical site of compression and the stability of the spine. If spinal metastases involve the vertebral body or threaten spinal stability, posterior decompression should always be accompanied by internal fixation with or without bone grafting.

Surgical palliation of cancer

The palliation of tumour-associated obstruction, fluid accumulation and bleeding may require surgical intervention, although the placement of shunts and stents is now more frequently undertaken by endoscopists and interventional radiologists. Plastic or metal stents are used to relieve obstruction of the bowel, oesophagus, bronchial tree, biliary ducts and ureters, and even patients with advanced malignancy benefit. Diathermy or laser coagulation of tumour-related haemorrhage similarly is a valuable palliative intervention which can often be undertaken endoscopically. Surgical relief of bowel obstruction may be indicated when stenting is not feasible but usually requires either colostomy or ileostomy depending upon the level of the obstruction. Fistulae are abnormal passageways connecting two epithelial-lined organs not normally connected and include rectovaginal, enterovaginal, colovesical and vesicovaginal or combinations of these. Fistulae may be either related to locally advanced disease or may be a consequence of radiotherapy. Fistula surgery is complex and demanding, requiring surgical expertise and often prolonged recovery, so it is usually reserved for cancer patients in remission. The surgical placement of shunts to prevent the reaccumulation of ascites (usually peritoneal–venous shunts, e.g. Leveen shunt) and pleural effusions (usually pleuroperitoneal shunts, e.g. Denver shunt) may be indicated for symptom palliation. Surgical oncologists may also be called upon to perform surgery for ulcerating and necrotic locally advanced cancers such as toilet mastectomy for fungating breast tumours. Orthopaedic surgeons frequently operate on pathological bone metastases either as a form of secondary prevention or following pathological fractures. Internal fixation of bones with lytic metastases are especially important in weight-bearing bones with large deposits occupying more than half the bone cortex that are at a high risk of fracturing. Surgeons thus have an important role in the palliation of symptoms in advanced malignancy and their input into the multidisciplinary team should not be seen as just to establish the diagnosis and surgically resect curable cancers.

Surgical reconstruction following cancer therapy

The aggressive treatment of bulky tumours often leaves major residual defects and, in combination with plastic surgeons, the discipline of surgical oncology has developed reconstructive surgery to reduce some of the effects of tumour resections. Plastic surgeons have developed a reconstructive ladder of increasingly complex wound management to deal with some of these residual deficits (Table 3.4). Reconstructive surgery is not, however, the exclusive responsibility of plastic surgeons. For example, orthopaedic surgeons have developed sophisticated procedures for limb reconstruction following sarcoma surgery using bone grafts and prostheses. Maxillofacial surgeons reconstruct mandibles with free-flap fibula transplants following surgery for oral cavity cancers. ENT surgeons medialize vocal cords with silicon injection to overcome the hoarse voice associated with recurrent laryngeal nerve palsy caused by mediastinal tumours. Breast reconstruction following mastectomy often involves the insertion of a tissue expander that is progressively injected with saline

Table 3.4 Reconstructive ladder of increasingly complex wound management coined by plastic surgeons.

1. Healing by secondary intent
2. Primary closure
3. Delayed primary closure
4. Split thickness graft
5. Full thickness skin graft
6. Tissue expansion
7. Random pattern graft
8. Pedicled flap
9. Free flap with vascular microsurgery

over the ensuing weeks until a suitable size and shape has been achieved, when it may be replaced by a more permanent implant. The second most common breast reconstruction procedure involves flaps of tissues from other parts of the body such as the back, abdomen, buttocks or thigh. These flaps may be pedicled, leaving the original blood supply, or may be free flaps with vascular microsurgery to connect to a new blood supply. A latissimus dorsi muscle flap can be performed without significant loss of function and retaining its original blood supply. Abdominal flaps usually take tissue from the lower abdomen, for example the TRAM (transverse rectus abdominis myocutaneous) flap which leaves the abdominal wall weakened. More recent abdominal flaps attempt to retain abdominal wall strength by using a muscle-sparing DIEP (deep inferior epigastric perforator) flap or SIEA (superficial inferior epigastric artery) flap. These require greater microsurgical skill. Other autologous tissue donor sites for breast reconstruction include SGAP (superior gluteal artery perforator) and IGAP (inferior gluteal artery perforator) flaps from the buttocks.

Radiotherapy

Radiotherapy involves the use of high-energy ionizing radiation to cause DNA damage and ultimately cell death. The damage induced by ionizing radiation may be lethal or sub-lethal to the tumour cells. In sub-lethal cell injury, damage to cellular proteins and organelles causes microscopic changes in the cell characterized down the microscope by swelling of mitochondria and endoplasmic reticulum and cloudiness of the cytoplasm known as hydropic degeneration. Cells may repair sub-lethal damage by removing damaged proteins and organelles by a cell stress response and autophagy and replace them with newly synthesized components. In contrast, lethal damage results in either cell necrosis or apoptosis.

Ionizing radiation acts by ejecting an electron from an atom to yield an ion pair. This may lead to direct damage to DNA via molecular excitation or indirectly via the hydrolysis of water into free radicals with an open electron shell configuration

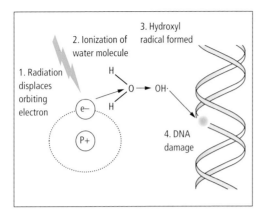

1. Radiation displaces orbiting electron

2. Ionization of water molecule

3. Hydroxyl radical formed

4. DNA damage

Figure 3.1 How radiation damages DNA.

characterized by the presence of an unpaired electron (Figure 3.1). These free radicals are highly reactive, usually short-lived chemicals such as the neutrally charged hydroxyl radical (OH·) derived from water which has an *in vivo* half-life of about 10^{-9} seconds. The other common free radical formed from water is superoxide (O_2^-) with one unpaired electron, which is responsible for the 'oxidative burst' or oxygen-dependent intracellular killing of ingested bacteria by phagocytes and is detoxified by the enzyme superoxide dismutase.

The dose of radiotherapy is defined as the amount of energy deposited in tissues and is measured in Grays (Gy) after Hal Gray, a British pioneer of radiation biology and physics who also established the Gray Laboratories at Mount Vernon Hospital. One Gray is the dose absorbed when 1 J (joule) is deposited in 1 kg of tissue. Each Gray per cell causes approximately 10 000 damaged DNA bases, 1000 damaged deoxyribose sugars, 1000 single strand breaks, 40 double strand breaks, 150 DNA–protein cross-links and 30 DNA–DNA cross-links. Radiation can have an effect at any point in the cell cycle, although it is only at the time of mitosis that cell death occurs. Therefore, there can be a time lag of days, weeks or even months between the radiotherapy and the full effects of the treatment becoming manifest. Typical radiotherapy doses for solid epithelial tumours are 60–80 Gy. This is delivered as multiple fractions over time for several reasons. Dose fractionation allows normal cells to recover from sub-lethal damage between fractions, whilst tumour cells are less efficient at repairing damage. Dose fractionation also ensures that tumour cells in different phases of the cell cycle are exposed to radiation since it causes greatest damage in the G2 and M phases. The exact scheduling and fractionation of radiotherapy varies but in general doses of around 2 Gy are delivered on a daily basis five days a week. In some circumstances more frequent dosing has been shown to be more efficacious but is of course more demanding on resources. For example, CHART (continuous hyperfractionated accelerated radiotherapy) involves radiotherapy delivered three times a day, every day of the week, usually for a fortnight.

Radiotherapy utilizes X-rays, electron beams and β- or γ-radiation produced by radioactive isotopes. X-rays are produced when a high-energy electron beam that is produced by heating an electrode in a vacuum, strikes matter. The energy of X-rays can be changed by altering the voltage input to the cathode of the X-ray tube that accelerates the electrons. Diagnostic radiology uses low-voltage equipment (e.g. 50 kV), producing X-rays of longer wavelength that are less penetrating. Therapeutic X-rays are produced by higher voltage machines (30–50 MeV) producing shorter wavelength, more penetrating X-rays.

Radiotherapy is delivered in three ways: external beam radiotherapy, brachytherapy and radioisotope therapy. External beam radiotherapy involves the use of isotope sources or linear accelerators to deliver radiation from a distance. In the case of brachytherapy, the radioactive source is a solid radioactive nuclide emitting γ-rays which is placed within the tumour or closely applied to the tumour. Finally, radioactive isotopes that are preferentially taken up in the target organ may be administered orally or intravenously; for example, oral iodine-131 is given for the treatment of thyroid tumours and intravenous strontium-89 in palliative treatment of bone metastasis.

External beam radiotherapy

Superficial voltage machines operate at 50–150 kV and their energy does not penetrate more than

1 cm below the surface of the skin. They are used chiefly to treat superficial skin cancers. Orthovoltage machines that yield X-rays of 200–300 kV energy penetrate to a depth of 3 cm. Metastases in bones close to the skin surface (ribs, sacrum) are frequently treated on these machines. Megavoltage radiotherapy machines usually use a cobalt-60 source that produces X-rays of 1.25 MeV on decaying to nickel-60. The cobalt-60 sources are contained within a protective lead shield and an adjustable window in this shield allows regulation of the γ-ray beam. However, there is considerable scatter of the beam, limiting the focus, and the relatively short half-life of the cobalt source means that it needs to be replaced every three to four years and that treatment times may become prolonged as the cobalt nears the replacement date. It is speculated that cobalt-60 sources could be used by terrorists to produce a 'dirty' bomb, a conventional explosive device to which radioactive material has been added.

Megavoltage machines have been replaced by linear accelerators that produce a high-energy electron beam by accelerating electrons down a cylindrical waveguide before they bombard a fixed target, resulting in a high-intensity electron beam (4–20 MeV) with greater penetration and less scatter. The advantages of this electron beam over X-rays lie in the penetration and decay characteristics that allow an electron beam to deliver its high energy to deep-seated tumours whilst sparing normal tissues in its pathway (Figure 3.2).

The accurate shaping of the radiation field to encompass the cancer but minimize damage to

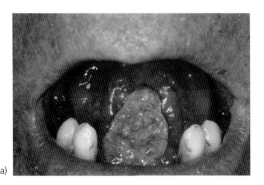
(a)

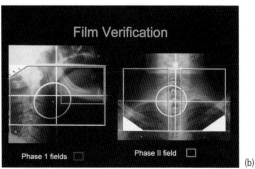
(b)

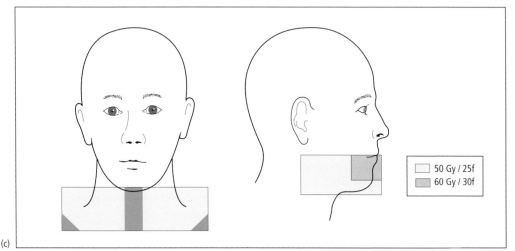
(c)

Figure 3.2 (a) Squamous cell cancer of the oral cavity. (b) Radiological verification of the radiotherapy fields. (c) The planned radiotherapy fields.

normal tissues really began with the introduction of the multileaf collimator composed of over 100 metal leaves, 5 mm thick and each aligned parallel to the radiation field. As each leaf may be moved independently to block part of the field, the resulting radiation field may be shaped and sculpted to suit the target. A further refinement of this process, known as intensity-modulated radiotherapy (IMRT), involves moving the multileaf collimator during the dose so that another level of fine tuning of the field can be achieved (Figure 3.3). One more recent development is image-guided radiation therapy (IGRT) that links the carefully shaped field with a continuous image of the patient. This process can overcome, for example, movement artefacts generated by the patient (hopefully still) breathing.

Brachytherapy

Brachytherapy employs sealed radionuclide sources that are implanted directly into a tumour or body cavity to deliver localized radiotherapy (Table 3.5). Examples of bachytherapy include radioactive iridium-192 needles or wires implanted into tumours of the breast, tongue and floor of the mouth. Sealed caesium-137 radioactive sources may also be placed into the vagina or rectum to treat cancers of the vagina, cervix, lower uterus, rectum or anus. Brachytherapy seeds are increasingly being used to treat localized prostate cancer (Figure 3.4). The major disadvantage of brachytherapy is the risk to staff handling the radioactive sources and caring for the patients. The radioactivity exposure of all staff involved with brachytherapy must be monitored. Another method used to reduce exposure is to place inactive source holders while the patient is anaesthetized, and once they have been correctly located (as determined by X-ray) the patient is allowed to recover from the procedure. With the patient in a shielded room, the live radioactive source is then introduced, either manually or by remote control using a selectron. This routine is termed manual or remote

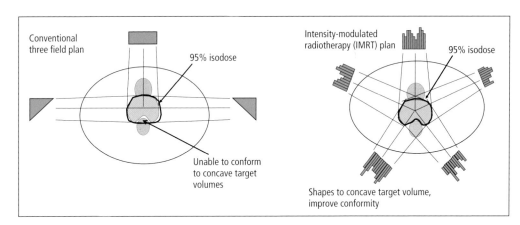

Figure 3.3 Comparison of conventional and intensity-modulated radiotherapy planning.

Table 3.5 Radionuclides used for brachytherapy.

Source	Half-life	Mean X-ray energy	Form
Cobalt-60	5.3 years	1.25 MeV	Pellets (beads, tubes, needles)
Caesium-137	30 years	0.66 MeV	Tubes, needles
Iridium-92	74 days	0.37 MeV	Wires, hairpins, cylinders
Iodine-125	60 days	0.03 MeV	Grains, seeds

Table 3.6 Table of systemically administered radionuclides used in oncology.

Radioisotope	Decay	Uses in oncology
Iodine-131	Beta: 192 keV Gamma: 364 keV Half-life: 8 days β- and γ-emitter	Used in treating thyroid cancer and in imaging the thyroid gland
Phosphorus-32	1.71 MeV Half-life: 14 days β-emitter	Used in the treatment of polycythemia vera
Rhenium-188	2.12 MeV Half-life: 17 hours β-emitter	Used to irradiate coronary arteries via an angioplasty balloon and in relieving the pain of bone metastases
Samarium-153	Beta: 825 keV Gamma: 103 keV Half-life: 47 hours β- and γ-emitter	Used in relieving the pain of bone metastases
Strontium-89	1.481 MeV Half-life: 50 days β-emitter	Used in relieving the pain of bone metastases

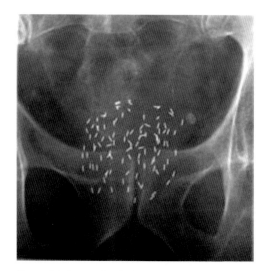

Figure 3.4 Prostate brachytherapy seeds *in situ* seen on pelvic X-ray.

after-loading and is frequently used for tumours of the upper vagina, cervix and endometrium.

Radioisotope therapy

Radioactive isotopes can be given by mouth or injection and are taken up by a particular tissue where they remain. Radioisotope therapy can only be used where a tumour is in a tissue that will preferentially accumulate a specific isotope, leaving other tissues unaffected. Examples are the thyroid, which will take up radioactive iodine and bone, that naturally accumulates phosphorus or will take up bone-seeking radiochemicals such as rhenium-186 hydroxyethylidine diphosphate (^{186}Re-HEDP) (Table 3.6). A disadvantage with this approach is that the source cannot be recovered, limiting the degree of control over the total exposure to radiation.

Toxicity of radiotherapy

External beam radiotherapy is usually given as repeated daily dose fractions rather than as a single large dose of radiotherapy, which would lead to severe damage to the normal tissues. Even with fractionation, normal tissues have a maximum tolerated dose as indicated in Table 3.7. The area to be irradiated is referred to as the radiation field. This is marked out on the skin before treatment and such markings often persist after treatment as tattooed dots. These radiotherapy tattoos are assiduously sought by clinical medical exam candidates but in

Table 3.7 Table of normal tissue tolerance of radiotherapy.

Tissue	Radiation effect	Dosage
Testis	Sterility	0.2 Gy
Eye	Cataract	10 Gy
Lung	Pneumonitis	20 Gy
Kidney	Nephritis	25 Gy
Liver	Hepatitis	30 Gy
Central nervous system	Necrosis	50 Gy
Gastrointestinal tract	Ulceration, haemorrhage	60 Gy

real life most patients will tell you that they have had radiotherapy if you ask them nicely. In general, radiation-related side effects occur within the field of treatment although a few systemic manifestations such as fatigue and nausea may occur. The toxicity of radiotherapy increases with both the volume of tissue irradiated and the dose given. The transient side effects that develop during treatment tend to reflect the acute damage to normal healthy tissue. Careful planning of the beam size and shielding of surrounding tissue, ensuring that radiation fields give effective tumour eradication with an acceptable level of toxicity, is, therefore, a prerequisite of successful therapy.

Radiotherapy-related side effects can be usefully divided into early and late toxicities (Table 3.8). Early toxicity occurs in hours to weeks and includes both systemic effects such as nausea, lethargy and myelosuppression (when a large volume of bone marrow is within the treated area, for example whole femur or pelvis radiation). Localized skin toxicity is a common early side effect that may be local erythema progressing to ulceration and desquamation in the more severe cases. Other early side effects depend on the anatomy of the radiotherapy field, e.g. alopecia with cranial irradiation (see Plate 3.1), oropharyngeal mucositis with head and neck radiotherapy, and diarrhoea, proctitis and cystitis with pelvic fields. These early reactions occur in tissues that are rapidly dividing and are usually present during or shortly after the course of radiotherapy and in most cases are reversible. Late side effects may take months or years to manifest themselves and once again depend upon the site being irradiated. These late tissue reactions occur when slowly dividing cells attempt division and are less frequently reversible. In some cases the effects are believed to be mediated by fibrosis of the vascular endothelium. Examples of late reactions include necrosis in the central nervous system leading to transverse myelitis and paralysis with spinal cord radiation fields, radiation-induced nephritis and osteomyelitis. Finally, radiotherapy is carcinogenic and may induce secondary tumours.

Radiosensitivity and radioresistance

Tumour resistance to radiotherapy appears to be an intrinsic property of that cancer, rather than an

Table 3.8 Table of adverse early and late reactions to radiotherapy.

Timing	Tissue	Reaction
Early reactions	Skin	Dermatitis
	Oral mucosa	Stomatitis
	Bladder	Cystitis
	Oesophagus	Oesophagitis
	Bowel	Diarrhoea, ulceration
	Bone marrow	Myelosuppression
Late reactions	Central nervous system	Necrosis
	Kidney	Nephritis
	Liver	Hepatitis
	Lung	Pneumonitis and fibrosis
	Vascular endothelium	Fibrosis

acquired attribute selected for by treatment, as in the case of chemotherapy. Indeed the radiation sensitivities of many types of tumour are relatively predictable. The response of tissues both malignant and normal to fractionated radiation depends upon the '5 Rs':

- Repair
- Reassortment
- Repopulation
- Reoxygenation
- Radiosensitivity.

In this context, repair is recovery from sub-lethal damage and is dependent on DNA repair mechanisms. Reassortment refers to the cell cycle phase of the tumour cells. Cells in G2 and M phases are most susceptible to radiotherapy and so after a first dose cells in G1 and S will make up a greater proportion of the live tumour cells. Depending on the timing of the subsequent fraction of radiotherapy these cells may have progressed or 'reassorted' to G2 and M phases with increased sensitivity. Repopulation is the ability of tumour cells to grow and divide between doses of radiotherapy; this is a particular problem with prolonged fractionation and delayed fractions. Hypoxic cells are relatively radioresistant and after the first fractions of radiotherapy, the death of sensitive cells reduces the competition for oxygen in the tumour and cells that were hypoxic previously become reoxygenated and hence more susceptible to radiation. Different cell lineages are more or less radiosensitive and these differences are in part intrinsic and independent of environmental factors. Amongst the factors that influence the radiosensitivity of tumours are the DNA repair genes, the production of free radical scavenging molecules (e.g. glutathione-S-transferases, superoxide dismutases, glutathione peroxidase), genes controlling apoptosis and cell cycle regulatory genes.

Chemotherapy

Drug discovery

The origins of chemotherapy for cancer lie in the use of biological warfare during the First World War, most hauntingly described in Wilfred Owen's

poem 'Dulce et decorum est'. Following the extensive use of chlorine gas in trench warfare, the German army first released mustard gas at Ypres on the night of 12–13 July 1917. Mustard gas had been synthesized in 1854 by Victor Meyer and was noted to be a vesicant in 1887. As a weapon of mass destruction, mustard gas or Yperite as it was then known, had the advantages over chlorine of requiring smaller doses, being almost odourless and remaining active in the soil for weeks. The British gas casualties from 1914–1918 reveal the greater fatalities with mustard gas. Mustard gas exposure causes a severe blistering rash and conjunctivitis followed by meyelosuppression after around four days. During the Second World War the only use of mustard gas resulted in an own goal when the Luftwaffe sunk the USS *John Harvey* off Bari harbour in southern Italy in 1943. The ship was carrying 2000 M47A1 bombs containing a total of 100 tonnes of mustard gas and the American sailors who survived developed conjunctivitis and skin blistering followed by a steep fall in their white cell counts, as documented by the naval surgeon Colonel Stewart Alexander. Meanwhile at Yale University, Alfred Gilman and Louis Goodman were using the closely related nitrogen mustard (mechlorethamine) initially in murine lymphoma models. In 1944 the first patient with lymphosarcoma (high-grade non-Hodgkin's lymphoma) was treated and although Mr J. D., a 48-year-old silversmith, achieved a temporary remission of his tumour, he later died of bone marrow failure.

The subsequent development of chemotherapy following this fortuitous finding as a by-product of biological warfare, owes much to luck and trial and error rather than design. One serendipitous discovery was made by Barnett Rosenberg, a physicist at Michigan State University in 1965. He studied the effects of electric currents on *Escherichia coli* using platinum electrodes in a water bath and found that they stopped dividing but not growing, leading to bacteria up to 300 times longer than normal. This was found to be due to cisplatin, a product from the platinum electrodes, which was interfering with DNA replication. By the end of the 1960s a number of cytotoxic drugs from natural sources had been identified. In 1971 President Nixon, losing a war in Vietnam, declared war on cancer, signing the Cancer Act and establishing a drug discovery programme at the National Cancer Institute (NCI). This project trawled though thousands of natural chemicals in search of potential cytotoxic agents. It was not until the 1990s that rational drug design targeting known tumour-related features emerged. Examples of this include trastuzumab, a monoclonal antibody raised against erbB2/neu/Her-2 in breast cancer, and imatinib, which inhibits the adenosine triphosphate (ATP) binding site of brc-abl fusion protein kinase in chronic myeloid leukaemia.

Mechanisms of cytotoxic drug

Amongst the many classifications of cytotoxic agents is a functional classification of cytotoxics (Table 3.9).

Alkylating agents

Alkylating agents transfer an alkyl group to purine (adenine and guanine) bases of DNA. Bifunctional alkylating agents form covalent bonds between two different bases resulting in interstand or intrastrand cross-links, whilst monofunctional alkylating agents cannot form cross-links but cause adducts. Both forms of DNA alteration inhibit DNA synthesis, so alkyating agents act chiefly during the S phase of the cell cycle. Bifunctional agents can act on more than one base and are more cytotoxic, whilst monofunctional agents are more mutagenic and carcinogenic. One of the mechanisms of tumour resistance to alkylating agents is enzymatic removal of alkyl groups from purine bases and enhanced repair of cross-links.

Antimetabolites

Antimetabolites are structurally similar to natural compounds and in general interfere with cellular enzymes. These agents inhibit the metabolism (usually synthesis) of compounds necessary for DNA, RNA or protein synthesis. They include: (1) purine analogues, (2) pyrimidine analogues, (3) folic acid analogues, and (4) others, e.g. hydroxyurea. Most antimetabolites have their greatest activity during the S phase.

Intercalating agents

Intercalating agents disrupt the steric integrity of the DNA double helix. The exact mechanisms of this action remain uncertain although anthracycline antibiotics intercalate into the DNA major groove between base pairs of the DNA double helix and this action is non-covalent with no base sequence specificity. Platinum agents also intercalate and form intrastrand links similar to those formed by alkylating agents.

Spindle poisons

Antimicrotubule drugs can be divided into two groups, those that stabilize microtubules by inhibiting depolymerization (e.g. taxanes) and those that are depolymerizing agents that inhibit polymerization of tubulin (e.g. vinca alkaloids). Spindle poisons inhibit the mitotic spindle function and therefore act in the M phase of the cell cycle. Tubulin exists as α-tubulin and β-tubulin monomers in dynamic equilibrium with tubulin polymers, or microtubules. Resistance to spindle poisons may occur by mutations of β-tubulin and these point mutations do not confer cross-resistance between taxanes and vincas. An early spindle cell poison included colchicine used for acute gout, familial Mediterranean fever and rarely psoriasis. Although colchicine, like vincas causes depolymerization, it binds to a distinct site and is not used as a cytotoxic.

Topoisomerase inhibitors

Topoisomerases prevent DNA strands from becoming tangled by cutting DNA and allowing it to wind or unwind. There are two mammalian classes of topoisomerases: topoisomerase I breaks single strands of DNA, whilst topoisomerase II breaks both strands of DNA. Topoisomerase I inhibitors act by inhibiting the re-ligation step of the nicking–closing reaction trapping topoisomerase I in a covalent complex with DNA. Topoisomerase I

Table 3.11 Cancers effectively treated by neoadjuvant and adjuvant chemotherapy.

Therapy	Tumour
Cancers effectively treated by neoadjuvant chemotherapy	Soft tissue sarcoma
	Osteosarcoma
	Locally advanced breast cancer
Cancers effectively treated by adjuvant chemotherapy	Wilms' tumour
	Osteosarcoma
	Breast cancer
	Colorectal cancer

(from a donor) bone marrow transplantation was developed to this end. Prior to high-dose chemotherapy, progenitor stem cells are harvested either from multiple bone marrow aspirations (bone marrow transplant or BMT) or now more often from peripheral blood following growth factor stimulation (peripheral blood stem cell transplant or PBSCT). These stem cells are immature haematopoietic cells capable of repopulating the bone marrow. The patient then receives the conditioning high-dose chemotherapy and/or radiotherapy and subsequently the stem cells are re-infused as a transfusion. This approach has an appreciable mortality of 20–50% in the case of allogeneic BMT and of 5% with autologous PBSCT. However, stem cell transplantation has a defined role in the management of a number of malignancies (Table 3.12).

Side effects of chemotherapy

The main actions of chemotherapy are focused on killing rapidly dividing cancer cells and hence many of their toxicities arise because of the effects on normal cells with high rates of turnover. Indeed the side effects of chemotherapy may be divided into the predictable toxicities that are common, often dose related and usually related to the mechanism of action of the drug. In contrast idiosyncratic side effects are usually rarer, unrelated to dose or mechanism of action but tend to be drug specific. The predictable effects of chemotherapy on fast dividing normal cells (bone marrow, gastrointestinal tract epithelium, hair follicles, spermatogonia) will be a consequence of inhibition of cell division and are especially found with cell cycle phase-specific cytotoxics. In contrast the side effects on slow-growing cell types will occur most frequently with drugs that are not cell cycle specific such as the alkylating agents that introduce DNA mutations into these cells resulting in secondary leukaemias and other tumours.

The side effects of chemotherapy may be divided into three time groups, immediate effects that occur within hours, delayed effects that occur within days, weeks or months but are generally manifested whilst the full course of chemotherapy treatment is on-going, and late effects that occur

Table 3.12 Cancers effectively treated by high-dose chemotherapy and stem cell transplantation.

Disease	Stage	Transplant	Approx. 5-year disease-free survival
CML	Stable phase	Allogeneic	30%
ALL	Second remission	Allogeneic/autologous	40%
AML	First remission	Allogeneic/autologous	50%
High-grade non-Hodgkin's lymphoma	Responsive relapse	Autologous	45%
Hodgkin's disease	Responsive relapse	Autologous	45%
Neuroblastoma	High risk first line	Allogeneic/autologous	50%
Neuroblastoma	Relapsed	Allogeneic/autologous	25%
Non-seminomatous germ cell tumour	Responsive relapse	Autologous	50%
Myeloma	First line	Allogeneic/autologous	30%

ALL, acute lymphoblastic leukaemia; AML, acute myeloid leukaemia; CML, chronic myeloid leukaemia.

months, years or decades after the chemotherapy has ceased. The top five side effects ranked by patients according to severity are nausea, fatigue, hair loss, concern about the effects on friends and family and finally vomiting. The immediate toxicities include nausea and vomiting, anaphylaxis, extravasation and tumour lysis. The delayed side effects are the most abundant and include alopecia, myelosuppression, stomatitis and the majority of the unpredictable toxicities. The late effects of chemotherapy include infertility and secondary malignancies.

Early side effects

Nausea and vomiting

Vomiting is a central reflex initiated in the vomiting centre of the medulla that co-ordinates the contraction of the diaphragm and abdominal muscles with relaxation of the cardiac sphincter and the muscles of the throat. There are four inputs into the vomiting centre: the labyrinths (e.g. motion sickness), the higher cortical centres (e.g. fear, anticipation), the vagus nerve sensory input from the gastrointestinal tract particularly the small bowel, and finally the chemoreceptor trigger zone (CTZ). The CTZ is located in the area postrema adjacent to the fourth ventricle where the blood–brain barrier is relatively deficient and chemicals in the blood and cerebrospinal fluid (CSF) are sensed, stimulating the vomiting centre. The different inputs to the vomiting centre rely on different neurotransmitters and this can be exploited pharmacologically in the control of symptoms (Figure 3.5). Chemotherapy chiefly acts on the gastrointestinal tract causing serotonin (5-hydroxytryptamine, 5HT) release and acting via the afferent vagus nerve. It also stimulates the chemoreceptor trigger zone which employs

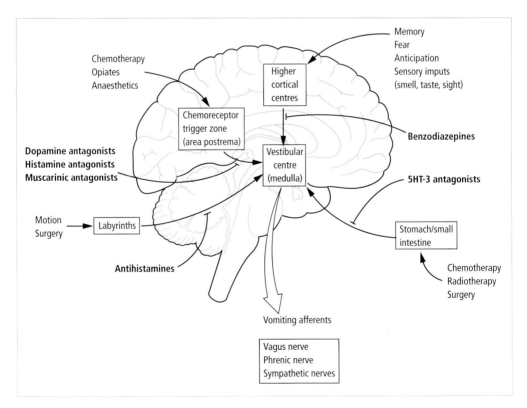

Figure 3.5 Neural pathways in vomiting.

dopaminergic and muscarinic pathways. Occasionally anticipatory vomiting is problematic and this acts through the higher cortical centres using γ-aminobutyric acid (GABA) neurotransmission. In contrast, the labyrinthine pathways utilize histamine-1 receptors and motion sickness is often successfully controlled with antihistamines.

The likelihood of being sick with chemotherapy depends upon the emetogenicity of the cytotoxics used as well as host-related factors. Cisplatin and mustine are amongst the most emetogenic whilst vinca alkaloids rarely cause nausea. Younger age, women, patients who have been sick previously with chemotherapy, and patients with a low alcohol intake are all more likely to suffer with chemotherapy-induced vomiting. Acute vomiting within six hours of chemotherapy is best controlled by a combination of steroids and 5HT-3 receptor antagonists. Delayed vomiting occurring up to five days after the chemotherapy is best treated with steroids and dopamine antagonists. Anticipatory vomiting that occurs prior to receiving chemotherapy is treated with benzodiazepines.

Anaphylaxis

As with all medicines, anaphylaxis may occur with chemotherapy and the most common culprits are taxanes and asparaginase. The incidence of hypersensitivity with paclitaxel is so high that routine prophylaxis with steroids and antihistamines (H1 and H2) is administered to all patients receiving paclitaxel.

Extravasation

Extravasation is the inadvertent administration of chemotherapy into subcutaneous tissue. This leads to pain, erythema, inflammation and discomfort, which if unrecognized and untreated can lead to tissue necrosis with the possibility of serious sequelae. The position, size and age of the cannulation site are the factors that have the greatest bearing on the likelihood of problems occurring (Figure 3.6) and the experience of the specialist administering the chemotherapy is crucial in this aspect. The likelihood of damage occurring is determined by the

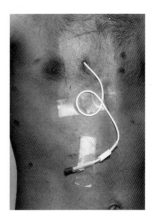

Figure 3.6 A patient with a Hickman line, a skin-tunnelled, long-term silicon catheter with a dacron cuff about 2 cm above the exit site that acts as a barrier to micro-organisms and prevents catheter dislodgment. Hickman lines are used for continuous infusional chemotherapy or for patients with poor venous access. Hickman lines are placed in the radiology department using ultrasound guidance or in theatres under general anaesthetic.

cytotoxic drug, with anthracyclines being especially likely to cause severe injury.

Tumour lysis

The rapid cytolysis of a large volume of cancer cells at the start of chemotherapy occasionally results in the tumour lysis syndrome or metabolic chaos. The destruction of tumour DNA leads to hyperuricaemia from the breakdown of nucleotide bases. The cytolysis causes hyperkalaemia by releasing intracellular potassium and the breakdown of proteins and DNA causes hyperphosphataemia and secondary hypocalcaemia. Acute renal failure may be a consequence of the high levels of urate and phosphate, whilst the high levels of potassium may lead to cardiac arrthymias. Tumour lysis only really occurs with acute leukaemias and high-grade lymphomas including Burkitt lymphoma. Bulky tumours, poor renal function and high levels of urate before chemotherapy increase the risk of tumour lysis.

Uric acid is soluble at physiological pH but precipitates in the acidic environment of the renal tubules, leading to crystallization in the collecting ducts and ureters, leading to obstructive uropathy.

Similarly calcium phosphate is precipitated in the renal tubules and microvasculature producing nephrocalcinosis. The most important issue in the management of tumour lysis is its prevention by a combination of hyperhydaration, allopurinol and urinary alkalinization to pH >7 with sodium bicarbonate to reduce urate precipitation in the renal tubules. Allopurinol is an inhibitor of xanthine oxidase, the enzyme that catalyzes the conversion of soluble xanthine (a product of purine catabolism) to uric acid. The treatment of established tumour lysis is an oncological emergency. The majority of patients who develop tumour lysis have chemosensitive tumours and are receiving potentially curative treatment. These patients should be considered candidates for urgent haemodialysis. A relatively new addition to the treatment is recombinant urate oxidase (rasburicase) which converts insoluble urate to soluble allantoin (Figure 3.7).

Delayed side effects (predictable)

The main predictable delayed side effects of chemotherapy are alopecia, bone marrow suppression and gastrointestinal mucositis.

Alopecia and onychodystrophy

Hair loss with chemotherapy is both drug and dose dependent and is related to the frequency of cycle repetition. Long-term therapy may result in loss of pubic, axillary and facial hair in addition to scalp hair. The loss of scalp hair often occurs in an acute episode while washing, usually two to six weeks after starting chemotherapy. It should be emphasized to patients that alopecia from chemotherapy is reversible, with hair regrowth beginning one to two months after completing chemotherapy. The hair may regrow a lighter or darker colour and is often curlier initially. Doxorubicin and cyclophosphamide are the commonest culprits. Patients should be offered wigs available on the NHS. Scalp cooling (below 22°C) may reduce alopecia by causing vasoconstriction and reducing circulation to hair follicles. The pharmacokinetic profiles of cytotoxics dictate that scalp cooling is only effective for anthracyclines. Concerns have been raised over the potential risk of developing scalp and cerebral metastases due to reduced drug circulation to these sites with scalp cooling. Along with alopecia, a frequent complication of chemotherapy is onychodystrophy or nail changes other than colour changes that usually make the nails brittle and prone to shedding (onycholysis) as well as fungal infection (onychomycosis). A common physical sign in patients who have received cyclical chemotherapy are Beau lines, horizontal grooves or lines on the nail plate that indicate cycles of arrested nail growth with chemotherapy cycles (see Plate 3.2).

Myelotoxicity of chemotherapy

The myelosuppressive effects of chemotherapy may affect the circulating red cells, white cells and platelets and the manifestations in these three series are in part related to their circulatory lifespans. In circulation the half-life of an erythro-

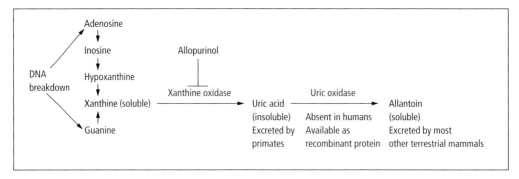

Figure 3.7 Purine catabolism pathway and the therapy of tumour lysis.

cyte is 120 days, of a leucocyte is six to eight hours and of a platelet is seven days.

There is a significant risk of severe myelosuppression if chemotherapy is initiated when the total white cell count is <3.0 × 10^9/l (or the neutrophil count is <1.5 × 10^9/l) and/or the platelet count is <150 × 10^9/l. These values are the usual cut-offs for administering a cycle of chemotherapy, however it may be given at lower values in patients with haematological malignancies or if supportive therapy is anticipated and when non-myelosuppressive regimens are employed. Myelosuppression is the dose-limiting toxicity for many cytotoxic agents; the main exceptions are vincristine, bleomycin, streptozotocin and asparaginase, which do not cause myelosuppression.

Thus anaemia is rarely a dose-limiting toxicity but is generally cumulative over successive cycles of chemotherapy. Anaemia is most troublesome with cisplatin since the nephrotoxicity of this agent may decrease erythropoietin production from the kidneys in response to anaemia. The symptoms of anaemia include fatigue, lethargy and exertional dyspnoea with haemoglobin levels in the range 8–10 g/dl. Reduced exercise capacity progresses to dyspnoea and tachycardia at rest and complications including cerebrovascular (e.g. transient iscaemic attacks) and cardiovascular (e.g. angina) ischaemia as the haemoglobin falls below 8 g/dl. The management of chemotherapy-induced anaemia is with transfusion and in the case of cisplatin-induced anaemia, at least, erythropoietin may be beneficial (Box 3.1).

Neutropenia (neutrophil count <1.0 × 10^9/l) is the commonest dose-limiting toxicity of chemotherapy and is a frequent cause of treatment delays and dose reductions. Neutropenia is most often manifest as infection (Figure 3.8) and neutropenic sepsis is a medical emergency, which if left untreated is potentially fatal. It is frequently overlooked by untrained medical staff and delays in starting intravenous antibiotics can be fatal. Neutropenic sepsis is defined as a fever of 38.0°C or higher for at least two hours when the neutrophil count is below 1.0 × 10^9/l.

The treatment of neutropenic sepsis includes a thorough clinical history and physical examina-

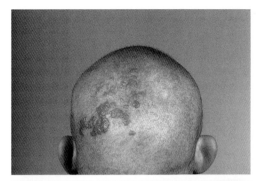

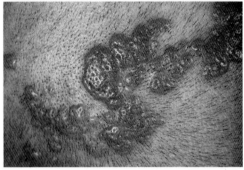

Figure 3.8 Herpes zoster scalp (with close up below): herpes zoster of left C2 distribution erupting as an opportunistic infection during a course of chemotherapy for Hodgkin's disease.

tion to identify possible sources of infection. Initial management must include resuscitation measures for shock if present. An infection screen should be performed, including blood cultures from peripheral veins as well as from any central access catheters, a urine sample for microscopy and culture, a chest X-ray and a throat swab for culture. Treatment should not be delayed awaiting the results of cultures. The most common organisms associated with neutropenic sepsis are common bacterial pathogens. Empirical antibiotic treatment should be instituted with broad-spectrum bactericidal antibiotics and policies will be dictated by local antibiotic resistance patterns. The most common initial treatment regimens are a parenteral combination of an aminoglycoside with either a cephalosporin or a broad-spectrum penicillin. Alternatively, monotherapy with a cephalosporin may be used. If there is no response within 36–48 hours, the antibiotic regimen should be reviewed

Box 3.1: Haematopoietic growth factors

The proliferation and maturation of blood cell lineages is determined by haemopoietic growth factors (Figure 3.9) or colony-stimulating factors (CSFs). Bone marrow stromal cells produce many of these growth factors. Recombinant haemopoietic growth factors are administered to ameliorate chemotherapy-induced cytopenias. They are given parenterally to avoid proteolytic degradation in the gastrointestinal tract.

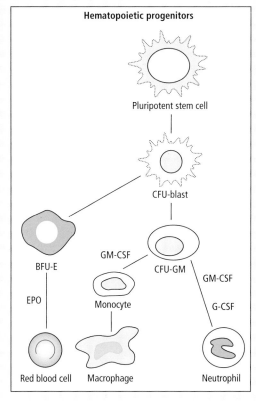

Figure 3.9 Haematopoetic pathway. BFU-E, blast-forming unit, erythroblast; CFU, colony-forming unit; CFU-GM, colony-forming unit, granulocyte–macrophage; EPO, erythropoietin; G-CSF, granulocyte colony-stimulating factor; GM-CSF, granulocyte–macrophage colony-stimulating factor.

Erythropoietin

This growth factor is naturally produced by the kidney in response to hypoxia and stimulates red cell proliferation. It may be overproduced in renal cell carcinoma leading to paraneoplastic polycythemia. As well as its role in the treatment of anaemia of chronic renal failure, erythropoietin may be used to treat cytotoxic-induced anaemia, particularly where cisplatin is implicated.

Granulocyte colony-stimulating factor (G-CSF)

G-CSF is a lineage-restricted growth factor promoting granulocyte differentiation whilst granulocyte–macrophage CSF (GM-CSF) is multifunctional, affecting granulocytes, monocytes, megakaryocytes and erythroid precursors but not basophils. Both CSFs are used in the treatment of chemotherapy- and radiotherapy-related neutropenia. Evidence-based guidelines are available that describe the rational use of G-CSF in four circumstances:

(continued on p. 63)

(continued)
1. Primary prophylaxis (i.e. with the first cycle of chemotherapy): not routinely used, occasionally used for pre-existing neutropenia, e.g. due to marrow infiltration.
2. Secondary prophylaxis: only for curable tumours with proven importance of maintaining dose intensity (germ cell tumours, choriocarcinoma, lymphoma).
3. Febrile neutropenia: data do not support routine G-CSF usage, but indicate use in the presence of pneumonia, hypotension, multiorgan failure and fungal infection.
4. Peripheral blood stem cell mobilization prior to harvesting for high-dose therapy and stem cell rescue.

Thrombopoietin (TPO)

TPO is constitutively produced by the liver and kidneys and acts on many stages of megakaryocyte growth and differentiation. It has yet to become incorporated into routine clinical use. Interleukin-11 however also raises platelet counts following chemotherapy and has been licensed for this indication in the USA.

in the light of culture results, and consideration given to adding antifungal cover (e.g. amphotericin B). For patients with severe neutropenic sepsis as defined by hypotension, pneumonia or multiorgan failure, granulocyte colony-stimulating factor (G-CSF) should be administered. Following an episode of neutropenic sepsis consideration should be given to reducing the chemotherapy dosage in subsequent cycles, or if dose intensity has been shown to influence the outcome (e.g. germ cell tumours, Hodgkin's disease) secondary prophylaxis with G-CSF to reduce the duration of neutropenia should be considered (Box 3.1).

Thrombocytopenia is a common side effect of chemotherapy, particularly with carboplatin, that rarely causes clinical manifestations unless it is severe. Although petechiae and bruising may occur, major haemorrhage is very rare unless the platelet count falls below 20×10^9/l. At platelet counts below 10×10^9/l there is an appreciable risk of gastrointestinal or cerebral haemorrhage and prophylactic administration of pooled platelets is warranted. Growth factor support for thrombocytopenia is currently investigational only (Box 3.1) and chemotherapy dose delays and reductions may be necessary following low platelet nadir counts.

Gastrointestinal tract mucositis

Mucositis is a frequent delayed side effect of chemotherapy occurring in 40–50% of patients, and is even more common in patients receiving chemo-

radiotherapy or radiotherapy alone for head and neck cancers. It is thought that chemotherapy and radiotherapy damage basal epithelial cells in the intestinal mucosa leading to apoptosis, atrophy and ulceration. Once ulceration occurs, bacterial and fungal infection and activation of macrophages leads to further inflammation. Mucositis is associated with significant morbidity and mortality risk, and chemotherapy dose reductions and delays. Sucking ice lollies during chemotherapy may reduce the incidence of mucositis with some cytotoxics by a mechanism analogous to the cold cap treatment for the prevention of alopecia. Various 'magic mouthwashes' (usually a mild local anaesthetic and antiseptic combination) may provide symptomatic relief from mucositis. The time course of mucositis closely resembles that of neutropenia, typically occurring 7–14 days after the administration of chemotherapy. Recent developments in the management of mucositis also hint at comparisons with the investigational study of keratinocyte growth factors as treatment for mucositis. In a few cases specific antidotes reduce the incidence of mucositis, such as folinic acid rescue after methotrexate.

Delayed side effects (idiosyncratic)

Many delayed side effects of chemotherapy are drug specific and are not immediately predictable from their mechanisms of action. The organs most frequently affected include the skin, nerves, heart, lungs and blood vessels.

Dermatological side effects

Dermatological complications include the already mentioned acute complications of extravasation and anaphylaxis as well as idiosyncratic delayed toxicities. These include hyperpigmentation, which occurs commonly with 5-fluorouracil and bleomycin and may follow the lines of the veins into which the chemotherapy has been administered. A hand and foot syndrome of painful redness, scaling or shedding of the skin of the palms and soles may occur with continuous infusions of 5-fluorouracil chemotherapy and also with liposomal anthracycline chemotherapy. In the latter case, the cytotoxics are delivered in a liposome to dramatically prolong their half-life, mimicking the pharmacokinetics of a continuous infusion regimen. A third unusual dermatological side effect of chemotherapy is radiation recall, an erythematous reaction of skin in the area of a previous radiation field. Indeed this may occur even when the radiation treatment was decades earlier and is most commonly seen with gemcitabine chemotherapy.

Cardiological side effects

Acute arrythmias can occur during chemotherapy infusions or shortly thereafter and this rare occurrence happens most frequently with taxanes. Similarly, 5-fluorouracil rarely precipitates chest pain and acute myocardial infarction, pericarditis and cardiac shock. However, the most common cardiotoxicity of chemotherapy is a dose-related dilated cardiomyopathy seen with anthracyclines. This usually presents with heart failure within 8 months of the last anthracycline dose. Diuretics improve symptoms and the early use of an angiotensin-converting enzyme inhibitor can increase the left ventricular ejection fraction, improving prognosis which, however, remains poor. This side effect limits the total cumulative dosage of anthracyclines that can be administered. The maximum cumulative lifetime doses of the anthracyclines have been established although cardiomyopathy may be seen at lower total doses.

Neurological side effects

Although only a few cytotoxics penetrate the cerebrospinal fluid, many cytotoxics cause neurotoxicity. Peripheral neuropathy, the most frequent neurotoxicity of chemotherapy, is commonly seen with vinca alkaloids, taxanes and platinum derivatives. The longest nerves are most affected so it presents as a symmetrical sensory loss over the feet and hands. This may progress to worsening paraesthesia, loss of tendon reflexes and eventually motor loss. Features usually slowly improve over several months following cessation of chemotherapy, although residual deficits may persist indefinitely. The same cytotoxics may be responsible for an autonomic neuropathy leading to abdominal pain, constipation, paralytic ileus, urinary retention, bradycardia and postural hypotension. Acute encephalopathy most commonly is associated with ifosfamide and symptoms include confusion, agitation, seizures, somnolence and coma. Cerebellar toxicity may follow cytarabine therapy and 5-fluorouracil. Cisplatin-induced ototoxicity is characterized by the progressive loss of high-tone hearing and tinnitus.

The inadvertent intrathecal administration of vinca alkaloids is fatal and this catastrophic clinical error has arisen because of confusion of the drug with a cytotoxic agent intended to be given intrathecally (usually methotrexate). Five such incidents have occurred in NHS hospitals in the past decade, representing an estimated rate of about three per 100 000 intrathecal chemotherapy treatments and recently resulting in the jailing of a junior doctor. A number of strict guidelines surrounding the administration of intrathecal chemotherapy are now in place to prevent this occurrence.

Pulmonary side effects

Chronic pulmonary toxicity and fibrosis occurs with a number of cytotoxics and the outcome is generally poor. Bleomycin is the most common culprit and the risk increases with dose. The cardinal symptom of drug-induced pulmonary toxicity is dyspnoea associated with non-productive cough,

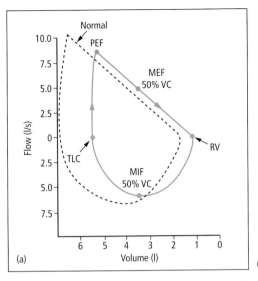

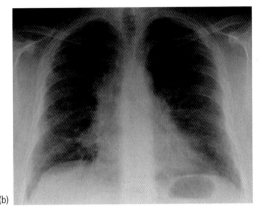

Figure 3.10 (a) Lung flow loop and (b) chest radiograph of a 35-year-old man treated with combination chemotherapy including bleomycin for advanced germ cell tumour of the testis. The chest radiograph demonstrates diffuse interstitial shadowing most prominent in the lower zones. The lung flow loop shows a restrictive deficit typical of bleomycin fibrosis. MEF, mid expiratory flow; MIF, mid inspiratory flow; PEF, peak expiratory flow; RV, residual volume; TLC, total lung capacity; VC, vital capacity.

fatigue, fever and malaise. Symptoms usually develop over several weeks to months. The chest X-ray classically shows reticulonodular infiltration at the bases and occasionally pleural effusions (Figure 3.10a). Lung function tests demonstrate a reduced diffusing capacity for carbon monoxide and restrictive ventilatory defects (Figure 3.10b). The usual treatment is with corticosteroids although there is little to support this and the mortality is high.

Hepatic side effects

Many cytotoxics cause elevated serum transaminases and bilirubin, and fatty infiltration and cholestasis may occur as the toxic effect progresses. Hepatic veno-occlusive disease (VOD) results from the blockage of venous outflow in the small centri-lobular hepatic vessels following damage to cells in the area of the liver surrounding the central vein. This rare side effect occurs with high-dose chemotherapy often as part of stem cell transplantation. The clinical features are painful hepatomegaly, ascites, peripheral oedema, marked elevations in serum enzymes and bilirubin, and hepatic encephalopathy. The onset is often abrupt, occurring during the first post-transplant week, and the clinical course is fatal in up to 50%.

Late side effects

Gonadal side effects

Chemotherapy causes a variety of toxic effects on male and female gonads leading to infertility. Moreover, cytotoxic drugs given during pregnancy may have teratogenic effects on the fetus. If fertility is maintained or restored, there are concerns about the heritability of the cancer and at least a theoretical risk of mutagenic alterations to germ cells.

Adult male gonadal toxicity
Male germ cells lie within the seminiferous epithelium and include stem spermatogonia, differentiating spermatogonia, spermatocytes, spermatids and sperm. The differentiating spermatogonia actively proliferate and are therefore highly susceptible to

cytotoxic agents. In contrast, the Leydig cells, which are in the interstitium and produce androgens, and the Sertoli cells, which provide support and regulatory factors to the germ cells, do not proliferate in adults and so survive most cytotoxic therapies. Because later stage germ cells (spermatocytes onwards) do not proliferate they are not susceptible to chemotherapy – sperm counts do not fall immediately on starting chemotherapy, but may take two to three months to decline; although minor falls in testosterone production may occur, only testicular radiation will produce significant testosterone deficiency. Men due to start chemotherapy should be offered sperm storage in order to enable them to father children in the future. Modern developments in *in vitro* fertilization are particularly relevant to the cancer patient. For those patients who were considered to be unsuitable for semen storage and remain azoospermic post treatment, the technique of intracytoplasmic sperm injection (ICSI) may be appropriate. Just remember, only one sperm is required to fertilize one ovum.

Adult female gonadal toxicity

In women, unlike men, the germ cells do not proliferate whereas the somatic cells do and this accounts for the different gonadal toxicity of chemotherapy in women and men. Female germ cells proliferate before birth as oogonia that arrest at the oocyte stage. At birth, a woman has 1 million oocytes, which are reduced to 300 000 at puberty. Oocytes are progressively lost by atresia, development and ovulation, until almost all are lost and menopause is reached. The interval from recruitment of primordial follicles to ovulation is 82 days and when cytotoxics destroy maturing follicles, temporary amenorrhea results. However, if the number of remaining primordial follicles falls below the minimum number necessary for menstrual cyclicity, irreversible ovarian failure occurs with permanent amenorrhea. This accounts for the increased risk of chemotherapy-induced menopause in older patients. Permanent ovarian failure is often accompanied by vasomotor symptoms, whilst temporary amenorrhoea, which may last up

to 5 years after chemotherapy, is usually asymptomatic. As in men, alkylating agents are the major culprits causing permanent gonadal failure in women. At present ovum storage remains an unreliable method for routine usage and requires ovarian stimulation prior to egg harvesting, which introduces a delay prior to starting chemotherapy and is relatively contraindicated in breast cancer. The storage of fertilized eggs (embryos) is more successful. The Roman Catholic Church opposes all forms of *in vitro* fertilization and under the papacy of Benedict XVI has condemned the practice in the 2008 magisterial instruction *Dignitas Personae*.

Teratogenicity of chemotherapy

Many cytotoxics are teratogenic in murine models although data in humans are thankfully limited. All alkylating agents are teratogenic with limited information suggesting a significant risk of malformed infants if exposed in the first trimester but no increased risk during the second and third trimesters. Methotrexate is, of course, a potent abortifactant during early pregnancy. No clear evidence is available to support the timing of pregnancy following chemotherapy although most clinicians advise a two to five-year gap before pregnancy

Carcinogenicity of chemotherapy

Many cytotoxic agents are genotoxic and this accounts for their antitumour activity but also carries the risk of inducing cancers; alkylating agents are the most potent carcinogens in this group (Table 3.13). The risk of induced malignancies depends not only on the cytotoxics administered but also on the initial cancer diagnosis, with greatest risks in patients with Hodgkin's disease where the second malignancy rate is 10–15% after 15 years. Two forms of secondary acute leukaemia following chemotherapy are widely recognized. Alkylating agents are carcinogenic with acute leukaemias occurring in up to 5% three to five years after exposure and associated with chromosome

Table 3.13 Table of carcinogenic medicines.

Carcinogenic drug	Associated tumour
Cytotoxics (especially alkylating agents and topoisomerase II inhibitors)	Acute myeloid leukaemia
Cyclophosphamide	Bladder cancer
Immunosuppression	Kaposi's sarcoma, post-transplantation lymphoproliferation
Oestrogens (unopposed)	Endometrial cancer
Oestrogens (transplacental)	Vaginal adenocarcinoma
Oral contraceptive pill	Hepatic adenoma
Androgenic anabolic steroids	Hepatocellular carcinoma
Phenacetin	Renal pelvis transitional cell cancer
Chloramphenicol	Acute leukaemia
Phenytoin	Lymphoma, neuroblastoma

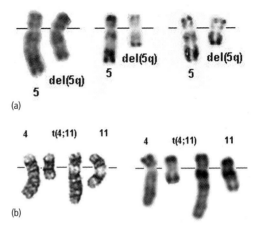

Figure 3.11 Chromosome translocation in secondary leukaemia. Partial karyotypes from patients with secondary acute leukaemia follow chemotherapy. (a) Deletions on the long arm of chromosome 5 are characteristic of alkylating agent-related secondary acute myeloid leukaemias that typically arise three to five years after chemotherapy and may be preceded by myelodysplasia. (b) The t(4:11) reciprocal chromosomal translocation commonly found in acute leukaemias that occur two to three years after chemotherapy with topoisomerase II inhibitors.

5q or 7 deletions (Figure 3.11a). Survival after secondary acute myeloid leukaemia (AML) is poor, usually only a few months. There is also an increased incidence of solid tumours after alkylating agents. Secondary acute leukaemia also occurs in patients treated with topoisomerase II inhibitors (Figure 3.11b). These leukaemias occur early, two to three years after therapy, and are associated with translocations of 11q23 (MLL gene) or 21q22 (AML1 gene). Data on the development of secondary solid tumours are less clear although cyclophosphamide is linked to a four-fold relative risk of bladder cancer and appears to be related to cumulative dose. Antimetabolites are generally not thought to be carcinogenic.

There is something quite horrible about the development of second cancers after curative treatment of a first cancer and for this reason effort has been expended in developing alternative treatment programmes that are not associated with increased cancer risk. The development of second cancers used to be a problem of particular poignancy in patients with Hodgkin's disease. This tumour commonly occurs in younger people who are returned to a normal life expectancy until the unpleasantness of their presentation with a second cancer. The alternative programme, which is in current use for the treatment of Hodgkin's disease, is called ABVD. This was originally introduced by a group of Italians, whose pronouncements about the effectiveness of ABVD chemotherapy were regarded with some scepticism by the medical community. However a randomized trial organized in North America showed that the Italians were right.

Psychiatric dysfunction

It is generally thought that patients who have cancer would tend to be more depressed than the population without malignancy. However, this is far from the truth. So far from the truth that it is a completely incorrect view. There is no difference in the incidence of mental illness in people affected with cancer than in a normal population. There is controversy around the association between pre-morbid psychiatric conditions and the development of cancer. The only malignancy in which there has been shown to be an association is breast cancer, where early work described a link between pre-morbid depression and breast cancer. The link is slight. Patients with cancer go through a series of mental changes around the time of their diagnosis. Each of these stages may be protracted, even to the extent that the patient remains unable to grow beyond that particular phase. These symptoms are symptoms of a grief response as seen in many other situations. Initially patients deal with malignancy by denial. They next move to a grief response, progressing from there to acceptance of their own situations.

Delayed side effects in children

Growth disorders in children

Both growth disorders and mental changes are problems that come chiefly as a result of the use of radiotherapy in childhood. Irradiation of the chest in the treatment of Hodgkin's disease is associated with destruction of the growing plates of the vertebrae and ribs, and dysmorphic appearance in later life. For this reason treatment with spinal radiotherapy is generally avoided in leukaemia and lymphoma occurring in childhood, with chemotherapy the preferred option.

Mental change in children

Cerebral radiotherapy given as part of prophylaxis for central nervous system recurrence of leukaemia may also cause significant problems. These problems are not generally of growth or of hormonal function, as the pituitary is relatively resistant to radiation. However personality defects are described with increased incidence, as are global loss of cerebral function manifesting as a less than expected IQ, personality change and occasionally fits. Although relatively resistant to radiation therapy, pituitary function can be damaged with loss of the gonadotrophs leading to failure to achieve puberty. Loss of thyroid-stimulating hormone (TSH) production occurs with high dosage radiotherapy and loss of posterior pituitary

function with even higher dosages of radiation therapy.

Gonadal toxicity in children

The germinal epithelium in the prepubertal testis does not appear to be any more resistant to cytotoxic therapy than in the adult and the sterilizing effects of chemotherapy on prepubertal boys may be predicted from data in adults. In contrast prepubertal girls are less susceptible to ovarian failure than adult women. Most chemotherapy regimens do not cause failure of pubertal development and menarche.

Endocrine therapy

Endocrine therapy (or hormonal manipulation) is an important part of managing cancers whose growth is dependent on hormones, namely, breast and prostate cancers. The aims of endocrine therapy for cancer are to reduce the circulating levels of hormones or block their actions on the cancers. The origins of endocrine therapy for breast and prostate cancer come from surgical oophrectomy and orchidectomy.

Breast cancer

In order to grow, many breast cancers that produce oestrogen receptors rely on supplies of oestrogen (Figure 3.12). Luteinizing hormone-releasing hormone (LHRH) agonists such as goserelin cause downregulation of pituitary LHRH receptors and, via a decrease in LH/FSH (luteinizing hormone/follicle-stimulating hormone), to a reduced plasma oestradiol. This is used in the neoadjuvant, adjuvant and palliative setting in premenopausal women. Tamoxifen binds to oestrogen receptors and prevents oestradiol binding. It is used in the neoadjuvant, adjuvant and palliative setting in postmenopausal women. Aromatase inhibitors, such as anastrozole, bind and inhibit aromatase enzyme in peripheral tissues including adipose tissue, which converts androstenedione and testosterone and other androgens into oestradiol and oestrone. This is the major source of oestradiol synthesis in postmenopausal women. They are used in

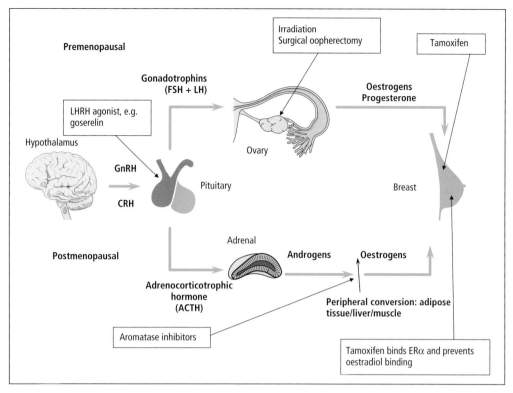

Figure 3.12 Hypothalamic–pituitary–gonadal axis in women and potential therapeutic interventions. CRH, corticotrophin-releasing hormone; ERα, oestrogen receptor α; FSH, follicle-stimulating hormone; LH, luteinizing hormone; LHRH, luteinizing hormone-releasing hormone; GnRH, gonadotrophin-releasing hormone.

the palliative setting for women whose disease progresses on tamoxifen. All the above drugs can cause menopausal symptoms, namely hot flushes, sweats and vaginal dryness. Specific and important adverse effects of tamoxifen are thromboembolic disease and uterine carcinoma.

Prostate cancer

The growth of prostatic carcinoma is under the control of androgens, hence the aim of hormonal therapy is to reduce testosterone levels or prevent it binding to the androgen receptor. LHRH agonists cause downregulation of pituitary LHRH receptors and via a decrease in LH to a reduced serum testosterone and tissue dehydrotestosterone (Figure 3.13). The adverse effects are impotence, loss of libido, gynaecomastia and hot flushes.

Tumour flare, an increase in tumour size which can cause symptoms such as increase in bone pain and spinal cord compression, can occur with the initial use of these drugs, due to an initial increase in testosterone. Therefore an anti-androgen such as bicalutamide, cyproterone and flutamide should be prescribed for a few weeks before LHRH agonists to prevent this happening. Anti-androgens act by blocking and preventing testosterone from attaching to the receptors in prostate cancer cells (Figure 3.13). The adverse effects of anti-androgens are hepatotoxcity, gynaecomastia, diarrhoea and abdominal pain. Combined androgen blockade (or maximal androgen blockade) is a term used to describe the use of an LHRH agonist and androgen receptor antagonist together. These agents are used alone or in combination for either locally advanced or metastatic prostate cancer.

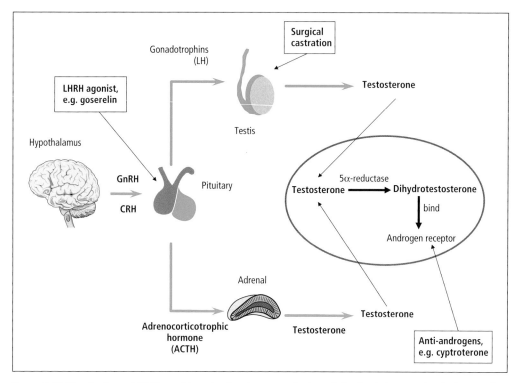

Figure 3.13 Site of actions of LHRH agonists and anti-androgens on the hypothalamic–pituitary–testis axis. CRH, cortico-trophin-releasing hormone; LH, luteinizing hormone; LHRH, luteinizing hormone-releasing hormone; GnRH, gonado-trophin-releasing hormone.

Immunological therapy

As far back as the 1700s, it was recorded that certain infectious diseases could exert a beneficial thera-peutic effect upon malignancy. Most prominent among the clinicians aiming to take advantage of these observations was a New York surgeon, William B. Coley. He used a bacterial vaccine to treat inoperable cancers and in 1893 reported high cure rates. Although a central role for the immune system in the surveillance and eradication of tumours has been postulated since then, immuno-therapy has only a minor place in the treatment of cancers. Support for any role of immunity in the control of cancer comes from a number of observa-tions. For some malignancies, a dense infiltration of lymphocytes in the tumour imparts a better prognosis. Cultivating and re-infusing these tumour-infiltrating lymphocytes occasionally results in some regression of the tumour. Con-versely, people with immunodeficiencies have higher rates of cancers, however in general these tumours are less common cancers that are caused by oncogenic viruses. Both passive and active spe-cific immunotherapy and non-specific immuno-therapy have a limited role in the management of cancer.

Passive specific immunotherapy

Passive immunotherapy with monoclonal anti-bodies is an established treatment for breast cancer and non-Hodgkin's lymphoma. Monoclonal anti-bodies are produced by a single clone of B cells and may be humanized to reduce their immunogenic-ity. In 1975, Georges Kohler and Cesar Milstein developed a procedure to fuse myeloma cells with B-lymphocyte cells from the spleen of immunized mice. These fused hybridoma cell clones retained the ever-living characteristics of myeloma cells and

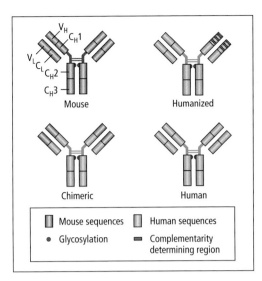

Mouse

Humanized

Chimeric

Human

| Mouse sequences | Human sequences |
| Glycosylation | Complementarity determining region |

Figure 3.14 Nomenclature and structure of chimeric and humanized monoclonal antibodies.

the ability to secrete monoclonal antibodies against the antigen that the mouse was immunized with. Milstein and Kohler shared the 1984 Nobel Prize with Niels Jerne for this work. Cesar Milstein had left his native Argentina for Cambridge in 1963 following the military coup that deposed the moderate President Frondizi. He joins a long list of distinguished British Nobel laureates in physiology and medicine who arrived in Britain as political asylum seekers, including Max Perutz (discoverer of the structure of haemoglobin), Hans Krebs (who described the citric acid cycle) and Ernst Chain (who, with Florey, developed the clinical application of Fleming's discovery of penicillin).

Several monoclonal antibodies are currently widely used in oncology and have been genetically modified to reduce the murine origins to prevent the development of host antibodies against the mouse sequences of the anibodies (Figure 3.14), for example rituximab and trastuzumab (Box 3.2). Rituximab is a chimeric monoclonal antibody directed against CD20, a protein expressed on pre-B and mature B cells. This is non-specific as it will ablate both normal and malignant B cells. However, the normal cells are subsequently regenerated by the bone marrow from normal stem cells. It is effective in low-grade and follicular non-Hodg-

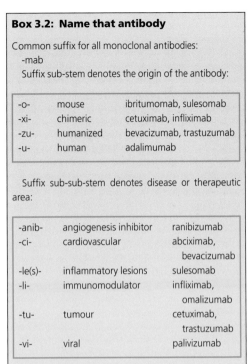

Box 3.2: Name that antibody

Common suffix for all monoclonal antibodies:

-mab

Suffix sub-stem denotes the origin of the antibody:

-o-	mouse	ibritumomab, sulesomab
-xi-	chimeric	cetuximab, infliximab
-zu-	humanized	bevacizumab, trastuzumab
-u-	human	adalimumab

Suffix sub-sub-stem denotes disease or therapeutic area:

-anib-	angiogenesis inhibitor	ranibizumab
-ci-	cardiovascular	abciximab, bevacizumab
-le(s)-	inflammatory lesions	sulesomab
-li-	immunomodulator	infliximab, omalizumab
-tu-	tumour	cetuximab, trastuzumab
-vi-	viral	palivizumab

However, there are inconsistencies. For example, bevacizumab, which according to the sub-stem -ci- was perhaps originally expected to be used in cardiovascular disease, is used to treat patients with colorectal cancer and macular degeneration; bevacizumab, cetuximab and ranibizumab all inhibit angiogenesis but have different sub-stems.

kin's lymphoma. Trastuzumab is a humanized monoclonal antibody directed against human epidermal growth factor receptor 2 (HER2), which is overexpressed in 30% of breast cancers and is associated with a poorer prognosis. It is used in metastatic breast cancer that is HER2 positive. Both these drugs can cause flu-like symptoms on infusion, such as chills and pyrexia. In addition, trastuzumab has been noted to be cardiotoxic, especially when given with anthracyclines.

Active specific immunotherapy

Active cellular immunotherapy involves the harvesting and *ex vivo* activation (in the test tube) of lymphokine-activated killer (LAK) cells (cytokine primed immune cells) and is an experimental treatment for renal cancers and melanoma. Other trial active immunotherapies include tumour vaccines and this technology is most often studied in the tumour types where occasional spontaneous regressions have been documented.

Non-specific immunotherapy

Global stimulation of the host cellular immune system in order to promote tumour rejection was probably the basis of Coley's adjuvant therapy. This has been replaced with the use of bacillus Calmette–Guerin (BCG), which is administered intravesically (via a catheter into the bladder) to prevent recurrence of superficial bladder cancers, and interferons and intereukins.

Interferon

There are three human interferons:
- Interferon alpha (IFN-α) produced by leukocytes
- Interferon beta (IFN-β) produced by fibroblasts
- Interferon gamma (IFN-γ) produced by T lymphocytes.

IFN-α is licensed for use currently and may act by enhancing the expression of human leucocyte antigen (HLA) antigens by tumour cells leading to increased recognition and lysis by cytotoxic T cells and natural killer cells. Only IFN-α is used in the treatment of cancers, including hairy cell leukaemia, chronic myeloid leukaemia, melanoma, renal cell cancer and Kaposi's sarcoma. The adverse effects of IFN-α are flu-like symptoms, fatigue and myelosuppression.

Interleukin-2

Interleukin-2 (IL-2) is a cytokine produced predominantly by activated CD4+ helper T lymphocytes that have been stimulated by antigen. It acts via a cell surface receptor expressed also on activated T cells thus behaving as an autocrine growth factor. In response to IL-2, CD4+ helper T cells are capable of differentiating from an initial common state (T_H0) into one of two apparently distinct types called T_H1 and T_H2. The T_H1 pathway

is essentially cell-mediated immunity, with the activation of macrophages, natural killer cells, cytotoxic T cells and a prolonged inflammatory response. The T_H2 pathway is essentially a humoral pathway, with the production of cytokines, which promote B-cell growth and the production of antibodies. IL-2 causes the growth and proliferation of activated T cells thus expanding tumouricidal LAK cells and may be used to treat melanoma and renal cell cancers. The adverse effects of IL-2 are fluid retention, multiorgan dysfunction and bone marrow and hepatic toxicity.

Protein kinase inhibitor therapy

Protein kinase enzymes phosphorylate the amino acid residues of their substrates, usually tyrosine, serine or threonine. The human genome includes about 500 protein kinases and perhaps 30% of all human proteins may be modified by phosphorylation, which may result in functional changes. Phosphorylation of substrate proteins may alter their enzyme activity, cellular location or association with other proteins and this is especially important in cellular pathways such as signal transduction that are dysregulated in cancer cells. Protein kinase inihitors are a relatively new and rapidly expanding class of drugs used in cancer treatment and include both monoclonal antibodies (-mabs) and small molecules (-nibs) (Table 3.14). In general, nibs target tyrosine kinase domains whilst mabs target the ligand-binding domains of receptors. Many of these novel agents have been developed using knowledge of the biology of tumours to target specific pathways in cancer cells. It was anticipated that this would have the added benefit of minimizing toxicity although some unexpected side effects have emerged such as the cardiotoxicity of trastuzumab.

Clinical trials

As new cytotoxic drugs are developed and other novel agents are found it is essential to evaluate their potential in a structured fashion in clinical trials. A stepwise progression has been introduced that includes three phases of clinical trials. Phase I

Table 3.14 Table showing the common protein kinase inihitors used in oncology.

Name	Target	Class	Clincal uses
Bevacizumab	VEGF	Monoclonal antibody	Colon cancer and NSCLC
Cetuximab	EGFR	Monoclonal antibody	Colon cancer and head and neck cancer
Dasatinib	BCR/ABL	Small molecule	CML
Erlotinib	EGFR	Small molecule	NSCLC
Gefitinib	EGFR	Small molecule	NSCLC
Imatinib	BCR/ABL	Small molecule	CML and GIST
Lapatinib	EGFR and Her2	Small molecule	Breast cancer
Sorafenib	Multiple target kinases	Small molecule	Kidney cancer and liver cancer
Sunitinib	Multiple target kinases	Small molecule	Kidney caner and GIST
Trastuzumab	Her2	Monoclonal antibody	Breast cancer

BCR/ABL, breakpoint cluster region/Abelson murine leukaemia viral oncogene homologue; CML, chronic myeloid leukaemia; EGFR, epidermal growth factor receptor; GIST, gastrointestinal stromal tumour; NSCLC, non-small cell lung cancer; VEGF, vascular endothelial growth factor.

trials determine the toxicity, including the dose-limiting toxicities and the dose scheduling of a new agent. They enrol a small number of patients with resistant tumours. Phase II studies are designed to identify promising tumour types using the dosing regimens established from the phase I trials. Phase III trials are larger randomized comparisons that allocate patients either to the new treatment or the established standard therapy. In all phases of clinical trials evaluations of response and toxicity are according to well-established standards. The side effects are measured using the Common Toxicity Criteria scale that rates the severity of side effects on a four point scale. The response to treatment is assessed using the RECIST (response evaluation criteria in solid tumours) criteria which are largely radiological and clinical measurements of the tumour size before and after treatment. A complete response is defined as the complete disappearance of all known disease, whilst a partial response roughly equates to a greater than 50% reduction in the size of measurable lesions with no new ones appearing. Although there is considerable debate as to whether these response criteria are appropriate for some of the novel therapies such as anti-angiogenic treatments, they are currently necessary for licensing approval of cancer drugs. The aims of clinical trials of a new agent include proving that it works, obtaining a license from the Food and Drug Administration (FDA) in the USA and the European Medicines Evaluation Agency (EMEA) as well as making money. In most cases all the goals are complementary, however there are examples from the biotechnology boom of the 1990s where making money appeared to be the sole objective and venture capitalists made fortunes without a drug ever achieving clinical use or benefiting any patients.

Randomized clinical trials are needed to establish evidence-based treatment protocols as well as determining the value of new agents. Large clinical trials are a major focus of clinical activity in oncology and patients are actively encouraged to participate in studies. The principles that underlie clinical trial management are outlined within Box 3.3.

Palliative care

Although it is widely held that palliative care is only offered when there is no chance of cure, this attitude risks denying patients adequate analgesia and supportive care irrespective of their prognosis. The concept that palliative care to provide optimal symptom control and enhanced quality of life should only be available to those patients with advanced disease is ridiculous. The integration of palliative care into the early management of patients with cancer is recognized as benefiting

Box 3.3: Does it work?

The value of a diagnostic test in clinical medicine depends upon whether the result means what you think it does and nowhere is this more relevant than in screening tests. The usefulness depends upon three factors, the sensitivity and specificity of the test and the population prevalence of the condition.

Sensitivity
The sensitivity of a test is the ability of a test to pick up a condition:
- Sensitivity = number of true cases detected/all true cases.
  A test that is 95% sensitive will detect 95% of all cases (or, put another way, miss 5% of cases).

Specificity
The specificity of a test is the probability that a negative test is a true negative:
- Specificity = number of true negatives detected/all true negatives.
  A 75% specificity means that 75% of all negative tests are true negatives, or conversely that 25% of negative tests are actually positive for a condition.

Usefulness
The practical usefulness of a test in a given population can be summarized using:
- Positive predictive value (the chance that a positive will be a true positive in that population) = true cases detected/all positive test results (true positives and false postitives)
- Negative predictive value (the chance that a negative will be a true negative in that population) = true negative results/all negative test results (true negatives and false negatives).

Prevalence and incidence
- Prevalence = frequency of a condition in the community at a given point in time (e.g. the prevalence of cancer in children in the USA is one in 330 children <19 years)
- Incidence = frequency of a disease occurring over a period in time (e.g. the incidence of breast cancer in England in 1998 was 131/100 000 females).

Running a trial

Ethics
The Declaration of Helsinki outlines an international basis of ethical clinical research. It describes the rights of patients including the right to abstain from a study, access to adequate information about both potential benefits and hazards of involvement, the right to withdraw from the trial at any time and finally the desirability of giving written informed consent prior to enrolment. In the UK, research trials must be submitted to research ethics committees for review.

Trial design
- Phase I trials determine the relationship between toxicity and dose schedules of treatment
- Phase II trials identify tumour types for which the treatment appears promising
- Phase III trials assess the efficacy of treatment compared to standard treatment including toxicity.

Randomization
Proper randomization should ensure unbiased comparisons. It achieves control for both known and unknown confounding factors.

Control
Controlled trials compare a 'new' test therapy with an existing treatment – either active or placebo.

Blinding
In double blinded trials neither the patient nor the doctor knows which treatment is being administered.

(continued on p. 75)

(continued)

Sample size

The number of patients (sample size) required in a trial will depend on the number of events (deaths or relapses) predicted in each arm and the difference that you wish to be able to demonstrate between the two arms of the trial. If you wish to detect a small difference between the two groups, more patients are needed.

Analysis

Intention to treat analysis compares outcomes between all patients originally allocated one treatment with all patients allocated to the other treatment.

Endpoints

Clinical trial endpoints include overall survival duration, disease-free survival, time to disease progression, response rate, quality of life measures, adverse effects and treatment toxicity. The efficacy of treatment may be measured using the response evaluation criteria in solid tumours (RECIST) criteria, which evaluate response in terms of radiological and clinical tumour shrinkage. The definitions broadly are:

- Complete response: disappearance of all known disease
- Partial response: >50% reduction in measurable lesions and no new lesions
- Stable disease: lesions unchanged (<50% smaller or <25% larger)
- Progressive disease: new lesions or measurable lesions >25% larger.

CTC toxicity scales

Grading scales exist to compare the side effects of treatments in trials including the common toxicity criteria (CTC).

Interpreting the results

Evidence-based medicine

Over the last two decades there have been numerous advances in evidence processing, including the production of streamlined guides to aid critical appraisal of the literature, evidence-based abstraction services, online and other forms of electronic literature searching, growing numbers of high-quality systematic reviews, and frequently updated textbooks in paper and electronic formats. All these initiatives have contributed to the emergence of evidence-based medicine as the optimal framework for clinical management.

Meta-analysis

Combining published data into a meta-analysis to provide an evidence base for clinical management is widely advocated. A meta-analysis may provide a more precise, less biased and more complete assessment of the available information than individual studies. However, the preferential publication of striking results in small studies and non-publication of larger negative studies ('publication bias') may skew meta-analyses. Thus the reliability of a meta-analysis depends on the quality and quantity of the data that go into it.

Bias

Bias in a study is a design flaw that results in an inevitable likelihood that the wrong result may be obtained. Bias cannot be controlled for at the analysis stage.

Potential biases in screening for cancer

Screening should reduce mortality but the following should be considered:

1. *Lead time bias*: the diagnosis of disease is made earlier in the screened group, resulting in an apparent increase in survival time, although the time of death is the same in both groups.

(continued on p. 76)

(continued)

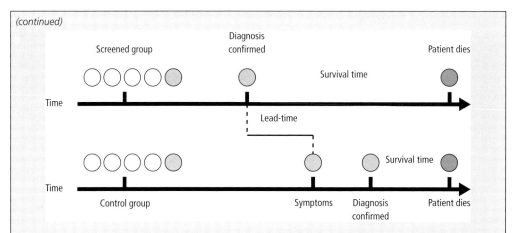

2. *Lag time bias*: the probability of detecting disease is related to the growth rate of the tumour. Aggressive, rapidly growing tumours have a short potential screening period. More slowly growing tumours have a longer potential screening period and are more likely to be detected when they are asymptomatic, causing an apparent improvement in survival.

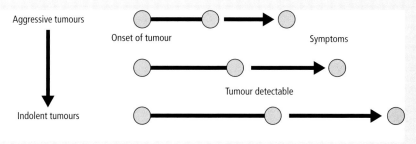

3. *Overdiagnosis bias*: The detection of very slow growing tumours in the screened group produces an apparent increase in the number of cases. In contrast these indolent tumours may remain silent in the control population as they may never cause symptoms. In this diagram, two patients in the control group died with undiagnosed cancer that did not affect their natural lifespan.

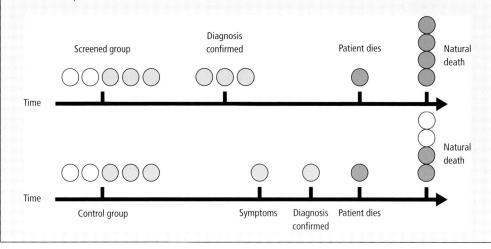

patients and encouraging a more holistic attitude to their care. The discipline of palliative care throughout the globe owes much to the pioneering work of Dame Cecily Saunders. She started life as a nurse during the Second World War and subsequently worked as a social worker before training in medicine, which she viewed then as the only route to change the care of the dying. She advocated above all else listening to patients as the best way to care for them. In 1967 she established the first hospice in the world, St Christopher's Hospice in London, in order to meet the needs of the dying patient, which are so often left unmet in a hospital. The hospice movement developed a comprehensive approach to dealing with the variety of symptoms experienced by patients with progressive debilitating illness including promoting the safe use of opiate analgesia. This attitude has been developed to deliver whole person care and to view the patient not in isolation but as part of a social unit that includes also family and friends.

Pain is the most feared and most common symptom of advanced malignancy and emotional, spiritual and psychological components may intensify physical pain. In Mother Teresa's Home for the Dying, the homeless of Kolkata (formerly Calcutta) were denied any analgesia other than aspirin and often suffered unnecessarily with great pain in the pursuit of austere religion. The relief of pain should therefore be viewed as part of a comprehensive pattern of care encompassing all aspects of suffering. The physical component of pain cannot be treated in isolation, nor can a patient's anxieties be effectively addressed whilst they are suffering physically. It is obvious under these circumstances that a multidisciplinary approach is required. In addition to pain relief, expertise in the management of other common symptoms is essential including constipation, diarrhoea, nausea, vomiting, dyspnoea and fatigue. In some circumstances surgery or radiotherapy may provide valuable symptomatic palliation, for example for the relief of spinal cord compression. Moreover in selected circumstances palliative chemotherapy is indicated even if the term seems to be a clinical oxymoron.

The delivery of palliative care until recently has been hospice based. However, the hospice concept has now extended to both the acute hospital and community settings, where specialist teams work in partnership with primary care teams in the delivery of palliative care. Community-based palliative care may enable patients to die at home or at least remain at home for as long as possible, which has long been known to be the favoured option of most patients.

Chapter 4

Cancer and people

Social and psychological aspects of cancer

Psychological carcinogenic risk factors

There is a great deal of speculation and anecdotal evidence connecting psychological factors and both the risk of developing cancer and its prognosis. Much of the research on the relationship between stressful life experiences and the onset of cancer has been poorly designed. However, the few well-conducted trials have failed to establish a link. A large study of women with newly diagnosed breast cancer found that women who have a severely stressful life experience in the year before the diagnosis or in the five years afterwards, do not seem to be at increased risk of developing a recurrence of the disease. Moreover, a meta-analysis addressed the influence of psychological coping strategies (including fighting spirit, helplessness/hopelessness, denial and avoidance) on cancer survival and recurrence. This meta-analysis found that there was little consistent evidence that psychological coping styles play an important part in survival from or recurrence of cancer.

Psychological distress in cancer patients

Psychological distress is frequent in patients with cancer and is often overlooked or even deliberately neglected by clinicians. However, over the last few decades, more oncologists have appreciated that psychological distress and psychiatric disorders such as anxiety, depression and delirium (in hospitalized patients) are frequent co-morbid conditions. Increasingly, the outcome measures in clinical trials of new therapies have included quality of life evaluation and not just assessed survival endpoints. A number of factors have been found to be associated with an increased risk of psychological distress in patients with cancer (Table 4.1). Clinical features of anxiety include anorexia, fatigue, loss of libido, weight loss, anhedonia, insomnia and suicidal ideation. Many of these key symptoms are at times attributed to the cancer and as few as one-third of cancer patients who might benefit from antidepressants are prescribed them.

As well as pharmacological treatments, psychological interventions are frequently employed in the care of people with cancer. These interventions have a positive effect on psychological morbidity and functional adjustment and may ameliorate disease and treatment-related symptoms. The most useful psychological intervention appears to be a group of treatments termed cognitive-behavioural psychotherapy. These include behaviour therapy,

Lecture Notes: Oncology, 2nd edition. By M. Bower and J. Waxman. Published 2010 by Blackwell Publishing Ltd.

Table 4.1 Factors increasing the risk of psychological morbidity in cancer patients.

History of mood disorder
History of alcohol or drug misuse
Cancer or its treatment associated with visible deformity
Younger age
Poor social support
Low expectation of successful treatment outcome

Table 4.2 Top tips for communicating with patients.

Clarify patient's statements
Use open questioning (not leading)
Note verbal and non-verbal clues
Enquire about patient's psychosocial problems (e.g. depression)
Keep patients to the point
Prevent needless repetition
Provide verbal and visual encouragement
Obtain precise information
Use brief questions
Avoid jargon

behaviour modification and cognitive therapy in various combinations. In behavioural therapy, a formal analysis of the patient's problem leads to an individualized programme of techniques aimed at changing their behaviour. Cognitive therapies explore how thoughts influence feelings and behaviour and aim to modify thought processes directly. These therapies consist of identifying maladaptive thought patterns (such as hopelessness in depression) and teaching patients to recognize and challenge these. Probably the most widely employed psychosocial intervention for cancer patients is supportive counselling that along with information and patient education empowers patients.

Psychosocial problems in cancer survivors

Even after successful curative treatment of cancer, patients continue to suffer psychological morbidity. The psychological sequelae in cancer survivors may relate to the illness and its treatment as well as family and personal issues. The majority of children who survive cancer cope well with long-term adjustment although adults generally fare less well. Three well-recognized scenarios in this context are:
• The Lazarus syndrome (difficulty with returning to normal life)
• The Damocles syndrome (fear of recurrence and terror of minor symptoms)
• The survivor syndrome (guilt about surviving where others have died).

Cancer survivors also suffer social problems including financial difficulties, particularly with insurance and mortgages. They have also been found to have greater problems in obtaining employment and keeping jobs and these may be compounded by frequent follow-up clinic visits.

Breaking bad news

Medical students have identified breaking bad news as their greatest fear in terms of communicating with patients, and in the first half of the 20th century it was routine practice to hide the diagnosis from patients with cancer. It is uncertain whether this was a paternalistic policy to protect the patient or because physicians avoided a difficult task that many found unpleasant (and one that might lead them to question their practices). Although many students believe that good communication skills are innate, it is clear that like so many things the techniques can be taught and learnt (Table 4.2). The way in which the diagnosis is communicated to patients is an important determinant of subsequent psychological stress and, even if patients recall little of the conversation that followed, they state that the competence of the doctor at breaking bad news is critical to establishing trust. Why do doctors fear breaking bad news? Obviously the information causes pain and distress to patients and their relatives, making us feel uncomfortable. We fear being blamed and provoking an emotional reaction. Breaking bad news reminds us of our own mortality and fears of our own death. Finally, we often worry about being unable to answer a patient's difficult questions since we never know what the future holds for either our patients or ourselves. Breaking bad news to patients should not involve protecting them from the truth but rather imparting the information in a sensitive manner at the patient's own pace.

Breaking bad news to patients requires preparation and this aspect is very often overlooked. The setting for these discussions should be quiet, comfortable and confidential so that the whole ward does not eavesdrop and so that your bleep and mobile phone do not constantly intrude. An adequate period of time (at least 30 minutes) should be set aside and the patient should be asked if she/he wants someone else present. The conversation should open with a question to find out how much the patient already knows. An open question such as 'What have you already been told about your illness?' can reveal not only what has been said and how much has been understood but also the emotional state of the patient ('I'm so terrified it's cancer'). This opening gambit frequently takes care of much of the hard work for you ('I think it's cancer but the doctors do seem to want to say'). Under these circumstances the diagnosis can be confirmed in an empathetic fashion. If this initial question does not open up a useful avenue, a warning shot should be fired off ('I have the results of your biopsy and I'm afraid that the news is not good'). Following this warning shot, wait for the patient to respond and check if the patient wants to be told more. This cycle of warning shot, pause and checking should be repeated when elaborating on details of the diagnosis and treatment options. In this way the patient determines how much information is delivered. Certainly long monologues are overwhelming and confusing and it is hopeless and insensitive to use this opportunity to try and teach pathophysiology. Learning to identify and acknowledge a patient's reaction is essential to breaking bad news. In general, prognostication with respect to 'how long have I got Doc?' and the quoting of five-year-mortality statistics are rarely helpful. Few doctors can explain the implications of skewed distributions, medians and confidence intervals, let alone in a way that is accessible to patients. Many patients will ask for these predictions hoping for reassurance. In these circumstances it is always easier to give false reassurance but the temptation must be resisted as you will not be doing your patient a favour in the long run. After answering the patient's enquiries, it should be possible to synthesize their concerns and medical issues into a concrete plan. Even in the bleakest of situations setting short-term achievable plans leaves the patient with a goal for the future and hope. The plan should include an explicit arrangement for following up the conversation and a method for the patient to contact you if something arises before the next planned visit.

Coping strategies

Increased interaction and empathy with cancer patients has costs to health care professionals that need to be appreciated and addressed. Improved communications brings health care professionals closer to the patient and may increase feelings of inadequacy when faced with insoluble issues and of failure when patients die. Health care professionals dealing with dying patients and their families risk burn-out and although the medical profession is notoriously resistant to external help, a team spirit, adequate training through communication workshops and peer support are important elements in coping with these emotional stresses. Another technique that is frequently employed is distancing, which may protect the doctors from their feelings but often reduces their compassion and their capacity to care for patients. Although the burden of caring for people with cancer falls most heavily on doctors and nurses, other staff members may also be affected. Indeed, when patients are dying their distress and that of their care givers trickles down to everyone in the clinic or ward.

Medical burn-out

The depletion of physical and mental resources induced by excessive striving to reach an often unrealistic work-related goal is termed burn-out. Burn-out of staff working in cancer care is common and victims often describe themselves as workaholics. The Maslach burn-out inventory is a tool that measures burn-out and a quarter of consultant oncologists in the UK have scores that denote this. The consequences of medical burn-out include emotional exhaustion leading to psychological detachment from patients and the sensation that little is being achieved in terms of personal accomplishment. This may account for the high frequency of experienced oncologists changing roles in their 50s, taking on management positions or jobs with cancer charities or immersing themselves increasingly in research rather than patient contact.

Unconventional treatments

The unmet emotional needs of patients have been held responsible for the increasing use of unconventional treatments for cancer. The void that patients may feel at a vulnerable stage in their lives may be filled with complementary treatments, alternative therapies or quackery.

Complementary and alternative therapies

According to the Cochrane Project, complementary and alternative medicine (CAM) is a broad domain of healing resources that encompasses all health systems, modalities and practices and their accompanying theories and beliefs, other than those intrinsic to the politically dominant health system of a particular society or culture in a given historical period. Thus, whilst orthodox medicine is politically dominant, CAM practices outside this system and is, for the most part, isolated from the universities and hospitals where health care is taught and delivered. As some CAM disciplines (e.g. acupuncture) become increasingly incorporated into conventional medicine they therefore loose their 'alternative' status. Indeed it is this co-operation of health systems that led to the introduction of the term 'complementary medicine' rather than the title 'alternative medicine'.

Every year around 20% of the population in the UK use CAM and this is interpreted as a measure of disillusion with conventional medicine. In contrast, the prevalence of use in the USA is 40% and in Germany is >60%. There is a prolonged history in Germany of CAM use and indeed Samuel Hahnemann (1755–1843), who first described homoeopathy (Box 4.1), was a German physician. The pantheon of complementary and alternative therapies includes alternative therapies with

---

Box 4.1: Homoeopathy – does it work?

The underlying principle of homoeopathic medicine is the use of extremely low-dose preparations prescribed according to the belief that like should be cured with like (readers may wish to refer to the Mitchell and Webb sketch 'Homoeopathic A&E' on youtube). Treatments are chosen according to the symptoms that they elicit when administered to healthy people. Since raw onions cause crying, stinging eyes and a runny nose, *Allium cepa* (derived from onions) is used as a homoeopathic remedy for hayfever. The most notorious experimental trial that attempted to explain the mechanism of action of homoeopathy was undertaken by Jacques Benveniste. He hypothesized that water had the ability to remember solutes that had been dissolved in it after finding that very dilute solutions of allergens could elicit basophil responses. In a show trial experiment, the then editor of *Nature* Sir John Maddox brought a team of independent referees to observe the experiments in Benveniste's laboratory. The observers included James Randi, a magician and investigator of the paranormal, and under his scrutiny Benveniste's team were unable to repeat the findings. Since that failure, Benveniste has continued to pursue the storage of memory in water, claiming to be able to store an electronic record in water that can be transferred back into an email format. These claims have been met with even greater scepticism and have earned him an unprecedented second IgNobel Prize.

Despite these claims the most widely believed theory of the mechanism of homoeopathy remains a placebo effect and more effort has been focused on establishing the efficacy of homoeopathy. A meta-analysis, published in the *Lancet*, examined over 100 randomized, placebo-controlled trials and found a significant odds ratio of 2.45 in favour of homoeopathy. Homoeopathic medicines can be purchased over the counter at chemists and health stores. In contrast to other forms of CAM, homoeopathy is supported by the NHS through both the National Homoeopathic Hospital in London and the fact that homoeopathic remedies may be prescribed on the NHS by any doctor registered with the General Medical Council.

Box 4.2: Acupuncture

Acupuncture originated over 2000 years ago in China. It was used by William Osler, the celebrated Canadian-born physician who was both Chief of Staff at Johns Hopkins University and subsequently Regius Professor of Medicine at Oxford University at the start of the 20th century. The recent resurgence in popularity of acupuncture dates from President Nixon's visit to China in the 1970s. The stimulation of acupuncture points by fine needles is intended to control the Qi energy circulating between organs along channels or meridians. The 12 main meridians correspond to the 12 major functions or 'organs' of the body and acupuncture points are located along these meridians. The analgesic actions of acupuncture may be explained by a conventional physiological gating model and acupuncture is known to release endogenous opioids. There is convincing evidence supporting the value of acupuncture in the management of both nausea and acute pain. The evidence base for the use of acupuncture in chronic pain is less secure and current evidence suggests that it is unlikely to be of benefit for obesity, smoking cessation and tinnitus. For most other conditions the available evidence is insufficient to guide clinical decisions. Acupuncture appears to be a relatively safe treatment in the hands of suitably qualified practitioners, with serious adverse events being extremely rare. It has been estimated that 1 million acupuncture treatments are given on the NHS in England each year, at an estimated cost of £26 million, equivalent to all other complementary therapies combined. A further 2 million acupuncture treatments are given in the private sector annually.

Box 4.3: Herbalism

The most widely used herbalism in the UK is Chinese and derives from the Daoist concepts of balancing the yin and yang elements of Qi energy. The revenue from herbal products in the UK exceeds £40 million per year. Perhaps the most familiar example of herbal medicine is the use of St John's wort (*Hypericum perforatum*) for treating mild to moderate depression. Systematic reviews of randomized controlled trials confirm its efficacy over placebo and its equivalence to amitryptilline with fewer side effects. St John's wort is, however, not free of side effects and has important drug interactions caused by inducing hepatic microsomal enzymes. Other more severe toxicities have been described with herbal medicines including rapidly progressive interstitial renal fibrosis in several women after taking Chinese herbs containing powdered extracts of *Stephania tetrandra* prescribed by a slimming clinic.

recognized professional bodies (e.g. acupuncture (Box 4.2), chiropractic, herbal medicine (Box 4.3), homoeopathy, osteopathy), complementary therapies (e.g. Alexander technique, aromatherapy, Bach and other flower extracts, body work therapies including massage, counselling stress therapy, hypnotherapy, meditation, reflexology, shiatsu, healing, Maharishi Ayurvedic medicine, nutritional medicine, yoga), alternative therapies that lack professional organization but have established and traditional systems of health care (e.g. anthro-posophical medicine, Ayurvedic medicine, Chinese herbal medicine, Eastern medicine (Tibb), naturopathy, traditional Chinese medicine) and, finally, there are other 'new age' alternative disciplines (e.g. crystal therapy, dowsing, iridology, kinesiology, radionics).

Many doctors remain concerned about the use of complementary and alternative medicines. These concerns may be based on a number of factors including that patients may be seen by unqualified practitioners, may risk delayed or missed diagnosis, may decline or stop conventional therapies, may waste money on ineffective therapies and may experience dangerous adverse effects from treatment. Moreover, the scientific academic training in medicine leads many doctors to question the value of those therapies where a plausible mechanism of action is not available. At present practitioners of CAM in the UK are free to practice as they wish without clear regulation; greater co-operation and respect between conventional doctors and complementary therapists would improve patient care.

Quackery

The word quack is supposedly derived from 'quacksalver', a 17th century variant spelling of quicksilver or mercury, which was used in certain remedies that the public came to recognize as

---

Box 4.4: The Luigi Di Bella cure

This treatment is named after its proponent, Professor Luigi Di Bella (1912–2003), a retired physiologist who lived in Modena. It is based on a combination of somatostatin, vitamins, retinoids, melatonin and bromocriptine. ACTH (adreno-corticotrophic hormone) and low doses of the oral chemotherapeutic agents cyclophosphamide and hydroxyurea are sometimes also included. It was claimed that the treatment stimulated the body's self-healing properties without damaging healthy cells. No scientific rationale or supportive experimental evidence was provided, and despite claims to have cured thousands of patients no clinical results were published in peer-reviewed scientific journals. In December 1997 a judge in the southern Italian city of Maglie ruled that the health authority should fund this treatment for a patient and this pattern was followed elsewhere. Although the initial child died of cancer, unprecedented public interest in the unconventional therapy led to public demonstrations with the right-wing media in Italy championing the cause. The socialist Italian government under considerable pressure decided to carry out phase II open-label studies in several cancer centres. Scrutiny of Di Bella's own clinical records of 3076 patients revealed that 50% lacked evidence that the patient had cancer and a further 30% had no follow-up data. Adequate data were available for just 248 patients of whom 244 had in addition received conventional treatments for their tumours. These findings rattled Di Bella's credibility and in October 1998 the findings of the first clinical trial were published in the *British Medical Journal*. Of 386 patients, just three had shown a partial response. The findings, however, failed to shake Di Bella's confidence. He accused drug companies of conspiring against him, and suggested that the results were sabotaged by mainstream doctors. Even in 2003, some 3000 patients receive Di Bella-based cancer treatments paid for by three Italian regional health services.

---

harmful. Pseudoscience uses the language and authority of science without recognizing its methods. It produces claims that cannot be proven or refuted and often poses as the victim ('scientists are suppressing the truth'). A quack may reasonably be defined as a pseudoscientist who is selling something, and a charlatan as a cynical pseudoscientist who knows he or she is deceiving the public. It is a sorry monument to human greed and stupidity that more money is spent on health frauds every year than on medical research. Quacks are convincing because they tell people what they want to hear. Moreover it is almost impossible for the cancer quack to fail. When a patient deteriorates, the cancer quack resorts to lines such as 'if only you had come to me sooner'. However, we should appreciate that quacks can teach us a great deal whilst we retain an honest and informed practice of medicine. Their popularity is attributed to their patience and ability to listen carefully and show both interest and affection. As well as this, quacks encourage patients to take an active role in their health care thus empowering them. The internet appears to have made cancer quackery even easier. Whilst much health information on the web is evidence based and of high quality, the open access has also been abused. Entrepreneurs have recognized the value of the web as a free-for-all market and have used it to promote fraudulent cancer treatments ranging from £100 a pound shark cartilage powder (Box 4.5) to 'The Zapper', a 9 volt electrical device for zapping away cancers.

Euthanasia

Euthanasia is the intentional killing by act or omission of a dependent human being for his or her alleged benefit. The term assisted suicide is used when someone provides an individual with the information, guidance and means to take his or her own life with the intention that they will be used for this purpose. Although active euthanasia remains illegal in the UK it was legalized in Australia's Northern Territory in 1995, but this bill was overturned by the Australian parliament in 1997. In 1998 Oregan state, USA, legalized assisted suicide following a ballot of the population. There were 129 deaths under Oregon's Physician Assisted Suicide Act between 1998 and 2002. Euthanasia was legalized in 2000 in Holland and in 2002 in Belgium. A survey published in 1994 showed that half of a mixture of hospital consultants and general practitioners in England had been asked by a patient to take active steps to hasten death, and that a third of those asked had complied with the patient's request. The reason people choose

---

Box 4.5: Shark cartilage

In 1993, William Lane a marine biologist and entrepreneur published a book entitled *Sharks Don't Get Cancer* following the discovery that some species of sharks have lower than predicted rates of cancer. This was followed by a prime-time television documentary focusing on a Cuban study of 29 cancer patients who received shark cartilage preparations. This resulted in patients clambering for sharks' cartilage and a consequent devastation of North American shark populations. According to the National Marine Fisheries Service 'the Atlantic shark … is severely over-capitalized' and it is estimated that over 200 000 sharks are killed in American waters just for their cartilage every month. The powdered cartilage has modest anti-angiogenic activity *in vitro*, however oral administration results in the digestion of these proteins prior to absorption. An open-label phase II clinical trial, which was in part funded by shark cartilage manufacturers, found not a single responder amongst 58 patients although both nausea and vomiting were reported. Cartilage Technologies subsequently announced that it would support no additional research on shark cartilage as a cancer remedy. It is, however, intriguing that squalamine, an aminosterol antibiotic isolated from shark livers, inhibits angiogenesis and suppresses the growth of tumour xenografts in animal models. Squalamine is easily synthesized without the need to fish for sharks and is under clinical trial investigation in age-related macular degeneration as well as solid tumours.

---

euthanasia is mostly out of fear of losing autonomy and/or bowel/bladder control, and an increasing proportion of the British public wishes to allow euthanasia for patients in certain incurable disease scenarios.

Ethics

Four principles underpin medical ethics: respect for autonomy, non-maleficence, beneficence and justice. In health care decisions, respect for autonomy means that the patient is allowed to act intentionally, with understanding and without controlling influences. This is the basis of informed consent. The principle of non-maleficence requires that we do not intentionally cause harm or injury to a patient, either through acts of commission or omission. In common language this is avoiding negligence and is based on Hippocrates' (460–377 BC) original decree 'primum non nocere'. The principle of beneficence is the duty of health care professionals to provide benefit to patients and prevent harm befalling them. These duties apply not only to the individual patient but to society as a whole, and therein frequently lies the problem. In practice, double effect reasoning, first attributed to Thomas Aquinas (1224–1274), may apply when an action has two outcomes – one good and one bad – and allows a lesser harm for a greater good.

Justice in health care terms is defined as fairness in distribution of care particularly when allocating scarce resources. A number of political doctrines interpret this differently. Karl Marx (1818–1883), of course, believed in egalitarianism 'from each according to his abilities, to each according to his needs'. Modern health care is rarely provided on this basis but rather on a system that distributes care according to a number of factors including need, effort, contribution, merit and free-market exchanges. Utilitarian philosophers, on the other hand, advocate a system that balances benefit between the collective public and the individual.

Perhaps the most interesting example of the rationing of health care is the Oregon health plan. The Oregon health plan was set up in 1987 with the aim of serving more low-income people using federal funds through a system that prioritizes heath care. An extensive list of more than 700 physical health, dental, drug dependency and mental health services was drawn up and their priority publicly debated in order to reflect a consensus of social values of Oregonians. The list of 587 approved procedures went into operation in 1994. The innovation that most sharply and controversially characterizes this systematic approach is its commitment to providing a standard health benefit based on ranking the effectiveness and value of all medical treatments. To determine which conditions are to be covered, Oregon's Health Services Commission ranks diagnoses from the most important (treatment has the greatest impact on health status) to the least important. This prioritization introduces a transparent approach to health care rationing and was originally designed to use the savings achieved to extend coverage to more people. Moreover it requires public involvement in health policies and incorporates public values into the rankings. The top five ranked items were the diagnosis and treatment of head injury, insulin-dependent diabetes mellitus, peritonitis, acute glomerulonephritis (including dialysis) and pneumothorax. At the cut-off cusp, medical treatment of contact and atopic dermatitis and symptomatic urticaria are covered, as is repair of damaged knee ligaments, but the treatment of sexual dysfunction with psychotherapy or medical and surgical approaches does not make the cut, nor does the medical treatment of chronic anal fissure nor complex dental prostheses. The Oregon Health Services Commission also excluded treatment for hepatocellular cancer and widely disseminated cancer.

Sociology of oncology

Inequalities in health are not confined to the marked differences between wealthy and poor nations but are recapitulated within countries, such as the UK. Eight tube stations on the Jubilee tube line separate Westminster from Canning Town in Newham and the life expectancy of a child born in Westminster exceeds that of a child born in Newham by six years – almost one year lost for each stop travelled. How much of this disparity is attributable to differences in health care is uncertain, even in a state health monopoly that is free at the point of delivery. Certainly, Marxist health analysts such as Howard Waitzkin propose that doctor–patient encounters reproduce the dominant ideologies of wider society and that medicine is a tool for social control. Modern medicine stands accused of serving the interests of capital and of ensuring that people adhere to the norms of behaviour. Many oncological health inequalities are behavioural and medicine has branded these as self-inflicted, for example tobacco use and diet. Similar arguments have accused medicine of gender discrimination. Women are greater users of health care because they live longer and because of the medicalization of reproductive health. It is also worth noting that the only national cancer screening programmes are for women (mammogram and cervical smears). Medicine has a long history of reinforcing a subordinate role for women in society leading to both radical and reformist responses from the feminist movement. Equivalent oncological responses would be the alternative medicine movement, which wishes to overthrow the current practice of oncology, and complementary medicine, which wishes to change cancer medicine from within, encouraging the adoption of a wider vision and a more holistic approach.

The use of metaphors in cancer medicine has been attacked by both Susan Sontag and John Diamond, who use their personal experiences of cancer to describe the negative implications of these metaphors. Many of these metaphors are bellicose, 'the fight against cancer' belittles the patient as 'a victim'. The use of these figures of speech may render cancer socially as well as physically devastating and 'losing the battle against cancer' denigrates a patient's role in society.

Part 2

Types of Cancer

Chapter 5

Breast cancer

Diseases of the breast, including tumours, have been attracting medical interest for more than 5000 years. The earliest written records of breast cancer are in the Edwin Smith papyrus, from ancient Egyptian civilizations of 3000 to 2500 BC. Hard and cold lumps were recognized as tumours, whilst abscesses were hot. The next major advances in the management of breast cancer occurred during the golden age of surgery at the end of the 19th century, following advances in antisepsis and anaesthesia. William Halsted in Baltimore described radical mastectomy in 1894. Moreover, in an early example of surgical audit, he reported a local recurrence rate in 50 women of only 6%. The next major advance in the management of breast cancer occurred in 1896 with the development of surgical oophrectomy as a treatment strategy for advanced breast cancer, which was pioneered by George Beatson in Glasgow (the Beatson Institute for Cancer Research in that city is named after him). Geoffrey Keynes, the brother of Maynard, and an expert in the watercolours of William Blake, developed lumpectomy and radiotherapy as a breast conservation measure in the 1930s whilst appointed as surgeon at St Bartholomew's Hospital in London. In the 1960s and 1970s the radical women's movements in Europe and America took breast cancer as a campaigning point, and their

campaigns led to increased focus on breast cancer treatment and research. Copying the AIDS awareness red ribbons, breast cancer activists adopted pink ribbons and now there are a rainbow of different cancer ribbons. These campaigns directly led on to improvements in screening strategies, and screening programmes were introduced without a significant evidence base for efficacy and against the views of the medical establishment. As a consequence of increased screening, the survival rates of breast cancer have risen steadily over the last 30 years. A list of five-year survival of breast cancer patients by stage of disease can be found in Table 5.1. Breast cancer patients were largely viewed as the property of the surgeons. In the United Kingdom in the last few years central governmental directives have led to multidisciplinary working. This has directly led to a decrease in the use of mutilating surgery, and an increase in the use of adjuvant treatments.

Epidemiology

Breast cancer is a common disease. According to the most recent figures, 45 500 women are affected annually and 11 750 die in England and Wales as a result of this condition. The likelihood of the development of breast cancer is affected by a positive family history of breast cancer, increasing age, diet, social class and nulliparity. Breast cancer risk increases with age, plateauing during the menopausal years of 45–55. Women are at increased risk

Lecture Notes: Oncology, 2nd edition. By M. Bower and J. Waxman. Published 2010 by Blackwell Publishing Ltd.

Table 5.1 Five-year survival of women with breast cancer by stage of disease.

Tumour stage	Stage definition	5-year survival
Stage I	Tumour <2 cm, no nodes	88%
Stage II	Tumour 2–5 cm and/or moveable axillary nodes	69%
Stage III	Chest wall or skin fixation and/or fixed axillary nodes	43%
Stage IV	Metastases	12%

from breast cancer from non-vegetarian diets; it is not clear what the reason for this should be. Women who are more than two standard deviations above average height and weight are at a greater risk from breast cancer, as are women of social classes I and II. There is a protective effect of a full-term pregnancy, provided the pregnancy is achieved prior to the woman's 30th birthday. There is a minor protective effect of having more than five pregnancies, but probably no protective effect from breast feeding. A late menopause correlates with an increased risk of breast cancer, but there is little evidence that an early menarche predicates for increased risk. Oestrogen-only hormone replacement therapy (HRT), as well as combined oestrogen and progestogen HRT, increase the risk of breast cancer in proportion to the duration of HRT administration. Both the oral contraceptive pill and alcohol and coffee consumption have been linked to breast cancer, but the associations are controversial.

A family history of breast cancer is a very important risk factor for breast cancer. If more than two first-degree relatives are affected, the risk to other female family members increases by a factor of two. There are clear links between breast cancer and other cancers, with associations between ovarian and endometrial cancer, and colonic tumours. There are four relatively common genes that lead to an increased risk of breast cancer and these are: BRCA1 and 2, CHEK2 and FGFR2. Prevalence and penetrance of mutions in these genes are variables reported and lead to a lifetime risk of breast cancer of greater than 80% and up to 60% of ovarian cancer. BRCA1 has been located to chro-mosome 17q21 and is a tumour suppressor gene, the product of which is involved in cell cycle regulation. The BRCA product binds with Rad51, a major protein of 3418 amino acids, which is involved in sensing and directing the molecular response to double stranded DNA damage.

The detected incidence of breast cancer is increasing in England and Wales, almost certainly as a result of the introduction of the screening programme. Death rates have fallen by nearly 30% over the last 15 years and survival chance has increased from 65% to almost 80%. Survival rates have increased to those seen in the United States. They are almost certainly due to the successes of the screening programme, which has led to the earlier detection of tumours at an earlier stage, with the resultant better prognosis. There are also contributions to this fall in mortality rate from an increased use of adjuvant chemotherapy and hormonal therapy. This contribution to a fall in mortality rates is likely to be in the range 4–7%.

Presentation

Women with breast cancer generally present to their clinicians with a lump in their breast. On average, there is a delay of approximately three months between the woman first noting the mass in her breast and her seeing a hospital clinician. Alternative sources of referral are from breast screening programmes, where mammographic detection leads to diagnosis of a previously unnoted breast lump. As a result of governmental concerns over the care of patients with breast cancer, the investigation and treatment of this disease has been prioritized. Patients in whom this condition is suspected ought to be seen in 'outpatients' within two weeks of receipt of the referral letter.

Outpatient diagnosis

The current standard is for women to be seen in a multidisciplinary setting that offers a 'one-stop shop' for diagnosis. Surgeons, with a special interest in breast cancer are located in a clinic with oncologists, with access to same-day cytology and imaging services. A careful history should be obtained from the patient prior to examination when seen in outpatients. The mass may be thought to be benign or malignant. Benign lumps are more likely in younger women and tend to be painful, enlarging before menstruation. Malignant lumps tend to be more common in older women and are generally painless: only 30% of malignant breast lumps are painful, and just 10% of lumps seen in new patients are malignant.

Diagnosis is by clinical, mammographic (Figure 5.1), ultrasonographic, cytological and histological means. After clinical examination, mammography, that is, a soft tissue X-ray of the breast, aspiration cytology, which is removal of cells by means of a needle and syringe, and core biopsy should be performed to further assess the significance of the breast lump. In a younger woman, ultrasonogra-

phy rather than mammography is the radiological investigation of choice. If there is confirmed malignancy, all women should then proceed to surgery within two weeks of diagnosis, as recommended by government guidelines (Figure 5.2 and see Plate 5.1).

Staging and grading

There are two main pathological variants of breast cancer, ductal and lobular, and these are both graded as given in Table 5.2. This grading was first described by Bloom and Richardson, and bears their eponyms. This grading scheme depends upon the degree of tumour tubule formation, the mitotic activity and the nuclear pleomorphism of the tumour. As one might expect, poorly differentiated tumours have a worse prognosis than moderately differentiated ones, which in turn have a worse prognosis than well differentiated breast cancer. There may be pre-invasive changes, and these are

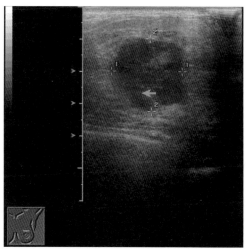

Figure 5.2 Breast ultrasound showing large, echo-dense, irregular, primary breast cancer lesion.

Table 5.2 Breast cancer grading and prognosis.

Grade	5-year survival
G1 Well differentiated	95%
G2 Moderately differentiated	75%
G3 Poorly differentiated	50%

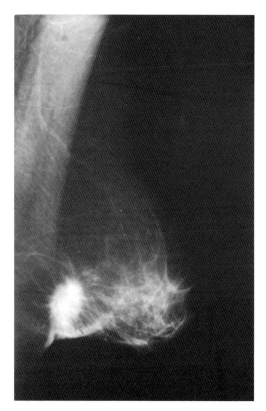

Figure 5.1 Lateral view of a breast mammogram showing a large, dense, speculated mass highly suggestive of breast cancer.

Table 5.3 TNM staging of breast cancer.

T stage (primary tumour)	N stage (nodal status)	M stage (metastatic status)
T0 No detectable primary tumour	N0 No nodes involved	M0 No metastases
T1 Tumour less than 2 cm	N1 Mobile axillary nodes	M1 Spread to distant organs
T2 Tumour measuring between 2 and 5 cm	N2 Fixed axillary nodes	
T3 Tumour measuring greater than 5 cm	N3 Involved supra- or infraclavicular nodes	
T4 Tumour of any size extending into skin or chest wall		

described as either ductal (DCIS) or lobular carcinoma *in situ* (LCIS). LCIS are additionally graded according to their microscopic features (see Plates 1.1 and 1.2).

Stage is defined according to the classification of the Union Internationale Contre Le Cancer (UICC), which is updated every 10 years or so (Table 5.3). The subscript 'P' denotes a pathological staging following surgery. There are many other staging systems.

Treatment

Surgery

Surgery for breast cancer depends upon the clinical stage of the disease. If the mass is less than 5 cm in size and not fixed, the preferred treatment is removal of the lump, which is termed 'lumpectomy'. Axillary lymph node dissection was conventionally performed, but now this has largely been replaced by sentinel lymph node biopsy which, if positive, may then be followed by an axillary clearance. The reason for this is that if the nodes are affected by a cancer, there is an advantage in this group of women to adjuvant chemotherapy. In the 'node-negative' woman there is a very much smaller advantage to adjuvant chemotherapy. In an older woman there may be an argument against routine axillary dissection. The reason for this is that adjuvant treatment with chemotherapy within this group of women is not dictated by lymph node status, because the advantage is much smaller than in younger women and the toxicity of the treatment outweighs these

modest gains. It is clear, however, that knowledge of the axillary nodal status does provide some prognostic information.

For a woman whose tumour measures 5–10 cm in size, the preferred surgical option is mastectomy, that is removal of the breast with axillary dissection. For more advanced breast cancer, the value of surgical treatment is much more contentious, and elderly women may be treated with hormonal therapy alone if the breast cancer expresses oestrogen receptors and/or progesterone receptors. In a younger woman, neoadjuvant chemotherapy may be given in the first instance, to reduce the size of the tumour, and this may be then followed by surgery and radiotherapy. There is a major role for reconstructive surgery and this may be carried out at the time of primary surgery or at a later date upon completion of adjuvant radiotherapy or chemotherapy. The psychological gain is tremendous and needs to be considered in older as well as younger women, for breasts are considered valued personal property in older just as much as in younger women.

Adjuvant radiotherapy

After lumpectomy, radiotherapy is given to the breast. This is done in order to reduce the risk of local recurrence of the tumour. Without radiation this risk is between 40% and 60%; whereas with radiation, the risk is reduced to approximately 4–6%, which is the same as that for more radical surgical procedures. Radiotherapy is generally given over a six-week period and requires daily attendance at hospital. The side effects of radiation include tiredness and burning of the skin, which is generally mild. More serious consequences of radiation are seen only rarely and include damage to the brachial nerve plexus and, with more old-fashioned treatment machines and plans, damage to the coronary blood vessels. Rarely, a second cancer, such as an angiosarcoma, may follow at the site of radiotherapy treatment.

Adjuvant hormonal therapy

Treatment with tamoxifen has been shown to have an advantage in terms of disease-free and overall survival in both pre- and postmenopausal women and is now given routinely to this group of patients. It is usually recommended that treatment should extend for five years. There is no advantage to adjuvant tamoxifen in oestrogen receptor-negative tumours. There have been changes in our understanding of the oestrogen receptor. Two different classes of oestrogen receptor (ER), described as α and β, have been identified. Tamoxifen is a selective ERα-antagonist, which in turn has effects on the progesterone receptor. In postmenopausal women, recent studies suggest that a newer group of drugs, the aromatase inhibitors, may be even more effective than tamoxifen as adjuvant therapy. The current standard is to give sequential therapy with tamoxifen and then an aromatase inhibitor. Treatment is given for a total of five years. Approximately 10% of circulating oestrogens derive from adrenal precursors, such as androstenedione, through the action of aromatase enzymes. The aromatase inhibitors block this action, limiting the synthesis of oestrone and oestrone sulphate produced by a second series of enzymes; the sulphatase system (Figure 5.3). Use of aromatase inhibitors is associated with osteoporosis. There have been reports of cases of endometrial carcinoma associated with the use of tamoxifen. The estimated risk is one case per 20000 women per year of use.

Adjuvant chemotherapy and receptor targeting therapy

Adjuvant chemotherapy has a significant place in the management of breast cancer. Although chem-

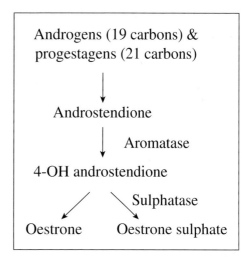

Figure 5.3 Peripheral oestrogen (18 carbons) synthesis pathway.

otherapy using the CMF (cyclophosphamide, methotrexate, 5-fluorouracil (5FU)) programme was the regimen first shown to be of benefit, and is widely used. A large international study showed that more intensive therapy using the FEC (5FU, epirubicin, cyclophosphamide) regimen is more effective than CMF. There has been recent interest in the use of taxane chemotherapy given in the adjuvant setting, with the possibility that survival may be further improved. Third generation adjuvant chemotherapy combining alternating FEC and taxane based treatment are now considered to be the standard. There is no evidence whatsoever that intensifying adjuvant therapy any further using, for example, high-dose treatments with bone marrow or peripheral blood stem cell support, improves the disease-free interval or the overall survival. About a quarter of breast cancers express the epidermal growth factor receptor 2 (EGFR2), also known as Her-2/neu, and c-erbB-2. This is the target for the monocloncal antibody trastuzumab (Herceptin). For patients with Her-2 receptor-positive tumours, treatment with adjuvant trastuzumab may be considered. Treatment is conventionally given for periods of 12–18 months. The advantage to treatment with trastuzumab is small, but is recommended in the context of the 60–70% five-year survival chance that patients with Her-2 strongly positive tumours have. The toxicity of treatment with trastuzumab is significant, and particularly of note are the direct cardiac effects that may manifest as heart failure.

Treatment of metastatic breast cancer

The treatment of metastatic breast cancer depends very much upon the age of the patient and the sites of metastasis. It is only rarely curable, and so life quality issues are immediately important. When we described this point to one patient, she replied: 'my dear, it's death quality issues that bother me'. In older women whose metastases are in the skin or bone, the preferred treatment option is hormonal therapy, provided that the tumour expresses oestrogen and/or progestogen receptor positivity. The agent of first choice is tamoxifen because of its lack of toxicity and efficacy. Approximately 70% of women aged 70 respond to this therapy. In a premenopausal woman, hormonal therapy is generally less effective, and at the age of 30, just 10% of patients overall will respond to treatment at all. But oophorectomy, (that is, removal of the ovaries by either radiotherapeutic, surgical or medical means), is generally the first therapeutic stratagem. Surgical oophorectomy is unnecessary, given that an equivalence of effect is provided by the use of medical treatment with an LHRH (luteinizing hormone receptor hormone) agonist. How much easier is it to provide a simple three-monthly depot injection than to expose a woman to laparoscopy and surgical oophorectomy. Radiotherapy is not a particularly successful way of causing gonadal failure. Ovaries are relatively radiotherapy resistant, and the conventional dosages of radiotherapy given to sterilize may not sterilize a younger woman, and certainly will not lead to an instant reduction in circulating ovarian steroid hormones.

In both pre- and postmenopausal women, radiation treatment is very effective in controlling bone pain. The addition of regular bisphosphonate therapy both relieves bone pain and reduces skeletal events such as fractures and spinal cord compression. If lungs or liver are affected, then chemotherapy is required. Overall, between 40%

and 60% of patients respond to chemotherapy, and this response is for a median duration of one year. The median survival of women with metastatic breast cancer ranges between 18 and 24 months, with 5–10% alive after five years. It should be noted that there are patients with very prolonged survival, and these include those women who have, for example, single sites of metastatic disease.

High-dose chemotherapy

Breast cancer responds to chemotherapy, but often after responding, patients relapse and die. There have been attempts to maximize response rates by intensifying chemotherapy. High-dose treatments were popular in the early 1980s. Response rates were found to be higher than for conventional treatment; toxicity, however, was significantly worse, and death rates reached 20% as a result of the side effects of treatment. Even more significantly, patients who responded and survived the toxicity, later relapsed, and the median duration of response was no better than that expected with conventional treatment.

In the 1990s, there was an increase in the numbers of patients receiving high-dose therapy for breast cancer. This was possible as a result of the improvement in supportive therapy, principally bone marrow rescue, either with stem cells or with marrow. Mortality has decreased and now is 5% in the best centres. Overall, there has been no significant improvement in the expectation for survival for patients with metastatic breast cancer, and only 20% of patients are alive two years after the transplantation. It has been recently argued that the relatively good results of intensive therapy reported in early studies are entirely the result of the selection of good-prognosis patients for treatment with high-dose therapy, and that the same effects could be achieved with less intensive, conventional therapy. It may be the case that early intensive therapy given as adjuvant treatment to patients with poor-risk tumours will lead to improved survival, but this has not been shown in any randomized study.

Carcinoma *in situ*

Carcinoma *in situ*, diagnosed by excision biopsy will progress to invasive cancer in 40% of patients over five years. Treatment with adjuvant radiotherapy will limit this progression rate to 1–4% per annum. An alternative to radiation therapy is mastectomy. Both radiotherapy and mastectomy are equally effective in local disease control. Lobular carcinoma *in situ* is associated with bilaterality, and mirror biopsy is recommended of the contralateral breast.

Paget's disease of the nipple

This is an eczematous condition of the nipple, associated in 80% of cases with an underlying ductal carcinoma, and in about 20% of cases with underlying ductal carcinoma *in situ*.

New treatment

Further hormonal therapies are also likely to become available with interest in the development of sulphatase inhibitors (Figure 5.3). Poor-prognosis breast cancer highly expresses EGFR. Therapy with gefitinib may be effective in these tumours. mTOR is a component of the P13K/Akt signalling pathway that mediates cell growth and proliferation. Inhibitors of this pathway, such as temsirolimus, have been shown to have activity in breast cancer.

Triple negative breast cancer, which is breast cancers ER, PR and HER2 negative, constitutes about 15% of all breast cancers and has an aggressive natural history. These triple negative tumours are highly sensitive to chemotherapy with DNA-damaging agents such as cisplatin, and the effects of these drugs can be potentiated by the use of PARP inhibitors which disable DNA base excision repair. In early clinical trials these agents have shown a highly significant improvement in response rates and overall survival.

Angiogenesis inhibitors, such as bevacizumab, have also been shown to have an effect in breast cancer, but this is likely to be of minor significance. Targeted therapies, in which an antibody to HER2+ or EGFR+ is tagged to a cytotoxic agent, have provided a way of delivering targeted chemotherapy to breast cancer, and have led, in a small randomized clinical trial, to have some efficacy, as have agents capable of inhibiting the tyrosine kinase linked to HER1 and -2 activation.

So, it is clear that there is hope that breast cancer will become a curable cancer within the next 10 years. There has been progress in the identification of susceptibility genes for breast cancer, and it is hoped that targeted therapy will lead to progress.

Chapter 6

Central nervous system cancers

The first recognized resection of a primary brain tumour was performed in 1884 by Rickman Godlee in collaboration with the Westminster Hospital neurologist Alexander Bennett. It should be remembered that the removal of the cerebral cortex tumour was performed before any diagnostic imaging was available, but even then the surgeon knew to operate on the contralateral side to the clinical signs! There are about 4500 people diagnosed with a brain tumour each year in the UK. That is the equivalent to an incidence of about seven in every 100 000 people each year. Brain tumours are slightly more common in men than in women. A further 300 children are diagnosed with central nervous system tumours in the UK each year.

Scientists use animal models to study genetics, development and oncogenesis and the most common models are mice (see onco-mice in Chapter 1), fruit flies (*Drosophila*) and nematode worms (*Caenorhabditis elegans*). However, fish have also turned out to be useful subjects – in particular zebrafish (*Danio rerio*), which are tropical freshwater minnows with five horizontal stripes running from their mouth to caudal fin. Zebrafish are the vertebrate model for studying the genetics of embryonic development because the embryos are transparent and the genome sequence is known

and can readily be modified by knockouts. A less well known fish model of cancer is the damselfish (*Pomacentrus partitus*) that lives on coral reefs and has several vertical stripes. Deb and Flo in *Finding Nemo* are damselfish, so that is an excuse to watch it again. Damselfish neurofibromatosis is a naturally occurring, neoplastic disease of these fish that consists of multiple neurofibromata and neurofibrosarcomas. It has been proposed as an animal model for neurofibromatosis type 1 in humans. However, whilst von Recklinghausen's neurofibromatosis type 1 is vertically transmitted as an autosomal dominant trait, damselfish neurofibromatosis is transmitted horizontally between fish and is thought to be due to an oncogenic retrovirus named damselfish neurofibromatosis virus (DNFV).

Epidemiology

Metastases to the brain are about ten times more common than primary brain tumours. The most common primary tumour sites amongst patients with brain metastases are lung, breast, melanoma and kidney. In addition, nasopharyngeal cancers may directly extend through the skull foramina. Meningeal metastases occur with leukaemia and lymphoma, breast and small cell lung cancers, and from medulloblastoma and ependymal glioma as a route of spread. Primary tumours of the central nervous system (CNS) account for 2–5% of all

Lecture Notes: Oncology, 2nd edition. By M. Bower and J. Waxman. Published 2010 by Blackwell Publishing Ltd.

cancers, and 2% of cancer deaths. Fewer than 20% of CNS cancers occur in the spinal cord. There appears to be a modest increase in the incidence of primary brain tumours over the last two decades, particularly amongst the elderly. A more dramatic rise in the incidence of primary CNS lymphomas is attributable to the AIDS epidemic.

Aetiology

Although the cause of most adult brain tumours is not established, a number of inherited phakomatoses are associated with brain tumours. Phakomatoses are a group of familial conditions with unique cutaneous and neurological manifestations and dysplasias of a number of organ systems. They include neurofibromatosis (von Recklinghausen's disease), tuberous sclerosis (Bourneville's disease), von Hippel–Lindau disease (cerebroretinal angiomatosis), Sturge–Weber syndrome (ezcephalotrigeminal angiomatosis), Osler–Rendu–Weber syndrome and Fabry's disease (angiokeratoma corporis diffusum). The first three of these are associated with brain tumours; von Reckinghausen's neurofibromatosis with cranial and root schwannomas, meningiomas, ependymomas and optic gliomas (see Plate 2.2); tuberous sclerosis with gliomas and ependymomas; and von Hippel–Lindau disease with cerebellar and retinal haemagioblastoma (Table 6.1). In addition, an increased incidence of brain tumours is a feature of Gorlin's basal naevus syndrome (medulloblastoma), Turcot syndrome (gliomas) and Li–Fraumeni syndrome (glioma). High-dose ionizing radiation to the head region administered in the past for benign conditions such as scalp tinea capitis fungal infection (ringworm) increases the risk of nerve sheath tumours, gliomas and meningiomas. There is much public concern that low-frequency non-ionizing electromagnetic fields such as those emitted by 60 Hz power cables may increase the risk of brain tumours, but there is no consistent evidence to support this hypothesis. Similarly, despite scares, there is no evidence to support an association with wireless radiofrequency devices such as mobile phones. This joins the long list of things that cause cancer according to the *Daily Mail*. It includes Facebook, deodorant, hair dye, talcum powder, mouthwash, tooth whitener, oral sex, chips and chocolate.

Pathology

Primary nervous system tumours may be glial tumours, non-glial tumours or primary cerebral non-Hodgkin's lymphoma. As you will recall from embryology, the early embryo has three distinct germ layers of cells; the innermost endoderm that gives rise to the digestive organs, lungs and bladder, the middle layer or mesoderm that gives rise to the muscles, skeleton and blood system, and the outer layer or ectoderm that gives rise to the skin and nervous system. Neuroectodermal tumours are classified on the basis of the predominant cell type and include all neoplasms with either central or peripheral nervous system-derived cell origins. After embryonic development ceases, neurons do not divide, but glial cells retain the ability to proliferate throughout life and thus most adult neurological tumours are derived from glial cells and are named gliomas. Seventy percent of primary brain tumours in adults are supratentorial, situated above the tentorium cerebelli, the tent of dura mater that lies between the cerebellum and the inferior portion of the occipital lobes. In contrast primary brain tumours in children are usually located below the tentorium (Table 6.2).

Gliomas account for 50% of brain tumours and are divided into grade I (non-infiltrating pilocytic astrocytoma), grade II (well to moderately differentiated astrocytoma), grade III (anaplastic astrocytoma) and grade IV (glioblastoma multiforme). The prognosis deteriorates with rising tumour grade. Other glial tumours include ependymomas, that arise from ependymal cells, usually lining the fourth ventricle, and oligodendrogliomas that arise from oligodendroglia. In the peripheral nervous system, neurofibromata and schwannomas are the most frequent glial tumours. Medulloblastoma is a glial tumour of childhood usually arising in the cerebellum, which may be related to primitive neuroectodermal tumours elsewhere in the CNS. Non-glial brain tumours include pineal parenchymal tumours, extragonal germ cell

Table 6.1 Phakomatoses associated with brain tumours.

Condition	Inheritance and genetics	Cutaneous manifestations	Eye	Nervous system	Brain tumours
Von Recklinghausen's neurofibromatosis (NF-1)	Autosomal dominant NF-1 gene (encodes neurofibromin that regulates GTPases in signal transduction)	Café au lait macules, axillary freckles	Lisch nodules (pigmented iris hamartomas)	Neurofibromata	Schwann cell tumours of spinal and cranial nerves, meningiomas, ependymomas, optic gliomas
Acoustic neurofibromatosis (NF-2)	Autosomal dominant NF-2 gene (encodes Merlin protein involved in cell adhesion)	Café au lait macules less common than in NF-1	Presenile cataracts	Bilateral acoustic neuromas Neurofibromata	Schwann cell tumours of spinal and cranial nerves, meningiomas, astrocytomas, ependymomas, optic gliomas
Tuberous sclerosis	Autosomal dominant TSC1 gene (encodes hamartin protein) and TSC2 gene (encodes tuberin protein)	Adenoma sebaceum, Shagreen patches, subungual fibromata, café au lait spots		Seizures, mental retardation	Giant cell astrocytoma of the foramen of Munro, gliomas, ependymomas
Von Hippel–Lindau	Autosomal dominant VHL gene (encodes VHL protein involved in ubiquination)	Skin hamartomas	Retinal angiomas		Cerebellar haemagioblastomas, ependymomas, phaeochromocytoma

Table 6.2 Brain tumours by age and site.

Adult	Child
Supratentorial	
Metastases	Craniopharyngioma
Glioma	Pinealoma
Meningioma	Optic glioma
Pituitary tumour	
Infratentorial	
Metastases	Medulloblastoma
Acoustic neuroma	Cerebellar astrocytoma
Cerebellar	Ependymoma of
haemangioblastoma	fourth ventricle

Table 6.3 Common presentation of brain tumours by site.

Tumour site	Common presentations
Frontal	Personality change
	Contralateral motor signs
	Dysphasia (dominant hemisphere)
Parietal	Contralateral sensory signs
	Visual field defects (optic radiation)
	Neglect
Occipital	Homonymous hemianopia
Temporal	Memory and behavioural disturbances
Posterior fossa	Raised intracranial pressure
	Ataxia and nystagmus
	Cranial nerve lesions

tumours, craniopharyngiomas, meningiomas and choroid plexus tumours. Meningioma is the commonest non-glial tumour and constitutes 15% of brain tumours. The majority of spinal axis tumours in adults are extradural, metastatic carcinoma, lymphoma or sarcoma. Primary spinal cord tumours include extradural meningiomas (26%), schwannomas (29%), intramedullary ependymomas (13%) and astrocytomas (13%).

Presentation

Glial tumours

Glial tumours may produce both generalized and focal effects, and these will reflect the site of the tumour and the speed of its growth. General symptoms from the mass effect, increased intracranial pressure, oedema, midline shift and herniation syndromes are all seen, including progressive altered mental state and personality, headaches, seizures and papilloedema. Focal symptoms depend upon the location of the tumour (Table 6.3). Although seizures are a feature of up to half of all glial tumours, fewer than 10% of first fits are due to tumours and only 20% of supratentorial tumours present with fits.

Meningioma

These tumours, which are more common in women, present as slowly growing masses produc-

ing headaches, seizures, motor and sensory symptoms and cranial neuropathies, depending on their site (Table 6.4 and see Plate 6.1). Meningiomas are some of the few tumours that produce characteristic changes on plain skull X-rays with bone erosion, calcification and hyperostosis.

Spinal axis tumours

For spinal axis tumours, the proportion of tumour sites is 50% thoracic, 30% lumbosacral and 20% cervical or foramen magnum. These tumours present with radicular symptoms due to nerve root infiltration, syringomyelic disturbance (dissociated sensory loss of pain and temperature sensation) due to central destruction by intramedullary tumours, or sensorimotor dysfunction (limb weakness and a sensory level) due to cord compression.

Investigation and staging

Neuroradiology has developed into the most important investigation in patients with suspected brain tumours, following the introduction of computed tomography (CT) in the mid-1970s by Geoffrey Hounsfield and magnetic resonance imaging (MRI) in the 1980s. Newer techniques, such as positron emission tomography (PET), single photon emission computerized tomography (SPECT) and functional MRI have also found roles in the diagnosis and management of patients with brain tumours. MRI with gadolinium enhancement

Table 6.4 Clinical features of meningiomas by site.

Tumour site	Clinical features
Parasagittal falx	Progressive spastic weakness
	Numbness of legs
Olfactory groove	Anosmia
	Visual loss
	Papilloedema (Foster–Kennedy syndrome)
	Frontal lobe syndrome
Sella turcica	Visual field loss
Sphenoid ridge	Cavernous sinus syndrome (medial)
	Exophthalmos and visual loss (middle)
	Temporal bone swelling and skull deformity (lateral)
Posterior fossa (foramen magnum, tentorium)	Hydrocephalus (tentorium)
	Gait ataxia and cranial neuropathies
	V, VII, VIII, IX and X (cerebellopontine angle)
	Suboccipital pain, ipsilateral arm and leg weakness (foramen magnum)

Parasagittal meningioma

Tentorial meningioma

Sphenoid ridge meningioma

Olfactory groove meningioma

Foramen magnum meningioma

Sella turcica meningioma

is the imaging technique of choice with advantages over CT particularly for posterior fossa tumours and non-enhancing low-grade gliomas (see figures in Chapter 1). PET with fluorodeoxyglucose-18, which accumulates in metabolically active tissues, may help to differentiate tumour recurrence from radiation necrosis (see Plate 6.1). Stereotactic biopsy is required to confirm the diagnosis, although occasionally tumours are diagnosed on clinical evidence, because biopsy might be hazardous, as in brain stem gliomas, for example.

Treatment

Some gliomas are curable by surgery alone and some by surgery and radiotherapy; the remainder require surgery, radiotherapy and chemotherapy, and these tumours are rarely curable. Surgical removal should be as complete as possible within the constraints of preserving neurological function. Radiation can increase the cure rate or prolong disease-free survival in high-grade gliomas and may also be useful symptomatic therapy in patients with low-grade glioma, who relapse after initial therapy with surgery alone (Figure 6.1). Chemotherapy with nitrosurea or temozolomide may prolong disease-free survival in patients with oligodendrogliomas and high-grade gliomas, although its high toxicity may not always merit this approach.

Therapy of meningiomas is surgical resection, which may be repeated at relapse. Radiotherapy reduces relapse rates and should be considered for high-grade meningiomas or incompletely resected tumours. Relapse rates are 7% at five years if completely resected and 35–60% if incompletely resected.

Unlike with other brain tumours, surgical resection does not have a useful role in primary cerebral lymphomas. In immunocompetent patients, the combination of chemotherapy and radiotherapy produces median survivals of 40 months. In contrast, in the immunocompromised patients, especially those with HIV infection, the prognosis is far worse, with a median survival of under three months. Palliative radiotherapy or best supportive care are the appropriate treatment options here.

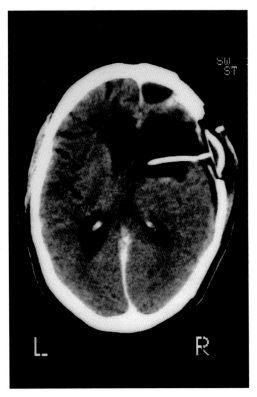

Figure 6.1 CT scan showing a patient with an Omaya shunt (a closed cerebrospinal fluid (CSF) shunt joining the lateral ventricle with a reservoir below the scalp) in place that is leaking, resulting in air seen in the right anterior brain and fluid accumulating around the shunt site. Omaya shunts may be placed to relieve non-communicating hydrocephalus caused by obstruction to CSF flow within the ventricular system, or to administer intrathecal chemotherapy.

Complications of treatment

Early complications of cranial radiotherapy which occur in the first three to four months are due to reversible damage to myelin-producing oligodendrocytes. This recovers spontaneously after three to six months. It causes somnolence or exacerbation of existing symptoms in the brain and Lhermitte's sign (shooting numbness or paraesthesia precipitated by neck flexion) in the cord. Late complications include radiation necrosis, causing irreversible deficits due to vessel damage. This may mimic disease recurrence, is radiation dose related and occurs in up to 15% of patients, with the

Table 6.5 Five-year survival rates of adult patients with brain tumours.

Tumour	5-year survival
Grade I glioma (cerebellar)	90–100%
Grade I glioma (other sites)	50–60%
Grade II (astrocytoma)	16–46%
Grade III (anaplastic astrocytoma)	10–30%
Grade IV (glioblastoma multiforme)	1–10%
Oligodendroglioma	50–80%
Meningioma	70–80%

highest frequency in children also receiving chemotherapy. SPECT and PET scanning may differentiate radionecrosis and relapse.

Prognosis

The prognosis of glial tumours depends upon the histology, the grade and size of the tumour, on the age and performance status of the patient and on the duration of the symptoms. The median survival for anaplastic astrocytoma is 18 months, and for glioblastoma multiforme is 10–12 months. Meningiomas, if completely resected, are usually cured, and the median survival is over 10 years.

New treatment

The treatment of brain tumours may well improve in the next 5–10 years. The most important recent advance has been with the use of adjuvant chemotherapy. It is hoped that the application of temozolamide, which crosses the blood–brain barrier, to radiotherapy for high-grade glioma will dramatically improve survival chances. Many high-grade gliomas express receptors for cErbB2/neu. Targeted antibody therapy delivered intravascularly may lead to further improvements in survival. Another recent advance is the use of biodegradable wafers implanted with chemotherapy that may be inserted at the time of surgery.

Newer radiotherapy delivery techniques that have been pioneered in the treatment of brain tumours include both gammaknife and cyberknife treatments, which have caught the attention and interest of the gently dozing neurosurgeon in the multidisciplinary team. Gammaknife radiotherapy is delivered by 201 cobalt-60 sources arranged in a ring in a helmet that is bolted to the patient's skull. Cyberknife radiotherapy uses a linear accelerator to deliver radiotherapy via a robotic arm that is linked to an image guidance system. Cyberknife radiotherapy does not need a skull frame because the real-time image linking means that if the patient moves, the robotic arm also moves so that the radiotherapy dose is delivered to the correct site.

Gene therapy has been adopted for trials in gliomas with viral vectors being administered either into the blood or directly into the tumour by surgeons. The genetically modified viral vectors may be non-replicating viruses that deliver a transgene that causes an anticancer effect, or replicating oncolytic viruses that directly lyse cancer cells by replicating. Gliomas are a good model to try these methods because they are pretty much the only cells dividing in the brain (apart from microglia and endothelial cells).

Chapter 7

Gastrointestinal cancers

Gastrointestinal malignancies have been attributed an important role in the history of Europe. Ferrante I of Arragon, the then King of Naples, was mummified and embalmed, following his death in 1494 and placed in a wooden sarcophagus at the Abbey of San Domenico Maggiore, Naples. In 1996, an autopsy was performed which revealed a large pelvic mass, and polymerase chain reaction (PCR) identified a mutation of the RAS oncogene, suggesting a colonic primary cancer. In 1821, Napoleon Bonaparte, the former Emperor of France, died in exile at Longwood House, St Helena. His health had been declining over a number of months with abdominal pain, weakness and vomiting, which he attributed to mistreatment by his English captors. An autopsy performed following his death concluded that the cause of death was stomach cancer; and indeed, there was a strong history of stomach cancer in his family, although

longstanding *Helicobacter pylori* infection may have contributed. Nineteen years later, Napoleon's grave was opened, and his body was returned to Paris to be finally interred in the magnificent tomb at the church of the Invalides, where it rests today. A popular alternative hypothesis proposed that his death was a consequence of chronic arsenic poisoning by his captors.

The gastrointestinal tract is one of the most frequent sites of cancer, and Table 7.1 shows the registration data for the most common tumours of the digestive system for southeast England in 2001 and the five-year survivals.

Gastrointestinal cancers include oesophageal cancer, gastric cancer, hepatobiliary cancer, pancreatic cancer and colorectal cancer, and these will be dealt with in more detail in the following five chapters.

Table 7.1 Gastrointestinal cancer registration data for southeast England for 2005

Tumour	Percentage of registrations		Rank of registration		Lifetime chance of cancer 1995–2005		Change in ASR		5-year
	Male	Female	Male	Female	Male	Female	Male	Female	Male
Oesophagus	3.4%	1.9%	7th	13th	1 in 75	1 in 95	+8.7%	−1.8%	8%
Gastric	3.6%	2.0%	6th	10th	1 in 44	1 in 86	−30%	−31%	13%
Pancreas	2.6%	2.7%	11th	8th	1 in 96	1 in 95	−2.0%	+5.1%	3%
Colorectal	14%	12%	3rd	2nd	1 in 18	1 in 20	−2.4%	−5.5%	46%

ASR, age-standardized rate.

Lecture Notes: Oncology, 2nd edition. By M. Bower and J. Waxman. Published 2010 by Blackwell Publishing Ltd.

Chapter 8

Oesophageal cancer

Epidemiology and pathogenesis

Cancer of the oesophagus is a relatively uncommon cancer in the UK, but the incidence is rising, at least in men (see Table 7.1). Worldwide, oesophageal cancer is the sixth most common cause of death from cancer. One-third are adenocarcinoma of the distal oesophagus and two-thirds are squamous cell cancers, with 15% in the upper, 45% in the mid and 40% in the lower portions of the oesophagus. Tobacco is a major risk factor for both histological types of oesophageal cancer, but the two types otherwise vary not only in their histology and anatomical distribution but also in their risk factors. Chronic irritation appears to be a major precipitant of squamous cell cancer and may be caused by alcohol, caustic injury, radiotherapy or achalasia. The Plummer–Vinson syndrome (also known as Patterson–Kelly–Brown syndrome) of chronic iron deficiency anaemia, dysphagia and oesophageal web is associated with squamous cell cancer of the oesophagus, particularly in impoverished populations. Tylosis is an autosomal dominant abnormality, characterized by hyperkeratosis (skin thickening) of the palms and soles. It carries a 95% risk of squamous cell cancer of the oesophagus by the age of 70. In contrast, the major precipitant of oesophageal adenocarcinoma appears to be gastro-oesophageal reflux disease (GORD). Related markers of reflux, such as hiatus hernia, obesity, frequent antacid and histamine H2 blockers, are also associated with an increased risk. Barrett's oesophagus (named after Norman Barrett, a thoracic surgeon at St Thomas' Hospital, London) develops in 5–8% of adults with reflux leading to metaplasia of the normal squamous epithelium of the lower oesophagus to columnar epithelium, which may become dysplastic. The annual rate of transformation to oesophageal adenocarcinoma is 0.5%, which is a hundred times greater than the normal risk. Over the last three decades, there has been a radical shift in the histology of oesophageal cancer in the industrialized world, with a marked decline in squamous cell cancers and a rise in adenocarcinomas. Adenocarcinomas are thought to take their origin from the stomach. Where they occur at the junction of the stomach and oesophagus, they are classified as carcinomas of the gastro-oesophageal junction, as the intelligent reader of this book might have concluded independently of the authors of this book. This may reflect alterations in the number of smokers and in the obesity and nutrition of patients.

Prevention

Half of all cases of oesophageal cancer could be prevented by giving up smoking, drinking less alcohol

Lecture Notes: Oncology, 2nd edition. By M. Bower and J. Waxman. Published 2010 by Blackwell Publishing Ltd.

and improving diet, substituting fresh fruit and vegetables for poorly preserved, high salt foods contaminated with nitrosamine carcinogens or microbial toxins. Endoscopic surveillance is recommended every two to five years for patients with Barrett's oesophagus but the evidence that screening is effective is absent. Low-grade dysplasia requires aggressive antireflux management, whilst multifocal or high-grade dysplasia should be treated by surgical resection.

Presentation

Patients present with dysphagia or odynophagia, weight loss and, less frequently, with haematemesis. At the time of diagnosis, more than half of the patients will have locally advanced, unresectable disease or metastases present. Left supraclavicular lymphadenopathy (Virchow's node), hepatomegaly and pleural effusion are common features of metastatic dissemination. The diagnosis is usually confirmed by upper gastrointestinal endoscopy and barium studies (Figure 8.1).

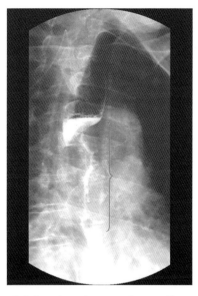

Figure 8.1 Oesophageal cancer. Gastrograffin swallow image showing a long tight stricture of the distal third of the oesophagus with shouldering that encroaches on the gastro-oesophageal junction. This malignant stricture was due to adenocarcinoma of the oesophagus.

Staging and grading

Although CT staging is most helpful in defining operability, additional information can be obtained from using endoscopic ultrasound. This allows the surgeon to have a better view as to the extent of the resection that is required.

Treatment

Only 40% of patients will have localized disease at presentation and are candidates for oesophagectomy with or without postoperative adjuvant chemoradiation. Surgery has a 5–20% mortality rate and may be complicated early by anastomotic

Table 8.1 Five-year survival rates of patients with oesophageal cancer, according to stage at presentation.

Stage	T stage (local tumour)	N stage (nodal status)	M stage (metastatic status)	5-year survival
0	Tis	N0	M0	>95%
I	T1	N0	M0	50–80%
IIA	T2–3	N0	M0	30–40%
IIB	T1–2	N1	M0	10–30%
III	T3–4	N0–1	M0	10–15%
IV	Any T	Any N	M1	<2%

Tis, carcinoma *in situ*; T1, invasion of lamina propria; T2, invasion of muscularis propria; T3, invasion of adventitia; T4, invasion of adjacent structures.

leaks, and later by strictures, reflux and motility disorders. At diagnosis, 25% of patients will have local extension and are treated with palliative radiotherapy, which may cause oesophageal perforation and haemorrhage, pneumonitis and pulmonary fibrosis, as well as transverse myelitis. The remaining 35% of patients will have metastases at presentation and are usually treated symptomatically. Although cancer of the oesophagus is sensitive to chemotherapy, the duration of response is typically short and may be measured in weeks. Cisplatin-based combination regimens have higher response rates, but this may be offset by their greater toxicity. Adjuvant chemoradiotherapy, either prior to surgery (neoadjuvant), or following resection, has yet to be proven as being beneficial. Over the last 30 years, there have been a large number of trials that investigated the benefit of chemotherapy given in the adjuvant setting for carcinoma that had arisen at the junction of the oesophagus and stomach. Until a short time ago, no benefit had been shown, but recent trials have led to the consensus that chemotherapy is probably of benefit in the adjuvant setting, though this benefit is small.

Prognosis

The five-year survival of patients with oesophageal cancer according to stage at presentation is detailed in Table 8.1.

New treatment

As we write, sadly, there are no new therapies that these authors know of for oesophageal cancer.

Chapter 9

Gastric cancer

Epidemiology and pathogenesis

Gastric cancer is the sixth most common malignancy in the UK and constitutes approximately 5% of all cancers. The male to female ratio is 1.5 to 1. In 2005 nearly 8000 people were diagnosed with stomach cancer in the UK and 5200 died of stomach cancer. The average age at presentation is 65 years. The survival for gastric cancer has tripled over the last 25 years but currently only 13% of patients are alive five years after diagnosis. Surprisingly, gastric cancer is the second most common cause of cancer deaths worldwide with 900000 new diagnoses in 2002. There are extreme geographical variations, with the incidence being five times higher in Japan than in the US.

The incidence of gastric cancer has fallen in the industrialized world over the last few decades. This is particularly the case for distal tumours of the stomach. It had been thought that one of the reasons for the decrease in the West is better food preservation. The reducing agents used to preserve food are thought to reduce the availability of free radicals within the stomach, a major cause of carcinogenesis, but this has not been proven in prospective studies. There is contradictory evidence for a protective benefit from fruit and vegetable intake, and also from the use of non-steroidal anti-inflammatory drugs.

In 1926 the Nobel Prize for medicine was awarded to a Dane, Dr Johannes Fibiger, who had described a nematode worm that he called *Spiroptera carcinoma*, which caused stomach cancers in rats that he caught in an infested sugar refinery. It was subsequently shown that the cancers were in fact only metaplasia and that the cause was vitamin A deficiency. Although Fibiger has been branded a fibber, it turns out that chronic infection is the cause of most human gastric cancers. The single most common cause of gastric cancer is infection with *Helicobacter pylori*: probably the most common chronic bacterial infection in man. This bacterium colonizes over half of the world's population. Infection is usually acquired in childhood and in the absence of antibiotic therapy persists for the life of the host. How *H. pylori* causes gastric cancer remains unclear. Strains that have CagA genes are more oncogenic and the products of these genes regulate protein secretion by epithelial cells. In addition, chronic *H. pylori* infection leads to the local production of inflammatory cytokines that are also thought to be involved in oncogenesis. Infection by *H. pylori* explains the aetiology of cancers developing in patients with atrophic gastritis. *Helicobacter* infection is more common in patients with gastric cancer than in 'controls', in particularly in younger patients.

Lecture Notes: Oncology, 2nd edition. By M. Bower and J. Waxman. Published 2010 by Blackwell Publishing Ltd.

Presentation

Patients with gastric cancer generally present to their general practitioner with symptoms of abdominal pain. Classically, the pain is epigastric and worse with meals. The differential diagnosis includes benign peptic ulceration. The routine prescription of protein pump inhibitors, without investigation by endoscopy, may lead to late diagnosis and the presence of advanced disease at diagnosis. Because the symptoms of gastric cancer are very similar to those of peptic ulceration, and because peptic ulceration is very common and not necessarily routinely investigated, early diagnosis of gastric cancer in the West presents a difficult problem. Fewer than 2% of patients with first time dyspepsia will have gastric cancer but the risk is greater in people over 55 years and those with dysphagia, vomiting, weight loss, anorexia or symptoms of gastrointestinal bleeding. Walk-in endoscopy clinics, however, are becoming much more widely available in the UK, and it is hoped that they will impact upon survival figures for gastric cancer.

Outpatient diagnosis

After initial assessment, which should include a full blood count, liver function tests and chest X-ray, more specialized investigations should be undertaken. These should include endoscopy with biopsy, ultrasonography and CT imaging of the abdomen and chest. There have been advances in endoscopic ultrasound that have allowed improvements in local staging of gastric tumours. These improvements are such that mucosal invasion can be distinguished from submucosal invasion. Twenty years ago, the vast majority of patients with gastric cancer presented with inoperable disease. Currently, approximately 50% of tumours are operable at the time of presentation although only 20% are curative resections.

Staging and pathology

The TNM staging system is widely used for staging gastric cancer, with the 'p' prefix denoting patho-logical confirmation of the staging. Ninety-five percent of all gastric tumours are adenocarcinomas. The remainder are squamous cell cancers and lymphomas. Small cell cancers are reported only rarely.

Treatment

Surgery

The only significant chance for a cure rests with surgery. Laparoscopic staging is carried out prior to definitive laparotomy. There is considerable debate concerning the operative procedures of first choice. Older retrospective data suggested that survival was improved with total gastrectomy compared with subtotal gastrectomy. Randomized trials, however, have since shown equivalent survival, with lesser complications for subtotal gastrectomy for carcinoma of the antrum, compared with total gastrectomy. One recent randomized study showed equal five-year survival of patients with either subtotal or total gastrectomy with lymphadenectomy. The operative mortality in the UK varies from 5% to 14% and is related to the number of these operations performed by the surgeon. Surgical developments have been led by the Japanese, who have to deal with the highest incidence of carcinoma of the stomach in the world. The current recommendation by the Japanese Society for Research in Gastric Cancer is for extensive lymphadenectomy, which involves the removal of the lymphatic chains along the coeliac axis and hepatic and splenic arteries. This sort of dissection also has the advantage of allowing more accurate staging for gastric cancer and has been associated with improved survival. For early-stage disease, advances in endoscopic techniques have led to curative mucosal resection techniques equivalent to subtotal gastrectomy, with clear evidence of reduced morbidity. Tumours of the gastro-oesophageal junction are increasing in the West and are treated surgically by subtotal resection of the oesophagus, along with the cardia and gastric fundus.

Adjuvant treatment

In 30 years of adjuvant therapy investigation, no significant role for adjuvant radiation or chemotherapy had been found. Despite this, active trial work continued with the hope of improving prognosis and recent trials have shown a benefit to adjuvant treatment. These benefits continue to be debated. However, neoadjuvant chemotherapy prior to surgery using ECF (epirubicin, cisplatin and infusional 5-fluorouracil (5FU)) or ECX (epirubicin, cisplatin, capecitabine) has been found to improve survival in patients with operable gastric cancer.

Treatment of metastatic or locally inoperable gastric cancer

Patients with inoperable local disease or metastases may be treated with chemotherapy. Over the years, many treatment programmes have been introduced, and the majority have contained 5FU. There is uncertainty as to whether or not combination therapy offers benefit. The response rates are higher but overall survival is similar for combination chemotherapy compared with single-agent 5FU treatment. In the 1970s, there was considerable enthusiasm following the introduction of a combination therapy containing 5FU, adriamycin (doxorubicin) and mitomycin C. This treatment schedule, known as the 'FAM regimen', was initially reported as leading to responses in 40% of patients, with a median duration of response of approximately nine months. Randomized trials have since shown that the same order of response can be obtained with single-agent 5FU, with the same expectations of survival. In recent times, there has been considerable support for combination chemotherapy using epirubicin and cisplatin with either continuous infusion 5FU (ECF) or its oral prodrug capecitabine (ECX). Initially, a 70% response rate was reported, and the median survival of patients responding was seven months. The programme is well tolerated and offers patients reasonable quality of life.

Survival

In the West, more than two-thirds of patients present with advanced tumours. The median survival of patients with advanced local disease or metastatic tumour is approximately six months.

Improving survival in gastric cancer

Patients with early gastric cancer have very good chances of survival, which can be in excess of 90%. For early-stage disease, surgery can be minimal, with advances in endoscopy, endoscopic ultrasonography and endoscopic surgery providing great improvements in limiting the morbidity of interventional therapies. Significant improvements have been seen in Japan as a result of the widescale implementation of screening endoscopy. In Japan, up to 40% of patients are found to have early-stage tumours, which contrasts with the situation in the West. One can only conclude that more widespread availability of endoscopic screening and earlier referral by GPs remains the only significant chance for improved survival. The development of effective therapies based upon any understanding of the biological basis of this tumour group seems to be a distant possibility at this point.

Chapter 10

Hepatobiliary cancer

Epidemiology and pathogenesis

Hepatobiliary cancer is the sixth most common malignant tumour in the world. The highest incidences are seen in South East Asia. In the United Kingdom, hepatobiliary cancer is relatively uncommon. There are approximately 3200 men and women registered with the condition each year, and sadly 3200 deaths. Generally, there are more women than men affected by these tumours. Liver cancer is divided into four main groups of tumour: hepatocellular cancer, which accounts for 75% of this group, and is more common in men than women; biliary tree cancers, also known as cholangiocarcinomas, which account for over 25%; and the rare hepatoblastomas and angiosarcomas which account for 1–2% of all liver cancers.

Hepatocellular cancer is associated with chronic infection with hepatitis B virus (HBV) infection. This is prevalent in up to 15% of males in certain populations. The lifetime risk of developing a tumour is 40% in this group of men. An epidemiological study of 22 707 Taiwanese male government employees followed over 10 years found that the relative risk of liver cancer was 98 for men with HBV. To put this risk into context, the relative risk for lung cancer amongst smokers is around 17. How HBV causes liver cancer is uncertain. The HBV

genome does include a weak oncogene HBX. However, since the greatest risk is amongst those with chronic infection it is thought that the constant proliferation of hepatocytes caused by the need to replace virus-damaged cells and the chronic inflammatory response in the liver are the main culprits. Support for this hypothesis also comes from hepatitis C virus (HCV) induced liver cancer. HBV and HCV are very different viruses genetically but both cause similar chronic infection and inflammation of the liver and both are associated with a high risk of liver cancer. In terms of the model for chemical carcinogenesis these viruses appear to act as tumour promoters rather than initiators. This is supported by synergism in risk between chronic HBV infection and mutagens such as aflatoxin B1. Aflatoxin B1 is derived from *Aspergillus fumigatus* which commonly infects foods such as peanuts that are stored in damp conditions and which causes mutation of p53. In one study from China the relative risk of liver cancer in people with HBV was 7, in those exposed to aflatoxin was 3, but in those exposed to both HBV and aflatoxin was 60. Hepatocellular cancers are also associated with alcoholism and other hepatitides causing cirrhosis such as haemochromatosis and acute and chronic hepatic porphyrias (acute intermittent porphyria, porphyria cutanea tarda, hereditary coproporphyria and variagate porphyria).

There is great interest in the role of the hepatitis-causing viruses in the aetiology of hepatocellular

Lecture Notes: Oncology, 2nd edition. By M. Bower and J. Waxman. Published 2010 by Blackwell Publishing Ltd.

cancer, and this is for three reasons. Firstly, a vaccine based on the surface antigen envelope protein of HBV (HBVsAg) protects against the acquisition of HBV. The widespread introduction f this vaccine in Taiwan has been shown to reduce the risk of hepatocellular cancer in children and a similar protection in adults is likely. Secondly, antiviral therapy against hepatitis B that is effective at lowering HBV titres may reduce the risk of liver cancer amongst people with chronic HBV. Similarly interferon-based therapy for chronic HCV may also reduce the risk of hepatocellular cancer in chronically infected individuals. Finally, screening people with chronic HCV and HBV may reduce the mortality of liver cancer by diagnosing patients earlier with surgically resectable disease. Liver ultrasound and serum α-fetoprotein (AFP) screening should be performed every six months in patients with chronic HBV or HCV. There are significant concerns with regard to the increasing infection rates with hepatitis C in Europe. It is thought that the risk of developing hepatobiliary cancer in the presence of chronic hepatitis C infection is even greater than that associated with hepatitis B infection.

The aetiology of hepatoblastoma is not known. Hepatic angiosarcoma is associated with exposure to polyvinyl choride (PVC) monomer. The mechanism for this is not clear, and the development of this tumour does not always occur in those men and women who have the heaviest exposure to PVC, as for example in those workers involved in autoclave cleaning in chemical works. When workers exposed to PVC are examined for their lifetime risk of developing angiosarcoma this is overall clearly four times higher than in the general population. Where there is a coincident HBV infection, the risk increases 25-fold compared with general population. PVC exposure is also associated with the development of brain and lung tumours.

Tumours of the biliary tree are divided into intrahepatic bile duct cancers (which are treated in the same way as hepatocellular cancers), perihilar cholangiocarcinomas (also known as Klatskin tumours) that occur at the bifurcation of the left and right hepatic ducts, and extrahepatic cholangiocarcinomas and gall-bladder cancers (Figures 10.1 and 10.2). They are seen at increased frequency in patients with ulcerative colitis and primary sclerosing cholangitis. In South East Asia, where these tumours are common, they are seen in association with biliary infestation with liver flukes (*Clonorchis sinensis* and *Opisthorchis viverrini*).

Presentation

Patients with hepatobiliary cancer generally present with advanced disease. Typical presentations are with jaundice, liver pain and weight loss.

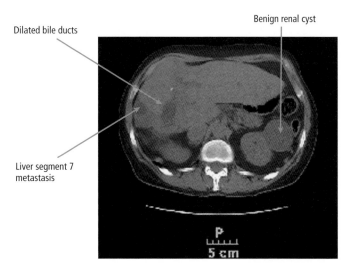

Dilated bile ducts

Benign renal cyst

Liver segment 7 metastasis

Figure 10.1 CT scan demonstrating intrahepatic dilated bile ducts that were due to cholangiocarcinoma. There is also a low attenuation metastasis in segment 7 of the liver and an incidental (benign) renal cyst.

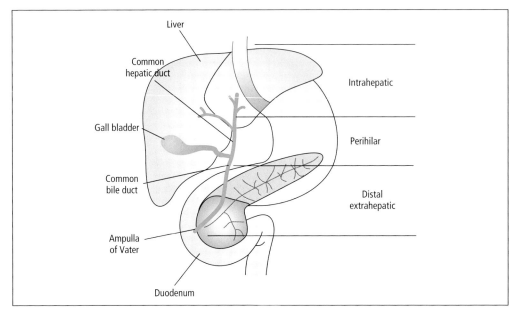

Figure 10.2 Anatomy of biliary tract cancers.

A patient with a suspected diagnosis of hepatobiliary cancer should be referred to the appropriate surgical unit for investigation. The management of these conditions is very complex and should only be in centres of excellence with highly specialized surgical units, who achieve significantly better results.

Standard investigations for patients with hepatocellular cancer should include blood counts, liver function tests, renal function tests, chest X-rays, ultrasound assessment and CT imaging. Ultrasonography has developed considerably over the last decade, and these technical improvements have been matched by improved standards in endoscopic assessment of the patient. Hepatobiliary cancers are associated with raised serum levels of AFP, which is characteristically raised to many thousands of ng/ml. In patients with cirrhosis, who may have AFP levels raised to a few hundreds of ng/ml, increasing levels are clues to the development of hepatobiliary cancer. CEA and CA199 are useful markers in the monitoring of hepatobiliary tumours.

Characteristically, patients with these tumours will commonly present with jaundice, and this presentation requires external stenting to stabilize the patient, enable investigations to take place and surgery to be considered. After staging, histological confirmation of the presence of a tumour should be obtained by percutaneous endoscopic retrograde cholangiopancreatography (ERCP) with needle aspiration or brush cytology or by liver biopsy.

Staging and grading

Hepatobiliary tumours are described as well, moderately or poorly differentiated. Staging for hepatic and billiary tract tumours is according to the TNM classification.

Treatment

Liver resection is the only treatment that offers a chance for cure for liver cancer. Surgery is limited by the degree of spread of the tumour and the presence or absence of background cirrhosis. The aim of surgery generally is to remove the lobe of the liver containing the tumour. It may be possible for patients with hepatobiliary cancer to be treated by

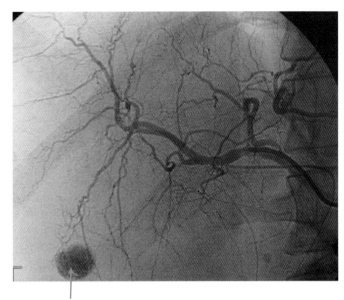

Figure 10.3 Selective angiography of the right hepatic artery showing a small area of hypervascularity due to hepatocellular carcinoma. As this was inoperable (there were four other lesions in different segments of the liver), it was treated by transcatheter arterial chemoembolization (TACE).

Hepatocellular carcinoma

liver transplantation and, if this is the case, the chance of survival increases dramatically. It is estimated that just 10% of patients with liver cancers have operable tumours. When curative surgery is not possible, hepatic embolization, sclerotherapy and chemotherapy may be appropriate (Figure 10.3). Tumours of the biliary tree are chemosensitive and very, very rarely operable. Similar treatment programmes are used in this condition as in hepatocellular cancer. Major problems have come for patients as a result of obstruction of the biliary tree, and this is actively treated by percutaneous or endoscopic stenting. This leads to relief of obstruction and to a useful, though limited, extension of life. Tumour embolization is now a much more commonly used procedure. Transcatheter arterial chemoembolization is performed, where a mixture of chemotherapy, with radio-opaque contrast and an embolic agent, is injected into the right or left hepatic artery (see Figure 10.2). Other approaches include radiofrequency ablation, which uses high-frequency radiowaves to heat up and destroy tumours, using electrodes inserted into the tumour under image guidance. A third treatment for localized unresectable tumours is percutaneous ethanol injection.

Table 10.1 Five-year survival rates of patients with hepatic and biliary tract cancers.

Tumour	5-year survival
Hepatocellular cancer	5%
Gall bladder cancer	5%
Cholangiocarcinoma	5%
Periampullary cholangiocarcinoma	50%

Prognosis

Five-year survival for patients with operable liver cancer is in the order of 33% when management involves partial liver resection. The five-year survival of patients transplanted is 80%. The median survival of patients who are not treated with curative intent is six to seven months (Table 10.1). The median survival of patients in the Far East is much poorer, and the vast majority die within two to three months of diagnosis.

New treatment

We have great hope that mortality from liver tumours will decrease significantly in the next few years. The reason for this is the development of

113

effective campaigns for vaccination against hepatitis B. However, there is considerable concern in Europe that the rising prevalence of hepatitis C, for which no vaccine is available, will lead to a rise in deaths from this condition.

There have been major changes over the last few years in our understanding of the molecular basis for hepatobiliary cancer, with the identification of cell surface receptors for VEGFR (vascular endothelial growth factor receptor) and EGFR (epidermal growth factor receptor). Treatments targeting these receptors and pioneered for patients with renal cell cancer have been found to be effective in hepatobiliary cancer. Responses are seen to sunitinib and sorafenib, but the use and value of these agents, though clear, has been, as ever, stymied by the action of the National Institute for Health and Clinical Excellence (NICE) in the UK. This action by NICE seems particularly bizarre in the context of a clear evidence base demonstrating a doubling of survival time with sorafenib in a large phase III clinical trial.

Chapter 11

Pancreatic cancer

Epidemiology and pathogenesis

Carcinoma of the pancreas has increased in incidence over the last decade. It is the tenth most common cancer, and is now the fifth most frequent cause of cancer deaths. There is an equal incidence between the sexes, and annually in the UK there are about 7700 deaths. It is very sad to note that registration figures virtually equal mortality rates. There is an increased risk of developing pancreatic cancer with age. In the 1980s it was suggested that excessive coffee consumption predisposed to the development of cancer of the pancreas, but this has subsequently been refuted. Smoking is also associated with an increased risk of this disease of between two- and five-fold. Diabetes, obesity and chronic pancreatitis all increase the risk of pancreatic cancer. Pancreatic exocrine cancers constitute well over 90% of all pancreatic malignancies and are adenocarcinomas. Pancreatic adenocarcinoma is believed to arise from ductal epithelial cells that progress through stages of pancreatic intraepithelial neoplasia with the sequential accumulation of somatic mutations in several genes including the oncogene K-RAS and the tumour suppressor genes P53, P16/CDKN2A and SMAD4/DPC4. Pancreatic adenocarcinoma cells express a wide variety of receptors that are potential therapeutic targets including epidermal growth factor (EGF) receptors, vascular endothelial growth factor (VEGF) receptors and insulin-like growth factor (IGF) receptors. Pancreatic adenocarcinoma also expresses a wide variety of hormone receptors, and these include receptors for somatostatin, gonadotrophin-releasing hormone, steroid hormones, insulin-like growth factors and VEGFs. It should be emphasized that these receptors are present in carcinomas, and that they are not present in the unusual secretory endocrine pancreatic tumours. The rare endocrine tumours of the pancreas are known as islet cell tumours or nesidioblastomas and include gastrinomas, insulinomas and pancreatic carcinoids. These tumours may be functional or non-secretory.

Presentation

Patients with carcinoma of the pancreas present with many different symptoms. These include abdominal and back pain, weight loss, anorexia and fatigue. In many patients the disease is asymptomatic, until they present with obstructive jaundice. Other, less common presentations include superficial venous thrombosis (Trousseau's sign), a palpable gall bladder in the presence of obstructive jaundice (Courvoisier's law states that this is unlikely to be due to gall stones) and diabetes. Because of the anatomical position of the tumour,

Lecture Notes: Oncology, 2nd edition. By M. Bower and J. Waxman. Published 2010 by Blackwell Publishing Ltd.

Pancreatic cancer

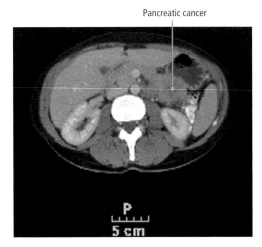

Figure 11.1 CT scan of a mass in the tail and body of the pancreas showing a low attenuation centre suggesting central necrosis of an adenocarcinoma of the pancreas.

late presentation is very common. The patient with a suspected diagnosis of pancreatic cancer should be referred by his or her GP to a general surgeon or a gastroenterologist and be seen in out-patients within two weeks of receipt of the GP's letter of referral. The clinician should organize a number of tests, which include full blood count, renal and liver function tests, a chest X-ray and a CT scan of the abdomen (Figure 11.1). Abdominal ultrasonography is also helpful but endoscopic ultrasound (EUS) is probably the most valuable diagnostic test when coupled with percutaneous needle biopsy. The measurement of serum levels of the carbohydrate antigen tumour marker CA19-9 is less helpful in the diagnosis of cancer of the pancreas as it may be elevated in most causes of obstructive jaundice (false positive) and may be normal in patients with pancreatic cancer (false negative). CA19-9 is, however, useful in monitoring cancer of the pancreas in patients with raised levels at diagnosis.

Investigation of the patient with pancreatic cancer is aimed at establishing the diagnosis and defining operability. After the initial tests have been carried out, the patient should proceed to EUS or, if not available, endoscopic retrograde cholangiopancreatography (ERCP). At ERCP, cytology specimens may be obtained from brush-ings, suction of the pancreatic duct or biopsy. ERCP is more invasive than other diagnostic imaging modalities and carries a significant complication rate so it is usually reserved for patients with biliary obstruction who require stenting. A failure to obtain a diagnosis by endoscopy should be followed by further investigation. Fine needle aspiration cytology under CT scan is usually successful at obtaining a tissue diagnosis.

Staging and grading

As with other cancers, numerous different staging systems are used including the TNM classification. The group staging system is summarized below:

- Stage I: cancer confined to the pancreas (T1N0M0 if <2 cm, T2N0M0 if >2 cm)
- Stage II: cancer has grown into the adjacent duodenum or bile duct but not spread to the lymph nodes (T3N0M0)
- Stage III: cancer has spread to the lymph nodes with (T3N1M0) or without (T1–2N1M0) direct tumour extension
- Stage IVA: cancer has invaded into the stomach, spleen, colon or nearby large blood vessels, and lymph nodes may (T4N1M0) or may not (T4N0M0) be involved
- Stage IVB: there is spread to distant organs by metastases (T1–4N0–1M1).

The vast majority of pancreatic cancers are exocrine adenocarcinomas of ductal origin and they are graded as either well, moderately or poorly differentiated tumours. The tiny minority of endocrine tumours are classified according to the products that they secrete.

Treatment

There is considerable nihilism attached, quite reasonably, to the treatment of a patient with pancreatic cancer. The initial management consists of relieving symptoms of pain and obstructive jaundice. For less than 20% of patients is there any hope for operability, as defined by imaging. No attempt should be made to proceed to surgery until the jaundice has completely resolved. Jaundice is dealt with by relief of biliary obstruction, either by endoscopic stenting or by percutaneous transhepatic stenting of the biliary system. Pain may be relieved by the use of opiates or may resolve with the relief of biliary obstruction. At laparotomy, just 30% of those 20% of patients with radiologically operable disease turns out to have surgically operable tumours.

Pancreatic surgery requires a considerable degree of specialization and should not be carried out outside of the setting of a specialist treatment centre. The reason for this is simple: specialist centres achieve better survival rates and lower morbidity and mortality rates. The operation of choice is Whipple's procedure, and this involves removal of the distal half of the stomach (antrectomy), gall bladder (cholecystectomy), distal common bile duct (choledochectomy), head of the pancreas, duodenum and proximal jejunum, and regional lymph nodes. Reconstruction consists of attaching the pancreas to the jejunum (pancreaticojejunostomy), the common bile duct to the jejunum (choledochojejunostomy), and the stomach to the jejunum (gastrojejunostomy), to allow bile, digestive juices and food to flow! There are modifications of this procedure, such as the pylorus-conserving pancreaticoduodenectomy, that are associated with less postoperative morbidity and equivalent efficacy.

Thirty years ago, surgery for pancreatic cancer was associated with a very high morbidity of approximately 25%. This has fallen in specialist centres to 5%, with the expectation that 20% of patients with operable disease will survive five years. Ampullary carcinomas of the pancreas generally present with early-stage disease because of their anatomical position. These tumours are associated with better prognoses than cancers of the rest of the pancreas. There is no role whatsoever for adjuvant chemotherapy or radiotherapy.

Treatment of inoperable disease

Patients with inoperable pancreatic cancer have a poor prognosis and the treatment of this condition is palliative. The median survival is four to six months. Active treatment with chemotherapy may be advised. The most successful chemotherapy

programmes have response rates of up to 40%, but the median duration of survival of these responding patients is just one month longer than might be expected without active treatment. Because pancreatic cancer is relatively common, a number of chemotherapy agents have been tried for this condition. The consensus view is that combination therapy using the more active agents, such as anthracyclines and taxanes, offers little benefit. The more drugs that are combined, the more toxicity, without an improvement in survival. The current consensus view is that single-agent gemcitabine probably offers as good an opportunity for disease palliation as does any combination regimen, although in practice it is often combined with cisplatin. Gemcitabine is easy to administer and has little toxicity. Quality of life issues are paramount in this condition because of the poor prognosis for inoperable disease.

An alternative approach to the management of pancreatic cancer is to treat symptoms. This is managed by stenting to relieve jaundice and by coeliac axis block. This procedure blocks the pain fibres originating from the pancreas and ensures good quality of life. The technique requires skill and is relatively well tolerated.

Prognosis

The outlook for patients with operable pancreatic cancer is unfortunately not particularly good, with a 20% chance of five-year survival. The outlook for those patients with locally advanced or metastastic disease is very poor, with a median survival of three to four months. It is for this reason that there is such an emphasis upon quality of life in pancreatic cancer, rather than on the prospects for cure.

New treatment

The expression by pancreatic cancer cells of numerous receptors and the poor results with systemic chemotherapy has led to strategies targeting these receptors. Epidermal growth factor receptor inhibitors including the protein kinase inhibitor erlotinib and the monoclonal antibody cetuximab have been studied with limited success. The VEGF pathway has also been targeted with the anti-VEGF monoclonal antibody bevacizumab and receptor tyrosine kinase inhibitors of VEGF receptors including sorafenib. Again the results have disappointed. The IGF pathway that is activated in pancreatic and other cancers is a novel target for therapeutic strategies and monoclonal antibodies targeting both the ligand (IGF1 and IGF2) and the receptor (IGF receptor 1, IGFR1) are under investigation along with receptor tyrosine kinase inhibitors of IGFR1.

The transfer of suicide genes to tumour cells by retroviral vectors has also been applied in pancreatic cancer cell lines. This approach is known as gene-directed enzyme prodrug therapy (GDEPT). The adenovirus vector that was used carried the herpes simplex virus thymidine kinase gene that phosphorylates the prodrug ganciclovir into deox-

yGTP that is incorporated into replicating DNA causing strand termination. This GDEPT strategy inhibited gene expression and cell growth of pancreatic cancer cell lines. The technique has been extensively modified with different viral vectors as well as different enzyme and prodrug combinations.

Pancreatic endocrine tumours

This is a fascinating group of tumours, interesting not only because of their biology, but also because patients with these tumours are expected to do well. Pancreatic endocrine tumours include carcinoids, insulinomas, glucagonomas, gastrinomas and Vipomas. The bizarre constellation of symptoms produced by carcinoids are well known even to medical students, as are the gastrointestinal

Table 11.1 Cinical manifestations of secretory endocrine tumours.

Tumour	Major feature	Minor feature	Common sites	Percentage malignant	MEN associated
Insulinoma	Neuroglycopenia (confusion, fits)	Permanent neurological deficits	Pancreas (β-cells)	10%	10%
Gastrinoma (Zollinger–Elison syndrome)	Peptic ulceration	Diarrhoea, weight loss, malabsorption, dumping	Pancreas Duodenum	40–60%	25%
Vipoma (Werner–Morrison syndrome)	Watery diarrhoea, hypokalaemia, achlorhydria	Hypercalcaemia, hyperglycaemia, hypomagnesaemia	Pancreas, neuroblastoma, SCLC, phaeochromocytoma	40%	<5%
Glucagonoma	Migratory necrolyic erythema, mild diabetes mellitus, muscle wasting, anaemia	Diarrhoea, thromboembolism stomatitis, hypoaminoacidaemia, encephalitis	Pancreas (α-cells)	60%	<5%
Somatostatinoma	Diabetes mellitus, cholelithiasis, steatorrhoea, malabsorption	Anaemia, diarrhea, weight loss, hypoglycaemia	Pancreas (β-cells)	66%	Case reports only

MEN, multiple endocrine neoplasia; SCLC, small cell lung cancer.

symptoms resulting from Vipomas, and the hypo- and hyperglycaemia from insulinomas and gluca- gonomas respectively (Table 11.1). Old school general physicians will expect that every medical student reading this book will be able to recount the ten skin conditions associated with carcinoid tumours, as well as describe the reasons for the effects of this tumour on the heart. They will take delight in quizzing you on their ward rounds so we suggest that you google them if there is an inpa- tient with carcinoid on your ward.

These endocrine malignancies are associated with enormously long natural histories, which may date back over decades.

The major treatment options for pancreatic endocrine tumours include octreotide to decrease hormonal secretion, and chemoembolization to reduce the symptoms that result from tumour bulk. Octreotide is an octapeptide mimic of soma- tostatin that inhibits the secretion of a whole host of peptide hormones including gastrin, glucagon, growth hormone, insulin, pancreatic polypeptide (PP) and vasoactive intestinal polypeptide (VIP). Octreotide also reduces pancreatic and intestinal fluid secretion, hence its use in the management of malignant bowel obstruction. Octreotide has a median period of effect of one year in carcinoids, but leads to no clinical evidence of disease regres- sion. Interferon may also lead to a reduction in secretory symptoms of carcinoid tumours. Where symptoms are significant and octreotide has failed, embolization is considered, both to the primary site and to hepatic metastases. Embolization is a significant enterprise and is associated in even the best centres with mortality rates of 3–5%. It should therefore be considered with great care before it is undertaken.

There has been considerable debate as to whether or not interferon causes a reduction in tumour mass. The balance of the evidence is in favour of interferon having a minor effect in reducing tumour bulk.

Chapter 12

Colorectal cancer

Epidemiology and pathogenesis

Colorectal cancer is a major cause of morbidity in the West. Each year in the UK approximately 37 500 people are diagnosed with colorectal cancer and 16 000 die of the disease. The incidence has risen modestly over the last quarter of a century and the five-year overall survival has doubled over the same time interval. In the 1960s and 1970s, there was increasing recognition of the possibility of a dietary basis to colorectal cancer. The disease was thought to be uncommon in the developing world, whilst the high red meat and low fibre diet and obesity in the more developed market economies were seen to be responsible for a higher incidence of colorectal cancer. Certainly the EPIC (European Prospective Investigation into Cancer and Nutrition) study revealed a 55% increase in risk for each 100 g/day increase in red meat consumption. This risk with red meat is supported by three meta-analyses that revealed significant, although smaller, risks. High fibre diets increase the transit time of the stool and decrease the colorectal epithelial exposure to carcinogens within the stool. The EPIC study also demonstrated a modest 20% reduction (mainly of left-sided colon cancers) in risk amongst the highest fibre eaters. However, this association has not been confirmed in meta-

analyses despite the constant advise to eat five fruits (or vegetables) a day. Nevertheless, the authors suggest that you do not tell young children this information as the reactions of their mothers is wholly unpredictable. Aspirin has been shown to have a protective effect against colorectal cancer, and epidemiological studies of prolonged aspirin use have shown a consistent reduction of up to 50% in the risk of colorectal cancers. This decrease in risk is thought to be due to the inhibitory effect of aspirin on cyclooxygenase-2, which is an enzyme found in high concentrations in colorectal tissue and promotes the growth of polyps. In randomized studies, aspirin has been shown to reduce the incidence of adenomatous polyps in patients screened after the excision of a primary colorectal tumour. There has, however, only been one single randomized trial of aspirin prophylaxis, which has shown no evidence for a reduction in colorectal cancer incidence and the toxicity, especially the risk of gastrointestinal haemorrhage, means that it is premature to recommend aspirin as chemoprevention. Patients with both Crohn's disease and ulcerative colitis are at risk from developing colonic tumours, and this risk rises to nearly 40% after 20 years follow-up.

Up to 20% of patients with colorectal cancer have a family history of colorectal cancer. There are two significant familial causes for colorectal cancer: familial adenomatous polyposis (FAP) and hereditary non-polyposis colorectal cancer (HNPCC). FAP is an autosomal dominant condi-

Lecture Notes: Oncology, 2nd edition. By M. Bower and J. Waxman. Published 2010 by Blackwell Publishing Ltd.

tion that accounts for 1% of all colorectal cancer. The gene for FAP was mapped to chromosome 5q21 in 1987 and the responsible gene APC was cloned in 1991. All patients with FAP develop colorectal cancer by the age of 40 years, so prophylactic colectomy is offered to teenagers with FAP. HNPCC, or Lynch syndrome, is responsible for 2–5% of colorectal cancers. HNPPC is characterized by colorectal cancers occurring at an early age and they are often sited in the right side of the colon. In addition, HNPCC is associated with endometrial carcinoma, and gastric, renal, ureteric and central nervous system malignancies. In this condition, the genetic abnormalities include microsatellite instability and mutated mismatch-repair genes (most frequently hMSH2 and hMLH1). In the vast majority of non-inherited colorectal malignancy, the molecular changes consist of a sequential accumulation of mutations in genes including p53, and deletion of the colorectal gene (DCC), K-Ras and APC.

Presentation

Patients with colorectal tumours present to their general practitioners with a history of altered bowel habit and rectal bleeding. This may also be accompanied by weight loss and abdominal pains.

These symptoms are suggestive of malignancy, and accordingly an urgent referral should be made to a specialist bowel surgeon. The patient should be seen within two weeks of receipt of the general practitioner's referral letter.

Outpatient diagnosis

In outpatients, the surgeon should take a full history from the patient and examine him or her. This should include a rectal examination, which may show the patient to have melaena. Proctoscopy and sigmoidoscopy should be performed in the outpatient setting. Blood tests should be organized, which should include a full blood count, renal function and liver function tests. A chest X-ray should be carried out and a barium enema or colonoscopy arranged as an outpatient procedure. The barium enema may show narrowing of the colon. In malignancy, this narrowing is typical and has the appearance of an apple core (Figure 12.1). Endoscopy may show a stenosing lesion or a polyp. Biopsies should be taken of the suspicious area.

Staging and grading

The tumour should be examined histologically. It is described as being either well, moderately or

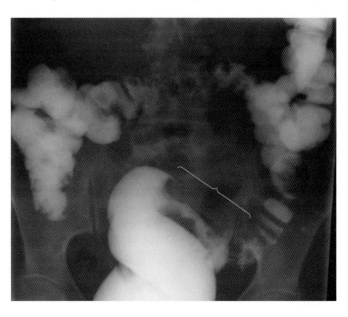

Figure 12.1 Barium enema investigation showing irregular stricture of the sigmoid colon with shouldering giving an apple core appearance typical of sigmoid colon cancer.

Table 12.1 TNM staging of colorectal cancer.

T stage (primary tumour)	N stage (nodal status)	M stage (metastatic status)
T0 No evidence of primary tumour	N0 No nodes	M0 No distant metastases
T1 Tumour invades submucosa	N1 Metastasis in 1–3 pericolic nodes	M1 Distant metastases
T2 Tumour invades muscularis	N2 Metastasis in 4 or more pericolic nodes	
T3 Tumour invades through the muscularis	N3 Metastasis in any lymph node	
T4 Tumour perforates the peritoneum		

poorly differentiated. The original staging system for colorectal cancer was reported by Cuthbert Esquire Dukes, a British pathologist, in 1932. With various modifications this system is still in use today. A Dukes' stage is given, and this reflects the degree of invasion of the tumour. Dukes' stage A is specified when a tumour is confined to the mucosa. Dukes' stage B is a tumour that perforates the serosa, and Dukes' stage C is given when lymph nodes are affected. Tumours of the colon are, furthermore, divided according to their anatomical sub-sites. These are the appendix, caecum, ascending colon, hepatic flexure, transverse colon, splenic flexure, descending colon and sigmoid colon. Finally, the tumour can be staged according to the TNM clinical classification system (Table 12.1).

Treatment

The suspicion of malignancy having been raised, the patient should be worked up for surgery including an assessment of operability by CT scanning. The CT scan will show whether or not there are enlarged lymph nodes within the abdomen and will define the possibility of further spread involving the liver. If there is no gross evidence of dissemination, the patient should be admitted to hospital for colectomy or an abdominoperitoneal resection. Removal of the primary is still considered in the presence of metastatic disease, to reduce the risk of perforation or obstruction.

The surgical plan depends upon the experience and practice of the clinician. There have been considerable developments in the area of laparoscopic surgery. If the patient is therefore considered to be an appropriate candidate, a laparoscopic colectomy might be performed. The results of rectal surgery are critically surgeon dependent, and much better results are obtained in centres where the surgeon specializes in this procedure.

Surgery for colonic cancer

At operation, a midline incision should be performed and the abdominal contents inspected. The tumour should be mobilized and removed together with a good margin of normal tissue. The tumour should be inspected and frozen sections performed, to ensure that the resection edges of the apparently normal gut contain no tumour. An end-to-end anastomosis is then made. If the patient is found to have three to five liver metastases at operation, these should be resected at an appropriate time, as successful resection is associated with a good prognosis and the possibility of cure. If there are more metastases, no operative action should be taken. Extensive resection of the lymph nodes should be performed, providing histopathological information which affects the patient's management.

Surgery for rectal cancers

The surgery that is performed depends upon the site of the carcinoma and a preoperative assessment of operability. Tumours of the upper and middle third of the rectum are treated by anterior resection. In this procedure, the rectum is mobilized from the sacral hollow, and the tumour is removed together with an adequate margin of normal tissue. This normal margin ranges between

2 and 5 cm. The mesorectum and lateral pararectal tissue should be removed. Lesions of the lower third of the rectum are treated by abdominoperineal resection, which requires a permanent colostomy. The rectum is mobilized, and the peritoneum at the base of the bladder or posterior vagina is incised. The lateral ligaments are divided and the anus excised. The quality of surgery in rectal cancer is critically important. Extensive lymphadenectomy is associated with significantly improved chances for survival.

Complications of surgery

A neurogenic bladder is very common after pelvic surgery but will usually recover within 10 days. Ureteric tears or transections may complicate surgery, but only rarely so. Sexual dysfunction in males is inevitable, and the most common problems are retrograde ejaculation and erectile impotence. Change in sexual function in women has not been assessed. Surgery is complicated by a mortality rate of 1–2%.

Adjuvant treatment for colonic cancer

Following recovery from surgery, no additional treatment is recommended for patients with Dukes' stage A disease. The value of adjuvant chemotherapy for Dukes' B disease remains controversial. This is because no major advantage has been shown for adjuvant chemotherapy within this group of patients. Patients with Dukes' C tumours, however, should receive adjuvant chemotherapy. The reason for this is that there is a survival advantage in this group of patients. Treatment should be with a 5-fluorouracil (5FU)-containing programme. There is considerable contention as to which is the optimal treatment schedule. In the late 1980s and early 1990s, the use of levamisole was prevalent, but treatment with this agent is no longer recommended. At present we have a plethora of agents that are active in metastatic colorectal cancer. The current problem is to know which agent or combination of agents are the most effective in prolonging survival in the adjuvant setting. The active agents, oxaliplatin, capecitabine, iri-

notecan and bevacizumab, which are all of benefit in this disease, may be considered with or without a 5FU and folinic acid-containing adjuvant treatment programme. Current recommendations are for treatment with 5FU, which may be administered intravenously, or as the oral analogue of 5FU, capecitabine. The patient might also be offered an oral combination chemotherapy regimen with the acronym UFT, containing tegafur and uracil. Treatment may be given in combination with folinic acid and irinotecan in the FOLFIRI regimen, or with folinic acid and oxaliplatin in the FOLFOX regimen.

Adjuvant treatment for rectal cancer

Patients with rectal cancer may receive preoperative radiotherapy. This has been shown to limit pelvic recurrence. It is disputed whether adjuvant radiotherapy improves survival. Alternatively, after the patient has recovered from surgery, he or she may receive pelvic radiotherapy. This has been shown in randomized studies to decrease the risk of pelvic recurrence by 5–10%. Patients with more advanced tumours (T3 and T4) may be treated with adjuvant chemoradiotherapy prior to surgery, in addition to radiotherapy. There is increased postoperative morbidity with chemotherapy given in conjunction with radiotherapy.

Management of metastatic disease

In the situation where there are limited metastases from colorectal cancer, consideration is given to the possibility of curative surgical treatment. If the patient is fit, and there are three to five hepatic metastases or less than three pulmonary metastases, resection may be considered to be appropriate. If surgery is successful, then the prognosis is relatively good, with survival chances ranging up to 40% at five years.

Generally, however, metastatic colorectal carcinoma has a poor prognosis, and the current recommendation for appropriate treatment is with 5FU-based regimens and radiotherapy. There is debate as to whether or not the addition of folinic acid is of an advantage to the patient. The current consensus is that there is a benefit at least in terms of remission rates, although no consensus has been reached regarding survival. The treatment regimen of first choice was called the 'De Gramont regimen' and includes fortnightly 5FU and folinic acid given for six months. A host of new treatments have recently become available for patients with colorectal cancer. The most commonly used chemotherapy regimens are FOLFOX and FOLFIRI. The addition of irinotecan and oxaliplatin to 5FU in these regimens has improved median survival from 9 to 18 months. Recently the addition of bevacizumab, a humanized monoclonal antibody against vascular endothelial growth factor (VEGF), to both the FOLFOX and FOLFIRI regimens has led to a further modest improvement in survival. Cetuximab, a partially humanized monoclonal antibody against the epidermal growth factor receptor (EGFR), and panitumumab, a fully humanized antibody against EGFR, have both been shown to prolong survival in patients with metastatic colon cancer that lack mutations in K-Ras. As a result of the use of these agents, survival in metastatic colorectal cancer has been extended from 18 months to almost 2 years. In this context, the cost of treatment becomes a significant political issue but, amongst the discussion on the politics of cancer care, little attention seems to be paid to the cost of not treating the patient. Dying from metastatic colorectal cancer without drug treatment is an expensive process, and the authors of this chapter are not merely considering financial cost when we make this statement.

Screening

It is estimated that there may be a genetic predisposition to colorectal cancer in more than 20% of patients with these tumours. In the vast majority of colorectal cases there is, however, at present no direct evidence of there being a genetic risk. Patients with a risk of developing colorectal tumours can be stratified as having low, low–moderate, moderate, moderate–high or high risk of developing malignancy. The criteria for proceeding to screening for these patients are defined as in Table 12.2.

Table 12.2 Screening scheme for colorectal cancer.

Risk	Action	Age
Low risk		
1 relative >45 years *or* 2 relatives >70 years	Reassure: no colonoscopy	
Low–moderate risk		
2 first-degree relatives, average age 60–70 years	Single colonoscopy	Aged 55 years
Moderate risk		
2 first-degree relatives, average age 50–60 years	5-yearly colonoscopy	Aged 35–65 years or starting
1 first-degree relative <45 years		5 years before age when youngest relative's tumour was diagnosed
Moderate–high risk		
2 first-degree relatives, average age <50 years	3–5-yearly colonoscopy	Begin age 30–35; refer to genetics
3 close relatives (not AC)		
High risk		
3 close relatives AC +ve (HNPCC) (FAP)	2-yearly colonoscopy Annual sigmoidoscopy from teens	Age 25–65; refer to genetics and counselling

AC, Amsterdam criteria; FAP, familial adenomatous polyposis; HNPCC, hereditary non-polyposis colorectal cancer.

In 2006, bowel cancer screening using faecal occult blood (FOB) tests was introduced in England. It is estimated that if the uptake of FOB testing reaches 60% by the year 2026, 20000 deaths from bowel cancer will be prevented. For every 1000 faecal occult blood tests completed, 20 will be abnormal and 16 patients will proceed to a colonoscopy, six of these will have polyps, two will have cancer, and eight a normal colonoscopy. The cost estimate equation for FOB testing is £1000 for each life-year saved. FOB testing will miss tumours and lead to a number of false positive findings. Colonoscopy is a more accurate means of detecting cancers but requires full bowel preparation, seda-

tion and carries a risk of perforation (around one in 1500). Although the costs of colonoscopy for screening normal populations is, unfortunately, not economic, it is the investigation of choice for high-risk populations (Table 12.2).

New treatment

This is one group of tumours where we are delighted to report that a host of golden opportunities for our patients have arisen. The development of drugs targeting angiogenesis such as bevacuvimab and the EGFRs such as cetuximab have led to real improvements is survival.

Chapter 13

Genitourinary cancers

The treatment of testicular cancer is one of the few solid cancers in adults that may be successfully cured even in the presence of metastases. This has only been achievable in the last 40 years, since the introduction of cisplatin chemotherapy. Cisplatin was discovered serendipitously by Barnett Rosenberg, a physicist at Michigan State University, in 1965. He studied the effects of electric currents on *Escherichia coli* using platinum electrodes in a water bath and found that they stopped dividing but not growing, leading to bacteria up to 300 times longer than normal. This was found to be due to cisplatin, a product from the platinum electrodes, which was interfering with DNA replication. Following this, Professor Sir Alexander Haddow, the then head of the Chester Beatty Institute in London, showed that cisplatin was active against melanoma in mice, and clinical trials with human patients began in 1972.

The genitourinary tract is one of the most frequent sites of cancer in men and includes prostate cancer, which has emerged as the most common tumour in men (excluding non-melanomatous skin cancers). Table 13.1 shows the registration data for these tumours for southeast England in 2001 and the five-year survivals.

Cancer of the genitourinary tract includes cancers of the kidneys, bladder, prostate and testes, which are discussed in more detail in the next four chapters.

Table 13.1 Genitourinary cancer registration data for the UK and five-year survival rates.

Tumour	Percentage of registrations		Rank of registrations		Lifetime risk of cancer		Change in ASR, 1997–2006	5-year survival
	Male	Female	Male	Female	Male	Female		
Prostate	25%	–	1st	–	1 in 14	–	+37%	61%
Testis	2%	–	17th	–	1 in 210	–	+5%	96%
Kidney	3%	2%	9th	11th	1 in 89	1 in 162	+12%	44%
Bladder	5%	2%	4th	12th	1 in 30	1 in 79	–30%	66%

ASR, age-standardized rate.

Lecture Notes: Oncology, 2nd edition. By M. Bower and J. Waxman. Published 2010 by Blackwell Publishing Ltd.

Chapter 14

Kidney cancer

Epidemiology and pathogenesis

Renal carcinoma is not a particularly common cancer and causes approximately 3% of deaths from malignancy in the UK. In 2006 about 7840 people developed renal cancers in the UK per year and there were approximately 3700 deaths. Renal cancers may arise from the kidney nephrons or from the collecting systems. The histology is different for these two tumours and is described, respectively, as 'renal cell' for tumours arising from the nephrons and 'transitional cell' for tumours arising from the transitional cell epithelium of the collecting system. There is evidence for a genetic predisposition to this disease in a small percentage of patients. Renal cell cancer has an increased incidence in patients with von Hippel–Lindau disease and tuberous sclerosis. Transitional cell tumours may be caused by tobacco.

There has been increasing interest in the molecular genetics of renal cell cancer. This is concentrated around the importance of the loss of heterozygosity at chromosome 3p and the inactivation of the von Hippel–Lindau gene. Both are associated with the development of renal cell cancers. In one recent study there was loss of het-

erozygosity around chromosome 3p in 96% of conventional histology renal cell cancers, although in tumours with less common pathologies, such as the papillary and chromophobe variants, these changes are far less frequent. It is therefore likely that the loss of heterozygosity represents the loss of a specific tumour suppressor gene for renal cell cancer, and this fits in with conventional models for the development of malignancy. There are chromosomal changes in non-clear cell tumours too. The PTEN/MMAC1 tumour suppressor gene is lost in up to 90% of patients with chromophobe renal cell carcinoma, and so the molecular pathology of renal cell cancer defines a specific phenotype. Other changes have also been noted, involving chromosome 16q and 14q. A stepwise progression of molecular changes similar to those that are well described in colorectal tumours seems to characterize renal cell cancer. These molecular changes are completely different from those seen in papillary tumours, which are characterized by loss of the Y chromosome and multiple trisomy. In clear cell renal cancer, 3p loss leads to inactivation of hypoxia-inducible factors. This in turn leads to activation of vascular endothelial growth factor (VEGFR) and epidermal growth factor receptor (EGFR), with resultant new vessel formation and tumour development. VEGFR and EGFR upregulation are features of renal cell cancer that have been exploited for treatment, and this will be discussed in more detail below.

Lecture Notes: Oncology, 2nd edition. By M. Bower and J. Waxman. Published 2010 by Blackwell Publishing Ltd.

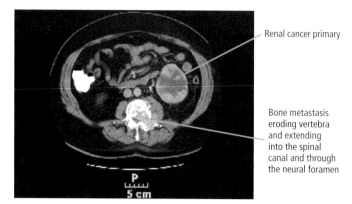

Renal cancer primary

Bone metastasis eroding vertebra and extending into the spinal canal and through the neural foramen

Figure 14.1 Renal cancer. This CT scan shows a left renal inferior pole mass. In addition there is erosion of the vertebral body and posterior elements of the third lumbar vertebra. This is associated with extension into the spinal canal causing cauda equine compression and through the neural foramen into the psoas muscle.

Presentation

Patients with renal cancers commonly present with pain in the loins or blood in the urine. Other symptoms include joint pains, symptoms due to anaemia, a varicocele, generalized symptoms of malignancy, such as weight loss and cachexia, and symptoms due to a spread of the disease to metastatic sites such as brain, lung or bone. If a diagnosis of renal carcinoma is suspected, the patient should be referred to a urologist. Renal cell cancers are characteristically associated with paraneoplastic syndromes, which include polycythemia and pyrexia of unknown origin.

Outpatient diagnosis

The urologist will assess the patient in the outpatient clinic, taking a full medical history and examining the patient. Investigations to be organized will include full blood count, liver and renal function tests and a chest X-ray. Further investigation will also include a CT scan of the abdomen (Figure 14.1) and the thorax to define operability. Angiography and an intravenous urogram (IVU) (Figure 14.2) may also have to be performed.

Staging and grading

The majority of renal tumours are adenocarcinomas of renal cell origin. Approximately 2% of renal

Filling defect in pelvicalyceal system

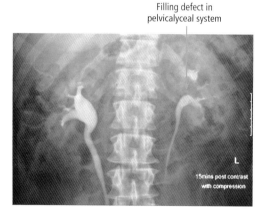

Figure 14.2 An IVU image demonstrating obstruction of the left pelvicalyceal system at the level of the pelviureteric junction with a filling defect. These appearances were due to a transitional cell carcinoma of the renal pelvis. Transitional cell cancer (TCC) of the renal pelvis arises in the collecting system and may be associated with TCC of the bladder and ureter. The biology, prognosis and treatment are similar to those of bladder cancer.

cancers are of transitional cell histology, arising from the collecting system rather than from the renal parenchyma. Both adenocarcinomas and transitional cell tumours are described as well, poorly or moderately differentiated. Nuclear grading, into four Fuhrman categories, is strongly correlated with prognosis. Only rarely is the kidney involved, either with a primary lymphoma or as the site of the spread of other cancers. The kidney can be the site of a rare non-metastasizing malignancy called an oncocytoma. The patient with renal cell carcinoma is staged according to the spread of the disease, using the TNM staging criteria.

Treatment

Surgery

If the patient has no evidence of spread of the disease, then the urological surgeon will arrange for the patient to be admitted for nephrectomy. At operation, the kidney and vascular pedicle and associated lymph nodes are removed, together with the ureter and adrenal. Renal tumours have a propensity to invade along the renal vein. This invasion may extend into the inferior vena cava (IVC) and right atrium. It does not represent a true invasion but a tumour thrombus. If this is suspected, then a combined approach involving a urologist and a vascular surgeon is advised in an attempt to fully resect the tumour.

Management of an inoperable primary tumour

Locally advanced, inoperable kidney cancer may cause significant symptoms, which may be poorly controlled by systemic palliative measures. These local symptoms can include haematuria, which may be so profound that regular blood transfusion is required, as well as loin pain, which may not respond to opiate analgesia. These symptoms can be treated by angioinfarction, where agents are introduced into the renal artery to occlude the tumour's blood supply. A number of different agents can be introduced into the renal artery. These include steel coils and chemotherapy pellets. By these means, successful symptom palliation is achieved in approximately 70–80% of all patients. The procedure does have significant morbidity, which includes a transient increase in pain, fever and, occasionally, shock due to the release of tumour products into the circulation. These symptoms peak a few hours after the procedure but may continue for up to 10 days. There is a specific mortality associated with the procedure, ranging up to

5%. In hospitals where it is not possible to treat by angioinfarction, radiation to the kidney may be given.

Adjuvant treatment

Local radiotherapy to the tumour bed following nephrectomy leads to no survival advantage in patients with adenocarcinoma and has morbidity. This is therefore not recommended. Similarly, adjuvant chemotherapy has no survival advantage. The value of adjuvant immunotherapy continues to be investigated; findings reported up to and including the year 2005, however, have shown no benefit. This includes treatment with interleukin 2 (IL-2) for poor prognosis tumours. The situation may possibly be different in transitional cell tumours. The outlook is very poor for these cancers, so adjuvant chemotherapy is given in some centres.

Management of metastatic kidney cancer

Where there are single sites or limited numbers of metastases, there is a surgical option that needs to be considered. The removal of limited numbers of pulmonary metastases, or brain or bone metastases, leads to a chance for cure. Where there are multiple metastases the situation is different. There have been significant changes in the management of metastatic disease as a result of our understanding of the molecular biology of this group of tumours.

Chemotherapy

Chemotherapy is generally ineffective in the treatment of adenocarcinoma of the kidney. The most active of the agents, which include the vinca alkaloids, produce responses in less than 10% of patients. Chemotherapy is given in the treatment of transitional cell tumours. The response rate of 60–70% is similar to that seen in patients with transitional cell cancer of the bladder. Unfortunately, these responses are transient and last for a median time of six to seven months.

Hormonal therapy

Initial reports of the efficacy of hormonal treatments in the management of renal cell cancer have proven to be incorrect. The use of hormonal therapies for renal cell cancer was based upon the observation over 30 years ago of a response to orchiectomy in Syrian golden hamsters bearing renal cell tumours. The leap of logic from this observation to the use of medroxyprogesterone acetate is rather dizzy, but response rates of up to 30% were described to medroxyprogesterone acetate. This order of response has, however, not been confirmed, and the true response rate to hormonal agents is probably less than 2%. A wide variety of hormonal treatments has been used in this condition, including tamoxifen and flutamide in addition to the progestogens. Transitional cell tumours do not respond to hormonal therapy.

Immunotherapy

Until recently, the most important therapy used for metastatic adenocarcinoma of the kidney was immunotherapy. The first agents used were bacillus Calmette–Guerin (BCG) and *Corynebacterium parvum*, but these have now been replaced by the interferons and interleukin 2. The overall order of response to interferon therapy is 15%. Approximately 5% of patients have a complete response, and the median duration of a complete response is 7 months. There is no incremental rise in response with dosages over three mega units weekly of interferon, merely increased toxicity. In 1985, the results of treatment with IL-2 were first published, and 60% of patients with kidney cancer were reported to respond to treatment. This high response rate was not confirmed in subsequent studies, which were nevertheless encouraging in that, overall, approximately 20% of patients were seen to respond to treatment.

The most significant aspect to IL-2 treatment is that responses are durable. Those lucky patients who achieve a complete response may be cured of their malignancy. In the original dosage regimen, treatment had significant toxicities. These toxicities are lower with subcutaneous low-dose scheduling of IL-2 treatments. Currently, IL-2 is given with interferon. Cytokine treatment may be improved by combination with chemotherapy, but this is controversial. Transitional cell tumours do not respond to immunotherapy.

New treatment

Unfortunately the effective treatment of patients with renal cell cancer has been held back in the United Kingdom by the action of the National Institute for Health and Clinical Excellence (NICE). The bureaucratic processes that regulate NICE have delayed by at least three years effective treatment for this condition, and caused the unnecessary and early death of many patients. In finally coming to a view as to the efficacy of modern therapies for renal cell cancer, false cost calculations were made, and the opinion issued by NICE was changed three times before final agreement to allow some effective treatment for renal cancer patients in the UK. Therapy targets VEGFR and EGFR and the tyrosine kinases that affect receptor activation using drugs such as sunitinib and sorafenib. Response rates approach 40%, and those patients who respond do appear to have responses that are sustained. Treatment does have toxicity, but these toxicities are generally mild. Because treatment targets VEGFR, gastrointestinal bleeding and bowel perforation may occur.

Other new treatments for renal cell cancer include temsirolimus and everolimus, which inhibit mTOR (mammalian target of rapamycin) that is integral to various signal transduction pathways. Unfortunately these agents, which are effective, have also been rejected for use by our patients by NICE as a result of what we and most of our colleagues believe to be false cost calculations. These agents appear to have the same order of efficacy as sunitinib and sorafenib, but are kept as second-line therapies for kidney patients after progression on sunitinib or sorafenib.

Prognosis

The prognosis for localized adenocarcinoma of the kidney is variable. The survival rate for patients with good prognosis tumours is 60–80%, but if there is vascular or capsular invasion, only 40% survive 1 year. The median survival for patients with metastatic disease is nine months. These statistics have significantly changed as a result of the development of new treatments for kidney cancer. Where treatment is allowed, the median survival for patients with metastatic disease has been extended to two years. Kidney cancer survival is significantly longer for those that live in the least deprived areas of the UK compared to those who live in areas of greater material deprivation. Overall, 10% of patients with metastatic renal cell cancer survive five years from diagnosis, and this group represents a curious feature of the malignancy. Even in the absence of metastases at presentation, the outlook for patients with transitional cell tumours is very poor, with 10% surviving for one year, and 5% for two years.

Chapter 15

Bladder cancer

Epidemiology and pathogenesis

Carcinoma of the bladder is common in the United Kingdom. Each year in the UK, approximately 1020 men and women are registered with the disease and 4900 die. Worldwide more than one-third of a million people are diagnosed each year with bladder cancer. The average age at which patients with this condition present to their clinician is 65 years. The most important cause of bladder cancer is cigarette smoking. Workers in the dye, paint and rubber industries are also at increased risk of bladder cancer.

There have been many developments in our understanding of the molecular biology of bladder cancer, and, although these developments have not translated directly into treatment advances, they do provide significant prognostic information. Bladder tumours are thought to progress from a localized, superficial tumour to invasive and then metastatic disease. They are often multifocal. In an attempt to define the molecular events categorizing progression, it was originally noted that there was identical loss of heterozygosity in multifocal bladder tumours. This original description, however, of what was thought to be a primary

genetic event in this cancer, has not been confirmed. Multiple loss of genetic material has been described, with the most common losses centred on chromosome 9q22, which is the site of a gene called *patched* (PTC). This is thought to be a tumour suppressor gene in basal cell carcinoma and medulloblastoma. There are other sites of chromosomal loss, particularly within chromosomes 3, 7 and 17. This loss of material can be used to follow up patients with bladder cancer, using fluorescence *in situ* hybridization (FISH) methodologies on urine cytology.

By far the most important of the recent findings in bladder cancer, however, has been the observation of overexpression of the human epidermal growth factor receptor (EGFR). This is reported in around 40% of the tumours of patients with bladder cancer. Overexpression correlates with a poor prognosis, and treatments directed against EGFR may well have some future role as therapies for this malignancy.

Presentation

The initial symptoms include haematuria, dysuria and frequency of micturition. These symptoms are, unfortunately, sometimes treated with antibiotics by GPs for a period of time, prior to referral to a specialist. New urinary tract infections in older women should always be investigated actively, and symptoms occurring in a man should always be

Lecture Notes: Oncology, 2nd edition. By M. Bower and J. Waxman. Published 2010 by Blackwell Publishing Ltd.

considered to be pathological and a referral made. There is of course a differential diagnosis, but one should have a very high index of suspicion of malignancy. Referral should be promptly organized to a specialist urological surgeon. The patient will be seen in an outpatient clinic. A careful history should be taken and an examination made. The patient's symptoms should be investigated further by performing a blood count, renal function tests, liver function tests and bacteriological and cytological examination of urine, to examine for the presence of infection and malignancy. An intravenous pyelogram (IVP) may be ordered to examine the urothelial tract radiologically or an ultrasound investigation carried out.

Outpatient diagnosis

These investigations should be organized promptly and the patient reviewed with the result within two to three weeks. A flexible cystoscopy is then generally organized and this takes place in the outpatient setting. If there is any suspicious appearance to the bladder, arrangements should then be made for a formal cystoscopy. The patient is anaesthetized for this procedure and the urethra and bladder carefully examined using a fibreoptic cystoscope. Any abnormal areas within the bladder should be biopsied together with areas of surrounding, apparently normal-looking bladder. The urologists at cystoscopy may describe a normal-looking bladder or the presence of a papilloma or solid tumour. The suspicious areas are treated by diathermy and the pelvis carefully examined in order to describe the clinical staging of the tumour.

Staging and grading

The tumour should then be examined pathologically and be given a grade according to differentiation. These grades are as follows:
- G1: well differentiated tumour
- G2: moderately differentiated tumour
- G3: poorly differentiated tumour.

Lesions are further characterized pathologically by their microscopic appearance as either transitional cell carcinoma or squamous carcinoma. Approximately 90% of patients in the UK have transitional cell carcinomas. The rest are squamous carcinomas or adenocarcinomas. There may be squamous metaplasia present within a transitional cell carcinoma, and this is indicative of a poor prognosis.

The tumour should also be staged according to the T (tumour), N (node) and M (metastatic categories) system (Table 15.1).

Table 15.1 TNMstaging of bladder cancer.

T (primary tumour)	N (nodal status)	M (metastatic status)
Tis Carcinoma *in situ*	N0 No lymph node involvement	M0 No evidence of metastases
TA Papillary non-invasive tumour	N1 Single regional lymph node involvement	M1 Distant metastases
T1 Superficial tumour, not invading	N2 Bilateral regional lymph node beyond the lamina propria involvement	
T2 Tumour invading superficial	N3 Fixed regional lymph nodes muscle	
T2A Tumour invading superficial muscle	N4 Juxtaregional lymph node involvement	
T2B Tumour penetrating through superficial muscle		
T3A Invasion of deep muscle		
T3B Invasion through bladder wall		
T4A Tumour invading prostate, uterus or vagina		
T4B Tumour fixed to the pelvic wall		

A subscript 'P' is given to describe the pathological staging of the tumour.

Treatment

Treatment of superficial bladder cancer

The majority of transitional cell carcinoma of the bladder present as superficial tumours. After resection by diathermy at cystoscopy, approximately 60% of these will recur. The recurrence rate is greater where there are multiple tumours, associated carcinoma *in situ* or poorly differentiated tumours. The outlook is best for solitary tumours, tumours with good histology and tumours without invasion of the lamina propria. There is controversy as to whether or not a solitary superficial but clearly non-invasive tumour should be followed up, because recurrence or further papilloma development is unusual. There is also debate as to whether or not these papillomas should be classified as malignant.

The recommendation for follow-up is slightly controversial, but in most practices cystoscopy is performed three-monthly until the patient is tumour free and thereafter six-monthly for two years and yearly for three years. Practice varies throughout the UK.

If tumours are poorly controlled by cystoscopic diathermy but remain superficial, agents may be instilled into the bladder to try and control the disease. A number of different compounds are used, including bacillus Calmette–Guerin (BCG), interferon, thiotepa, adriamcyin, mitomycin C, mitrozantrone and epodyl. BCG is the treatment of choice for carcinoma *in situ*, and mitomycin C is the most popular treatment of multifocal superficial tumours. Maintenance BCG reduces recurrence rates.

Treatment of invasive bladder cancer

The treatment of muscle-invasive carcinoma of the bladder is by radiation or with surgery. Both have similar efficacy in terms of the control of the disease. This varies according to clinical staging: 40–60% of T2 tumours, 25% of T3 tumours and 5% of T4 tumours are controlled by radiotherapy or surgery. In the UK, radiotherapy is the most widely practised treatment, because the patient keeps his or her bladder at the end of therapy. Radical cystectomy has a mortality of up to 3%, depending on which centre it is performed in. After cystectomy, patients must be nursed either in intensive care or in high-dependency beds. Continent bladders may be fashioned by the surgeon so that the patient does not require an ileostomy. Men are invariably rendered impotent by cystectomy. Little is known of the effects of cystectomy on female sexual function. There are well-known electrolyte disorders associated with ileostomies.

Radical radiotherapy is generally given to a total dose of 6500 cGy over a six-week period. Treatment may be given to the whole pelvis, focusing down upon the bladder towards the end of treatment, or may be given to the bladder alone. There is a clear rationale for treating the bladder alone. Treatment of the whole pelvis is given with the aim of shrinking nodal disease, but this is unlikely in the dosage regimens used. If nodes in the pelvis are involved, there is a significant chance of distant nodal spread and so radiation of pelvic node is pointless. Whole pelvis radiotherapy has significantly greater toxicity than treatment to the bladder alone, and there is no logical reason for using whole pelvis radiotherapy.

During radiotherapy, the patient may get cystitis or proctitis. At the end of treatment, he or she may suffer from a small, shrunken bladder as a consequence of radiation fibrosis. Both cystitis and proctitis are common after radiotherapy to the bladder, occurring in up to 30% of patients.

Chemotherapy has been given to patients with bladder cancer. Response rates seem to be similar to radiotherapy and surgery. The advantage to the patient is the avoidance of the long-term side effects of radiotherapy and retention of the bladder.

Treatment of metastatic bladder cancer

When bladder cancer has spread beyond the bladder it is conventionally treated with chemotherapy. Recent advances in the treatment of this disease mean that new hope is now offered to patients with metastatic cancer. A number of different treatment schedules are used for treatment, including regimes which have the acronyms CMV, MVAC and MVMJ. New agents have become available for the treatment of bladder cancer. These include gemcitabine. The standard treatment currently is combination therapy with gemcitabine and cisplatin, chosen for efficacy and comparative lack of toxicity (Figure 15.1).

Prognosis

The consensus view is that diathermy and intravesical chemotherapy prevent the progression of superficial to locally advanced or metastatic disease in 40% of cases. Overall, however, approximately 30% of patients with superficial tumours develop invasive disease. If there is associated carcinoma *in situ*, over 60% of patients will develop invasive cancer. Poorly differentiated superficial bladder cancers have a particularly poor prognosis and are treated aggressively. Despite treatment, just 20% of patients survive five years.

The results of treatment vary from centre to centre, but the overall expectation is for an initial response in approximately 50% of patients with metastatic disease, for a median duration of 9 months. During the terminal phases of illness,

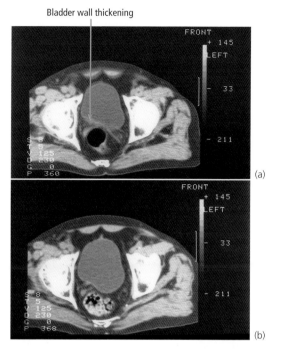

Figure 15.1 (a) CT scan demonstrating thickening of the posterior bladder wall due to invasive bladder cancer and (b) the same image after four cycles of platinum-based combination chemotherapy showing a reduction in bladder wall thickening.

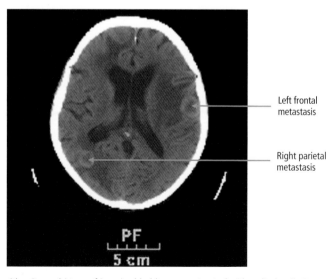

Figure 15.2 A man with a 3-year history of invasive bladder cancer treated with radical radiotherapy developed morning headaches and numbness of his right arm. His CT scan shown here shows two ring-enhancing metastases in the left frontal and right parietal regions with marked surrounding oedema.

patients require specialist care for symptom palliation. The disease may spread to bone, lung or liver, and opiate analgesia or local radiotherapy may be helpful in easing symptoms (Figure 15.2).

New treatment

The major prospects for the development of new treatments for bladder cancer are targeted at methods of inhibiting the activity of the epidermal growth factor receptor. The first in development is gefitib (Iressa), but this is just one of a family of at least six EGFR targeting therapies in development.

Chapter 16

Prostate cancer

Epidemiology and pathogenesis

Carcinoma of the prostate is the second most common cancer of men in the Western world. The latest incidence figures suggest that in the UK, 35 000 men were diagnosed as having prostate cancer and that there were over 10 000 deaths. Prostate cancer death rates have trebled in the last 30 years, and the incidence figures have increased so strikingly that the number of men affected by this cancer has overtaken lung cancer as the most common of all male cancers in the UK. This is also the case in the US, where prostate cancer has replaced lung cancer as the most common cancer of males.

How do we explain this increase in prostate cancer incidence? It is very unlikely that there is a genetic basis to this dramatic recent change in incidence. What is likely is that there is an environmental risk factor. This can be seen from studies on the incidence of cancer in the succeeding generations of migrating populations – as well as from dietary evidence, we believe. There were huge waves of migration from South East Asia to North America and Hawaii at the turn of the 19th century. Prostate cancer has a very low incidence in Asia. The incidence of prostate cancer in the generations that followed these waves of migration increased, so that in two generations the incidence of prostate cancer was almost equivalent to that occurring in their Caucasian neighbours.

The second line of evidence comes from dietary studies, where it has been clearly shown that the incidence of prostate cancer in vegetarians is 50–75% that of the incidence in omnivores. There are striking correlates between prostate cancer and diets containing smoked foods and dairy produce, and protective benefits from diets that are rich in yellow beans.

The genetic basis to prostate cancer has not been clearly elucidated and the reason for this is that it is unlikely that there is one. There are links between familial breast cancer and prostate cancer, and overall the risk of developing prostate cancer is increased by just 1.3-fold if you have an affected father with the condition and by 2.5-fold if you have a brother affected. No consistent genetic defect has been described in prostate cancer. Most have a multiplicity of observed changes. These include a loss of heterozygosity around a number of chromosomes, the most common of which is a loss of genetic material on chromosome 10p. The tumour suppressor genes are infrequently mutated in prostate cancer – for example, the retinoblastoma (RB) gene is mutated in just 5% of patients' tumours. No specific cell surface molecular identity has been demonstrated to occur consistently in prostate cancer. Epidermal growth factor

Lecture Notes: Oncology, 2nd edition. By M. Bower and J. Waxman. Published 2010 by Blackwell Publishing Ltd.

receptor (EGFR) positivity is described in up to 40% of tumours.

Prostate cancer is strikingly hormone dependent. This is because the growth of prostatic tumours is regulated by the androgen receptor, which is a member of the steroid superfamily of transcription factors, and the majority of treatments for prostate cancer have their effect through this receptor.

Presentation

Patients with prostate cancer commonly present with urinary frequency, a poor urine flow or difficulty with starting and stopping urination. Other associated symptoms on presentation include bone pain and general debility. Weight loss is rare. The patient with symptoms such as these should be referred by his GP to a urologist.

Patients with a potential diagnosis of prostate cancer are diagnosed in general practice as a result of prostate-specific antigen (PSA) screening and referred directly to oncology. In the UK between 2% and 6% of men are screened. PSA levels are not necessarily diagnostic of prostate cancer. Where levels are raised above the normal range of 4μg/l to between 4 and 10μg/l, the chance of the patient having prostate cancer is approximately 25%. At levels over 10μg/l, the chance of diagnosing prostate cancer increases to 40%. Levels of this antigen may be elevated in benign prostatic hypertrophy. PSA is a serine protease and acts like drain cleaner for the prostate, dissolving the prostatic coagulum.

In outpatients, a careful history should be taken, a full examination made, routine blood tests performed and levels of acid phosphatase and PSA assessed. In addition, plain X-rays of the chest and pelvis should be performed and a transrectal ultrasound and bone scan booked (Figures 16.1 and 16.2; see Figure 1.8).

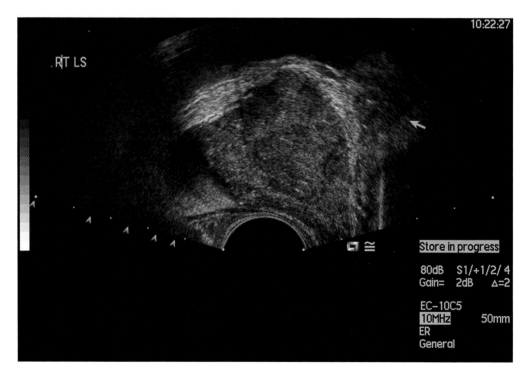

Figure 16.1 Transrectal ultrasound of the prostate gland showing extension of the primary tumour through the prostatic capsule (T3 disease).

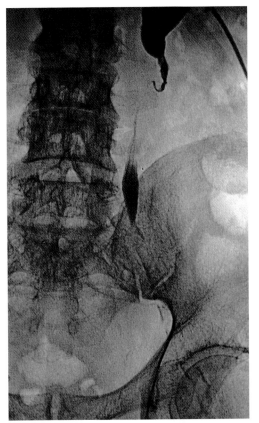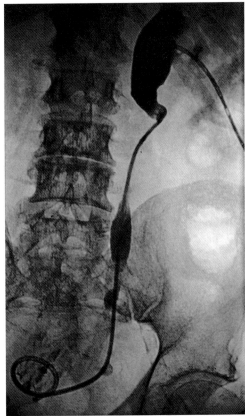

Figure 16.2 Antegrade nephrostogram showing irregular tapering and lack of contrast due to ureteric obstruction and hydronephrosis before and after the passage of a JJ stent to relive obstruction that was due to external compression by prostate cancer.

Staging and grading

From the clinical findings an assessment can be made of the degree of prostate enlargement. If the prostate is malignant, it is staged as in Table 16.1.

The tumour grade can be described as well, moderately or poorly differentiated. This is elaborated in the Gleason scoring system. The Gleason system scores prostatic tumours on a 1–10 scale, where 10 is the most poorly differentiated. The combined Gleason grade describes the appearances of the two most common areas of prostatic malignancy. High-grade PIN, an acronym that coasts off the tongue with greater ease than prostatic intraepithelial neoplasia, has been suggested as a premalignant condition leading to invasive cancer, as CIN leads to invasive cervical cancer. However, the evidence for this is very poor and surgeons should be discouraged from operative procedures in patients with this condition.

If the X-rays show no evidence of metastases, a bone scan should be carried out. Transrectal ultrasound has low specificity for defining malignancy but a high specificity for describing the integrity of the prostatic capsule. In many centres, magnetic resonance is used as an adjunct to this procedure and has a reasonable specificity for describing prostatic staging. A CT scan should be used to define lymph node spread. Transrectal ultrasonography should be combined with needle biopsy. As a standard, six cores are taken in general. Since diagnostic certainty is increased by carrying out more biopsies, 8 or even 12, needle cores are taken in many centres. Where the diagnosis is difficult and

Table 16.1 TNM staging of prostate cancer.

T (primary tumour)	N (nodal status)	M (metastatic status)
T0 No tumour palpable	N0 No nodes	M0 No metastases
T1 Tumour in one lobe of the prostate	N1 Homolateral nodes	M1 Metastases
T2 Tumour involving both prostate lobes	N2 Bilateral nodes	
T3 Tumour infiltrating out of the prostate to involve seminal vesicles	N3 Fixed regional nodes	
T4 Extensive tumour, fixed and infiltrating local structures	N4 Juxtaregional nodes	

PSA levels are high, saturation biopsies are carried out but this procedure, which may involve 20 or more biopsies, may lead to yet further difficulties in defining treatment if a focus of low-grade cancer is found.

Treatment

Treatment of early-stage prostate cancer

The treatment of prostate cancer depends upon clinical stage and is surrounded by controversy. Early-stage small bulk prostate cancer, that is T1 and T2 disease, may be treated by observation, radiotherapy or radical prostatectomy if there is no evidence of spread. The options for treatment depend upon the patient's overall state and preference. Observation involves regular follow-up without treatment. Radiotherapy involves approximately 6 weeks of attendance at hospital for prostatic irradiation, which is given in an attempt to sterilize the tumour. Radiotherapy has morbidity. Acutely, it may be associated with symptoms of cystitis and proctitis; post-treatment it may produce impotence in up to 70% of patients. Radical prostatectomy involves major pelvic surgery, with removal of the prostate and associated lymph glands. Modern anaesthetic techniques and surgical advances have meant that the morbidity is limited, but a degree of incontinence is reported in up to 25% of patients, and a degree of impotence, which is under-reported by surgeons, occurs in up to 90% of patients. It is agreed that morbidity has been reduced by the introduction of nerve-sparing techniques. There is an operative mortality of less than 1%. Surgeons delight in new

toys, and have been allowed to play with the Da Vinci robot; radical prostatectomy carried out by this procedure is said to lead to fewer problems with potency, and certainly less blood loss than with standard open surgery.

The reason the patient can be offered the prospect of choice in determining what therapy he should have for early-stage disease is that observation, radiotherapy and radical surgery have all been shown to offer the patient with good or moderate histology tumours the same overall chance of long-term survival. For younger patients, with poor histology, surgery offers a better survival chance than radiotherapy. The survival advantage is minimal. There has, however, been no randomized comparison of these three options involving significant patient numbers: hence this subject remains a matter for vociferous debate. A recent study of approximately 600 patients randomized to receive either watchful waiting or radiotherapy showed a better outlook for patients treated surgically.

In the early 1990s, investigations were initiated into the value of hormonal therapy given in addition to radiotherapy and surgery. No advantage to such 'neoadjuvant' hormonal therapy has been found in those patients proceeding to radical surgery. A number of randomized studies have shown an advantage to neoadjuvant hormonal therapy in patients receiving radiotherapy. The majority of studies have found a decreased risk of local relapse with hormonal therapy, and two major trials reported improved survival. There is controversy as to the suitable duration of treatment with adjuvant hormonal therapy.

Brachytherapy is a radiotherapy technique where the local intensity of radiation is increased by the

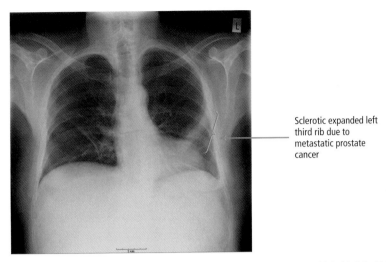

Figure **16.3** The chest X-ray shows a sclerosis and expansion of the anterolateral aspect of left third rib. This appearance was due to metastasis from prostate cancer, although the differential radiological diagnosis would include lymphoma, osteopetrosis and Paget's disease.

Sclerotic expanded left third rib due to metastatic prostate cancer

implantation of radioactive seeds or wires. This technique has been applied to localized prostate cancer. Excellent results have been claimed, but not proven in any randomized trial. Recent publications have shown that the incidence of major side effects of brachytherapy is the same as for conventional radiation, and the efficacy of brachytherapy is no doubt similar to conventional radiation treatment. Brachytherapy has additional side effects to radiotherapy and these include a 12% instance of urethral stricture requiring surgical intervention.

Treatment of locally advanced or metastastic prostate cancer

When patients have locally advanced, that is T3 or T4, prostate cancer or metastatic disease (Figures 16.3 and 16.4), the treatment involves the use of hormonal therapy. Again, this area is one of considerable debate and controversy. Hormonal therapy for this condition was first described in the 1940s, when the disease was found to be dependent upon testosterone. For this reason, the first treatments offered in the 1940s were orchiectomy, that is, removal of the testes, or oestrogen therapy.

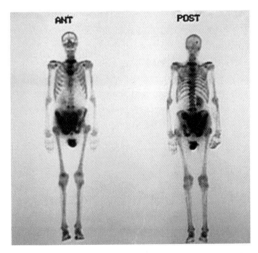

Figure **16.4** Bone scan showing multiple hot spots in the axial skeleton due to bone metastases and a non-functioning left kidney due to long-standing obstruction. The patient had locally advanced and metastatic prostate cancer.

The results of treatment were first analyzed in the 1960s by the Veterans Administration Cooperative Urological Research Group (VACURG). In their studies, the VACURG randomized patients to treatment with oestrogens or placebo, or with orchiectomy or placebo, respectively. The overall

141

survival of patients treated or untreated was the same, but there was an excess mortality rate from cardiovascular deaths in the oestrogen-treated group. The reason for this is that oestrogens cause an increased coaguability of blood and increased blood volumes.

Because orchiectomy is barbaric and oestrogen therapy is associated with morbidity and mortality, medical treatments for this condition have been sought which are not so invasive and have no side effects. The most effective of these new treatments, which has the least morbidity associated with its use, is a group of compounds called the gonadotrophin-releasing hormone agonists. These include leuprorelin acetate, goserelin acetate and buserelin. These are currently given subcutaneously by monthly or three-monthly injection.

Prostate cancer is very responsive to treatment, and 80% of patients improve subjectively. After a period of approximately one year, however, most patients with metastatic cancer on presentation have PSA evidence of relapse. In relapse, treatment is palliative and hinges upon the use of radiotherapy and steroids. Blood transfusion is often necessary. Chemotherapy is increasingly popular in patients with prostate cancer. The reason for this popularity is that patients respond to docetaxel chemotherapy. The median survival in patients starting treatment with docetaxel is 18.7 months, which provides a benefit of three months over conventional therapy using mitoxantrone, a regimen which was introduced in the late 1980s.

Effects of treatment delay

Later analyses of the VACURG study showed that all the patients who were initially given placebos were eventually treated with hormonal therapies by their primary care physicians. As survival of both groups of patients, 'treated' and 'untreated', was the same, the real conclusion of the study is that early, as compared with late, treatment offers the same prospect for survival. This important issue was investigated by the Medical Research Council (MRC) in a randomized prospective trial. The MRC trial was published, and initial analysis showed both an increased risk of disease complica-

tions and a more rapid rate of death in those patients who had delayed treatment. It would appear that this increased risk of complications and of death is confined to patients with metastatic cancer. In a review of the MRC trial in 2002, however, the principal author revised his conclusions and considered it to be uncertain whether or not there is a survival advantage and a reduced complication rate to early treatment.

Prognosis

Prognosis for small bulk localized disease

The outlook for small bulk localized disease depends upon grade. Observation, radiotherapy and surgery all lead to an equivalent survival of 80% at 10 years for patients with well or moderately differentiated tumours. Patients with poorly differentiated, high Gleason grade tumours have a worse outlook with observation and radiotherapy than with surgery. Only 15% of patients survive 10 years, compared with 60–80% undergoing the latter treatment. It is argued that patient selection influences this result, as fitter patients, who will invariably do better than less well patients, are selected for surgery.

Prognosis for metastatic and large bulk localized disease

It has been shown in clinical trials that the addition of an anti-androgen to gonadotrophin-releasing hormone agonist therapy leads to an improvement in survival rate. The median survival for patients with metastatic tumours treated with combination anti-androgen therapy is three years, as opposed to 2.5 years for patients treated with single-agent gonadotrophin-releasing hormone agonist or by orchiectomy. The prospects for survival for a patient with locally advanced disease without metastases are much better. The median survival of this group is 4.5 years. It is not known whether there is an advantage to combination gonadotrophin-releasing hormone agonist and anti-androgen therapy in this patient group.

Screening

There is controversy also regarding the value of screening. Two recent reports, one from the Institute of Cancer Research, and the other from the University of York Health Economics Unit, have published findings similar to each other. Both reports conclude that there is little value to screening because of the poor specificity of the diagnostic tools and the lack of a proven survival advantage to early treatment.

Recently two major trials results were published, one showing a survival advantage, the other, no advantage. Both trials involved many thousands of patients. The European study that showed a survival gain to screening, also demonstrated that one patient's life was 'saved' for every 48 cancers detected.

New treatment

When biopsies from patients with recurrent tumour are examined and compared with biopsies on presentation, it is striking that up to 50% will show androgen receptor mutations. This is in contradiction to the situation in breast cancer, where hormone receptor amplification is the most commonly observed change. Over 700 mutations of the androgen receptor have been described, and these changes are a clue to the probable reason for the response to second-line hormonal therapy. The most commonly used second-line treatment is the withdrawal of anti-androgen therapy. Cessation of treatment with flutamide, for example, given in combination with an LHRH (luteinizing hormone-releasing hormone) agonist will lead to a response in up to 40% of patients. This response is transient and is thought to occur because the mutation has led the tumour to depend upon the anti-androgen as a growth factor. New treatments will thus have as their basis a molecular design that takes advantage of known androgen receptor changes.

Chemotherapy has become more important in the treatment of recurrent disease, following work in the early 1990s that showed good symptom palliation from the use of mitoxantrone chemotherapy given with concurrent steroids. New treatments with drugs such as docetaxel have shown promise and become a standard. Newer taxanes are in development and are effective as second line chemotherapy. Responses have been seen to anti-angiogenesis agents such as thalidomide and to steroids such as calcitriol. Dendritic cell therapy and vaccination approaches are also being trialled.

Recent work has shown major responses to vitamin D given orally to patients in dosages normally used as food supplementation. The reason for response to vitamin D is of great interest, but at present is not known. The oncogene SRC is upregulated in prostatic cancer cell lines and, for this reason, trial work with a new drug, dasatinib, is under current investigation. The synthesis of androgenic steroids takes place most in the adrenal, where hydroxylase enzymes are responsible for the grand passage of cholesterol to androstenedione and 4-hydroxyandrostenedione. Treatments such as with ketoconazole were aimed at blocking this pathway. However, whilst doing so, transiently, ketoconazole also causes significant side effects. Abiraterone, a new steroid hydroxylase inhibitor, has been found to be an effective treatment of prostate cancer in relapse.

As time goes by, we have become more aware of the side effects of hormonal therapy. The use of anti-androgen treatment is associated with osteoporosis, loss of muscle bulk, anaemia and neurological change, which includes both dementia and Parkinsonism. At present, the consensus view is that osteoporosis is best managed with bisphosphonates.

Until recently, men with prostate cancer represented a rather passive but extremely brave group of individuals who accepted their fate. The last two decades have seen significant changes in the way that men deal with their cancers, and prostate cancer has now become, quite rightly, politicized with the cause championed to good effect.

Chapter 17

Testis cancer

Epidemiology and pathogenesis

The treatment of testis cancer represents one of the major and wonderful triumphs of oncology. The application of modern treatments has led to a fall in death rates by 70% over the last 10–15 years, and in 2007 only 58 men died of this condition in the UK compared to over 2000 patients that were diagnosed. The major predisposing factor to the development of testicular cancer is maldescent of the testes. There have been significant advances in the understanding of the molecular biology of adult male germ cell tumours. It is over 15 years since the original identification of the characteristic cytogenetic marker of adult male germ cell tumours: isochromosome 12p. An extra copy of chromosome 12p is present in 85% of all tumours, and in the remaining percentage there are tandem duplications embedded within other chromosomal material. The cyclin D2 gene, which is concerned with the regulation of the cell cycle, is mapped to this area. This suggests that the aberrant expression of cyclin D2 leads to the dysregulation of the normal cell cycle and tumour development. This abnormality is present in both seminoma and teratoma. Testicular tumours also express c-KIT, stem cell factor receptor and platelet-derived growth factor (PDGF) α-receptor gene. Mutations in the KIT gene occur in 8% of all testicular germ cell tumours but are seen in 93% of patients with bilateral disease. These changes in the KIT gene appear to be specific to seminoma. These molecular findings suggest possible therapeutic options.

Presentation

Media campaigns have led to public awareness of testicular cancer as a curable condition and of the importance of early diagnosis. Generally, patients noticing testicular masses present to their GPs and are referred immediately to urology outpatients. There remain, however, a number of alarming instances where GPs have treated patients with testicular tumours for epididymitis rather than referring them on. Patients with teratoma present during the second and third decades of their lives, generally with swelling of the testes and less frequently with pain. Men with seminoma may present in their third to fifth decades. Men with testicular cancer may have gynaecomastia. This is due to the production of steroid hormones by the malignancy, and clearly not to α-fetoprotein (AFP) or human chorionic gonadotrophin (HCG) synthesis.

In urology outpatients, after examination, the patient should proceed to initial staging by routine haematology, biochemistry and measurement of AFP and HCG. A chest X-ray should be requested and an ultrasound examination of the testes ordered. The ultrasound will show features sugges-

Lecture Notes: Oncology, 2nd edition. By M. Bower and J. Waxman. Published 2010 by Blackwell Publishing Ltd.

tive of testicular cancer, such as increased vascularity accompanying a mass. There may be additional features of microlithiasis, suggesting that the tumour has developed from carcinoma *in situ*. Carcinoma *in situ* is a bilateral condition with a 3% subsequent chance of development of a second testicular tumour.

Following these investigations, arrangements should be made for the patient to proceed to orchiectomy. This is performed through a groin rather than a scrotal incision, which would lead to an increased risk of the scrotal spread of testicular cancer, particularly in cases where there are embryonal elements to the tumour. The testis is removed by the surgeon, cut in half, examined and sent for pathological examination (Figure 17.1).

Staging and grading

There are four main types of testicular tumour: seminoma, teratoma, lymphoma and small cell. Teratoma constitutes approximately 75% of all testicular malignancies and appears cystic when examined by the naked eye. Pure seminoma constitutes 20% of tumours and is uniform in appearance. Approximately 5% of all testicular tumours are lymphoma, the appearance of which is generally uniform but with some areas of necrosis. Less than 1% of tumours are of small cell origin. These tumours have no specific macroscopic features.

Microscopically, teratomas constitute a variety of different elements which may include cartilage, muscle, bone and virtually any other tissue. Subtypes of teratoma are described, and they are called undifferentiated, differentiated or choriocarcinoma. Seminoma consists of uniform and large cells with darkly standing nuclei.

Having made a histological diagnosis, treatment is initiated and depends upon the stage to which the tumour has advanced. The following stages are described and determined by CT imaging of the chest, abdomen and pelvis:
- Stage I: tumour confined to testes
- Stage II: tumour spread to abdominal lymph nodes
- Stage III: tumour spread to lymph nodes above the diaphragm

- Stage IV: tumour invading organs other than lymph nodes such as liver or lung.

The disease is further sub-staged according to the size of the metastatic deposits and the number of pulmonary metastases. In the US, retroperitoneal lymph node dissection is undertaken to stage testicular cancer, although this practice is disappearing. In our view, node dissection is not indicated as a routine staging procedure because of the major morbidity of the operation and also because of the side effects, which include retrograde ejaculation. Node dissection for staging purposes is not part of medical practice in the UK, which relies on imaging.

Retrograde ejaculation is the ejaculation of sperm backwards into the bladder rather than forwards into the urethra. This phenomenon does not necessarily mean that the patient is functionally sterile, because sperm can be collected and artificial insemination techniques employed to successfully fertilize the patient's partner. In modern times, such IVF programmes require aspiration of sperm from the testes or testicular biopsy with sperm retrieval if collection of urine post-ejaculation with sperm retrieval is unsuccessful.

Treatment

Treatment of Stage I testicular cancer

The tumour stage of testicular cancer defines its treatment. If the tumour is localized to the testis, two actions are available to the clinician. The first activity for both seminoma and teratoma is observation without further therapy. If this policy is followed in the absence of poor prognosis pathology features, then the likelihood of any further treatment being required is 13% for testicular teratoma and 17% for seminoma. It should be noted that almost all patients who develop progressive disease during the period of observation without treatment are salvageable by chemotherapy.

In the UK, the majority of urologists refer patients with stage I seminoma for radiotherapy, following which the prognosis is excellent, with virtually no chance of relapse. The option of two courses of single-agent carboplatin might also be offered. A randomized trial has shown that

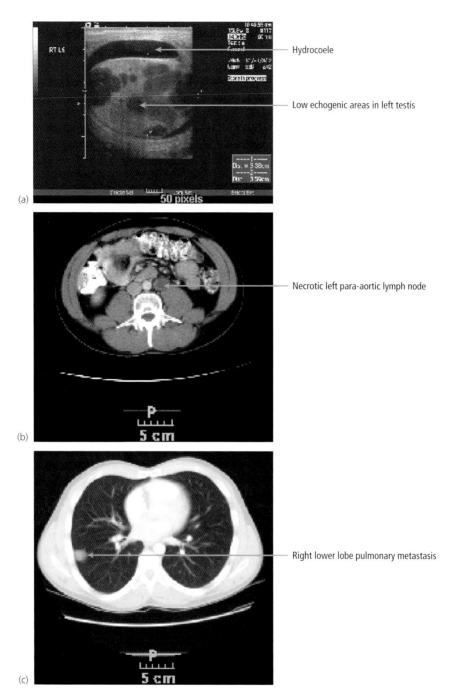

Hydrocoele

Low echogenic areas in left testis

(a)

Necrotic left para-aortic lymph node

(b)

Right lower lobe pulmonary metastasis

(c)

Figure 17.1 Testicular cancer. A 24-year-old Australian bar man presented with a swollen testicle. (a) His ultrasound examination showed an enlarged left testicle with multiple low echogenicity areas and a small hydrocoele. (b) His body CT scan showed an enlarged and necrotic left para-aortic lymph node, and (c) a right lower lobe peripheral lung nodule. His tumour markers were raised (serum AFP = 670 ng/ml; serum HCG = 56 IU/ml). Despite having metastatic disease at presentation, his chances of cure are over 80%.

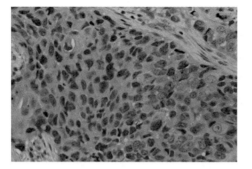

Plate 1.1 Histology of invasive ductal carcinoma of the breast with neoplastic cells invading the breast stroma.

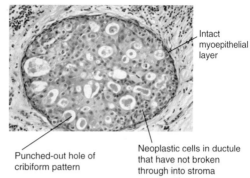

Intact myoepithelial layer

Punched-out hole of cribiform pattern

Neoplastic cells in ductule that have not broken through into stroma

Plate 1.2 Histology of intraductal carcinoma *in situ* of the breast, demonstrating neoplastic cells in a breast ductule with an intact myoepithelial layer.

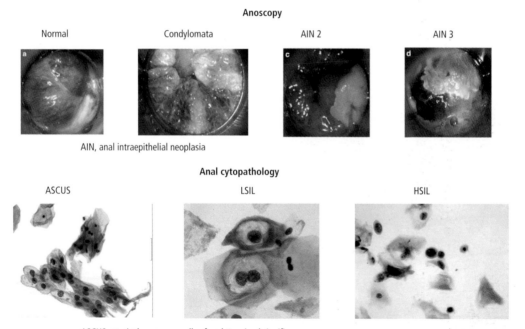

Anoscopy

Normal | Condylomata | AIN 2 | AIN 3

AIN, anal intraepithelial neoplasia

Anal cytopathology

ASCUS | LSIL | HSIL

ASCUS, atypical squamous cells of undetermined significance
LSIL, low-grade squamous intraepithelial lesions
HSIL, high-grade squamous intraepithelial lesions

Plate 1.3 Progression of pre-invasive anal cancer with associated cytopathology changes.

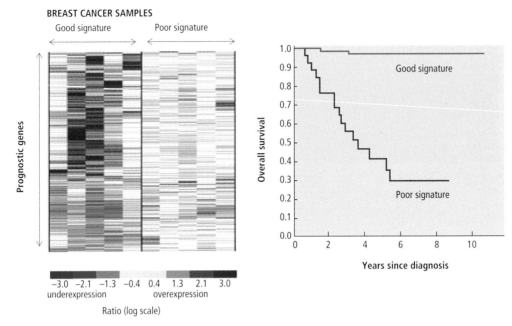

BREAST CANCER SAMPLES

Good signature   Poor signature

Prognostic genes

Overall survival

Years since diagnosis

−3.0 −2.1 −1.3 −0.4 0.4 1.3 2.1 3.0
underexpression   overexpression

Ratio (log scale)

Good signature

Poor signature

Plate 1.4 Gene expression profiles for breast cancer samples differentiate tumours into good- and poor-prognosis signatures that predict survival.

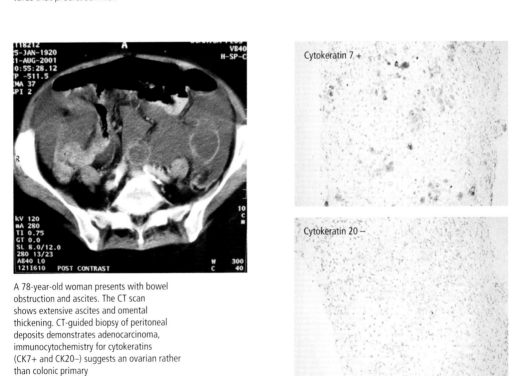

Cytokeratin 7 +

Cytokeratin 20 −

A 78-year-old woman presents with bowel obstruction and ascites. The CT scan shows extensive ascites and omental thickening. CT-guided biopsy of peritoneal deposits demonstrates adenocarcinoma, immunocytochemistry for cytokeratins (CK7+ and CK20−) suggests an ovarian rather than colonic primary

Plate 1.5 Cytokeratin immunohistochemistry in a patient with disseminated peritoneal metastases.

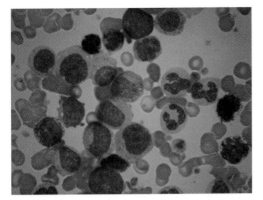

Plate 34.6 Peripheral blood film showing chronic myeloid leukaemia with a spectrum of myeloid cells including eosinophils, basophils, and segmented neutrophils as well as immature myeloid cells.

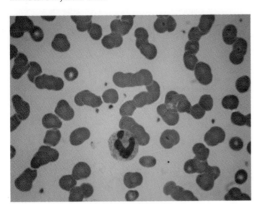

Plate 37.1 Peripheral blood film showing rouleaux formation with erythrocytes stacked up on each other, and a single neutrophil. Rouleaux are found at high levels in the blood of proteins such as fibrinogen or γ-globulin. They are particularly prominent in diseases that cause a very high erythrocyte sedimentation rate (ESR), such as multiple myeloma, cancers, chronic infections (e.g. TB) and connective tissue diseases.

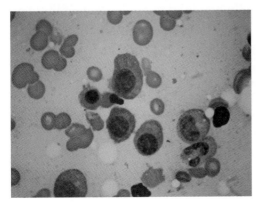

Plate 37.2 Bone marrow aspirate of myeloma showing plasma cells with large eccentric nuclei and basophilic cytoplasm.

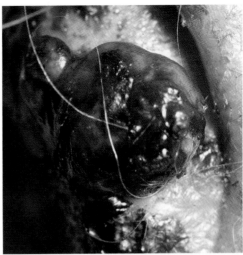

Plate 39.1 A large, raised, bleeding skin lesion on the pinna, a common site for squamous cell cancers of the skin. These tumours are related to UV exposure and may be preceded by actinic or solar keratoses.

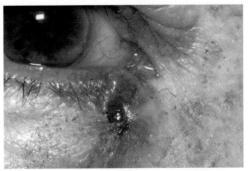

Plate 39.2 A pearly edged, ulcerated lesion characteristic of a basal cell cancer of the skin.

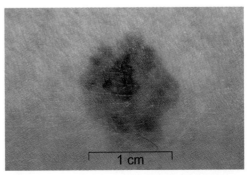

Plate 40.1 Atypical or dysplastic naevi are large naevi (moles) with irregular boarders and varied pigmentation. Atypical naevi are the precursors of melanomas.

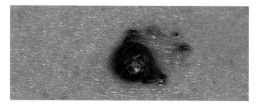

Plate 40.2 A pigmented nodular lesion with an irregular edge and adjacent satellite lesions. This was a nodular melanoma.

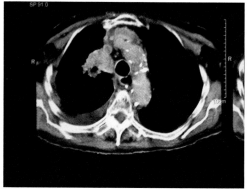

(a)

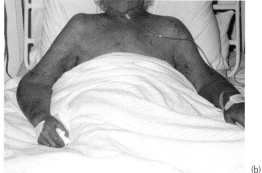

(b)

Plate 46.1 An 80-year-old woman presented with shortness of breath, headaches and swollen arms. (a) The CT scan shows a large right hilar mass that was small cell lung cancer compressing the superior vena cava and collateral circulation. (b) The clinical image also shows dilated veins on the anterior chest wall due to collateral circulation. The flow of blood in these veins will be from above as the blood is bypassing the obstructed superior vena cava to return via the patent inferior vena cava.

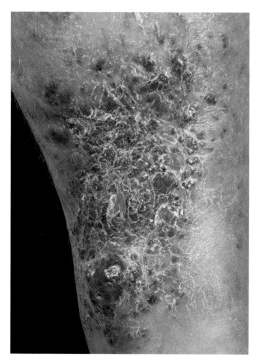

Plate 40.3 Irregular nodular pigmented lesion on the skin at the site of a previously excised malignant melanoma. This represents local recurrence of the melanoma.

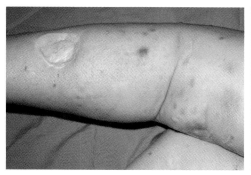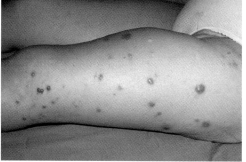

Plate 40.4 Multiple nodular skin metastases arising from a melanoma of the left calf that had been widely excised 2 years earlier, requiring a skin graft.

chemotherapy with carboplatin is as effective as radiation therapy and without the morbidity, two infusions being given at four-weekly intervals in contrast to three weeks of daily radiation therapy. Patients with stage I teratoma are generally referred for adjuvant chemotherapy using BEP (bleomycin, etoposide and cisplatin) chemotherapy: two to four courses are given. Treatment in certain circumstances might be modified, dropping bleomycin from the treatment programme to reduce the risk of lung damage.

Treatment of stage II testicular cancer

For stage IIa seminoma, that is, with a nodal mass of less than 2 cm in diameter as defined by CT scanning, many clinicians in the UK advise treatment with radiotherapy. A consensus of opinion is now emerging, which follows the view that two courses of cytotoxic chemotherapy are equally as effective as radiation treatment in the control of this stage of disease. For stage IIb seminoma, that is, for patients with a disease mass of less than 5 cm, some clinicians, particularly radiotherapists, still treat with radiotherapy, but this is not generally advised in view of the side effects of large field radiotherapy. Chemotherapy should be given using either single-agent or combination therapy.

For all patients with greater than stage IIb disease, whether it is seminoma or teratoma, cytotoxic chemotherapy is given. Before the advent of cytotoxic chemotherapy for teratoma, the disease was invariably fatal. The development of effective chemotherapy programmes has bought about a revolution in the management of patients with malignancy, and now virtually all patients are cured by treatment.

Treatment of advanced testicular cancer

Treatment with cytotoxic agents was originally introduced into medical practice by Li in the early 1960s. As a result, approximately 8% of patients with advanced disease were cured, using a combination of agents that included actinomycin and chlorambucil. In the early 1970s, Samuels treated patients with vinblastine and bleomycin and pro-

duced remissions in approximately 50% of men treated. This treatment was of considerable toxicity because of the large dosages of vinblastine and bleomycin used and the relative lack of support programmes for patients with neutropenic sepsis and thrombocytopenia, which occur as a result of the use of these agents. In 1976, Einhorn introduced the BVP (bleomycin, vinblastine and cisplatinum) programme for the treatment of malignant testicular tumours. This regimen was enormously successful, and 70% of patients with advanced disease were cured. By substituting etoposide for vinblastine, less toxicity resulted with equivalent effect.

Over the last decade, there have been further refinements in the way that treatment has been given. Drug treatment that initially required six courses of five-day treatments has now been reduced to four courses of three-day treatments. Substitution of drugs within this programme to produce the modern three-day JEB (bleomycin, etoposide and carboplatin) programme has meant that toxicity has been limited, and the expectation is that 95% of patients with good-prognosis tumour are cured with this regimen, and 48% of patients with poor-prognosis disease are cured with BEP chemotherapy. Extraordinarily, there has been further change in the collective view with regard to chemotherapy for testicular cancer, and many oncologists have reverted back to the original five-day BEP programme. This is based upon analyses of huge numbers of patients and the realization of the superiority of this standard programme.

Treatment of residual tumour masses

At the end of treatment, one problem may be that of a persistent mass. By this we mean a residual tumour at the site of the original metastatic disease. The approach to this problem is to proceed to surgery. Surgery may be very extensive and involve both thoracotomy and laparotomy. At surgery, the residual mass of tumour is excised as completely as possible, and this may require dacron grafting of major vessels or removal of a kidney in order to take away the tumour completely. This operative procedure is extremely intricate. Histological examination of the excised mass shows that in one-third of cases there is necrotic tumour, in one-third of cases there is differentiated teratoma and in one-third of cases there is undifferentiated cancer. If necrotic tumour is found, no further action is taken. If undifferentiated tumour is found, further chemotherapy is given and 30–40% of patients will be cured by a combination of chemotherapy and surgery. In those patients who have residual differentiated tumour, it is important to remove the residual mass of the disease because over a five-year period approximately 50% of differentiated tumours undergo further malignant change, transforming to undifferentiated malignancy.

Unfortunately, a significant number of patients still have progressive or unresponsive tumours, and for these patients there is still a possibility of cure, which is in the range of 20–40%. Treatment programmes such as VIP (vinblastine, iphosphamide and cisplatin) or high-dose therapy with stem cell rescue are used to treat such patients.

Monitoring treatment

The effects of treatment are very closely monitored by measuring the serum levels of AFP, PLAP and HCG. These are hormones secreted by teratoma and seminoma. If the tumour is being treated effectively, then the levels of these hormones in the blood will decay over a known period: 3–5 days for AFP and approximately 12–36 hours for HCG.

Side effects of treatment

There are specific toxicities that relate to treatment. Cisplatin will cause renal damage, deafness and a peripheral neuropathy, which may manifest as numbness in the fingers or toes or complete loss of motor and sensory function in the limbs. Bleomycin unfortunately causes pulmonary toxicity, that is, an irreversible and progressive loss of lung function, which is fatal in approximately 2% of patients treated (see Figure 3.13). Testicular cancer and the drug regimen that is used generally causes sterility; by this we mean loss of functional spermatogenesis. In 80% of patients, however, there is recovery of spermatogenesis, which generally occurs at 18 months from the completion of treatment.

Prognosis

The treatment of teratoma and seminoma is highly complex and requires patient management in centres of excellence, where the delivery of chemotherapy and the maintenance of patients during neutropenic and thrombocytopenic episodes can be successfully achieved. In the best centres, 95% of patients with good-prognosis tumours are cured, which is without doubt a significant advance in medical science, as young men with this malignant tumour can be returned to an active life within the community after treatment.

Prognostic indices have been described in detail by many authors. One of the more commonly used is described by the International Germ Cell Cancer Collaborative Group. Patients with non-seminoma are classified as having good-prognosis disease with a five-year survival of 92–95%, intermediate-prognosis tumours with a 72–80% five-year survival and poor-prognosis tumours with a 48% five-year survival. Patients with pure seminoma are described as having either good- or intermediate-prognosis disease. The classification into these categories is based on the presence or absence of non-nodal visceral metastases and serum levels of tumour markers. The influence of delay on prognosis is variably reported. Some authors link delay in excess of one year to a good prognosis, although this is described as being associated with a poor prognosis by other authors.

New treatment

Testicular cancer remains an exclusively chemo-sensitive disease even at progression, and for this reason almost every new drug that has been developed for oncology has been applied to this condition. Amongst this new group of chemotherapy agents, the taxanes and gemcitabine have shown promise. Imatinib (Glivec), a c-KIT antagonist, has been applied to the treatment of testicular cancer. There are case reports of activity but no major trial evidence for a response to imatinib.

Chapter 18

Gynaecological cancers

In 1951, George and Margaret Gey and Mary Kubicek developed HeLa, the first human cancer continuous cell line. It proliferates in tissue culture and has been the basis of a great deal of research into cancer biology and drug development. The sample originated from the cervical cancer of a young black woman, Henrietta Lacks of Baltimore. Many thousands of tons of HeLa cells are now found in the incubators and freezers of laboratories around the world. Unfortunately the patient died less than a year after the cell line was established, and her family are said to be shocked by the development and proliferation of the cell line, which was obtained presumably without consent at the time. Gynaecological tumours are not restricted to humans; female Asian elephants and rhinos are particularly susceptible to uterine fibromata.

Gynaecological cancers range from gestational trophoblastic tumours, which are associated with probably the highest survival of any malignant tumour, to ovarian cancers where fewer than a third of women will survive five years. The registration and prognosis data for the commoner tumours are shown in Table 18.1.

Gynaecological cancers include gestational trophoblastic disease, cervical cancer, endometrial cancer and ovarian cancer and will be discussed in more detail in the following four chapters.

Table 18.1 Gynaecological cancer registration data for UK and five-year survival rates.

Tumour	Percentage of female registrations	Rank of female registrations	Lifetime chance of cancer	Change in ASR, 1997–2006	5-year survival
Cervix	2%	12th	1 in 136	−16%	66%
Endometrium	4%	5th	1 in 73	+20%	77%
Ovary	5%	6th	1 in 48	−7%	41%

ASR, age-standardized rate.

Lecture Notes: Oncology, 2nd edition. By M. Bower and J. Waxman. Published 2010 by Blackwell Publishing Ltd.

Chapter 19

Gestational trophoblastic disease

Gestational trophoblastic tumours originate from placental tissues and are among the few human cancers that can be cured, even in the presence of widespread metastasis. The term gestational trophoblastic disease (GTD) covers hydatidiform molar pregnancies, invasive moles, choriocarcinomas and placental site trophoblastic tumours. Half of the women with choriocarcinoma develop GTD after a molar pregnancy; the remainder have previously had non-molar gestations. Since GTD is relatively rare but can be treated with very high cure rates, all patients should be referred to specialist national units.

Epidemiology and pathogenesis

The incidence of GTD varies geographically, with the highest rates reported from Asia, and the risk rises with maternal age and a history of prior molar pregnancy. In the UK, hydatidiform moles account for one in 1000 pregnancies and about 10% of these will progress to persistent trophoblastic disease requiring chemotherapy. Cytogenetic and molecular analysis of hydatidiform moles has provided a clue as to their origin (Figure 19.1). The majority of complete moles have a 46XX karyotype, with both X-chromosomes of paternal origin

(androgenetic). They are believed to originate from fertilization of an empty ovum by a haploid sperm that then underwent duplication. In contrast, partial moles contain both maternal and paternal DNA and are typically triploid 69XXY, presumably as a result of fertilization of a single ovum by two sperm. It is thought that this developmental abnormality affecting uniparental diploid cells (in this case androgenetic, 46XX) is due to genomic imprinting. The expression of some genes is determined by their parental origin – whether the allele was inherited from the mother or father – and this persists through multiple rounds of DNA amplification. This parent-of-origin effect is known as genomic imprinting and only affects a minority of genes. Genomic imprinting is an epigenetic phenomenon that does not rely on changes to the DNA base sequence but rather on methylation of individual bases. One example of imprinting in humans is the insulin-like growth factor 2 (IGF2) gene. Only the paternal copy of IGF2 is expressed in foetal life; the maternal gene is said to be 'imprinted'. The relaxation of this maternal imprinting results in congenital Beckwith–Weidemann syndrome: gigantism, macroglossia, exophthalmos, neonatal hypoglycaemia and predisposition to childhood cancers, including Wilms' tumour, rhabdomyosarcoma and adrenal tumours. Imprinting is also responsible for paired congenital syndromes on chromosome 15q11. This region is differently imprinted in maternal

Lecture Notes: Oncology, 2nd edition. By M. Bower and J. Waxman. Published 2010 by Blackwell Publishing Ltd.

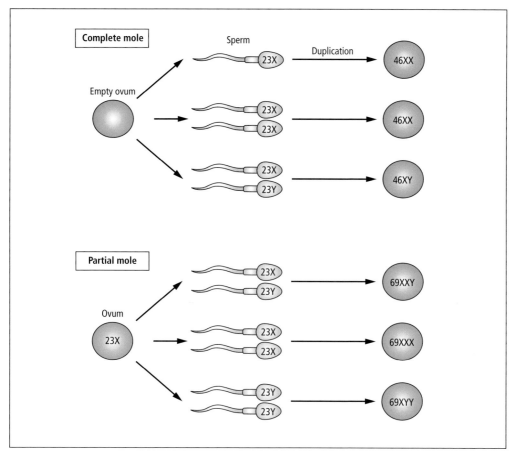

Figure 19.1 Possible chromosomal origin of complete and partial hydatidiform moles.

and paternal chromosomes, and both imprintings are needed for normal development. In a normal individual, the maternal allele is methylated, while the paternal allele is unmethylated. Some individuals fail to inherit a properly imprinted 15q11 from one parent, either due to deletion of the 15q11 region from that parent's chromosome 15 or rarely due to uniparental disomy (in which both copies have been inherited from the one parent). If neither copy of 15q11 has paternal imprinting, the result is Prader–Willi syndrome (characterized by hypotonia, obesity and hypogonadism). If neither copy has maternal imprinting, the result is the Angelman syndrome (characterized by epilepsy, tremors and a perpetually smiling facial expression).

Presentation

Women with trophoblastic disease usually present with antepartum haemorrhage, passing grape-like particles during early pregnancy, anaemia and hyperemesis. Hyperthyroidism may occur because human chorionic gonadotrophin (HCG) acts as a weak thyroid-stimulating hormone (TSH) receptor agonist, due to homology between β-subunits of HCG and TSH, which has been called molecular mimicry. Metastases are typically haemorrhagic. The most frequent sites are the lungs and brain, where they mimic pulmonary thromboembolic disease and subarachnoid haemorrhage. It is therefore always worthwhile performing a pregnancy test in women with these presentations, since normal serum or urine HCG levels exclude this diagnosis. Choriocarcinoma, although rare, is an important diagnosis, as the tumour is exquisitely sensitive to chemotherapy and over 95% of women with this diagnosis can be cured. The definitive diagnostic investigations are a quantitative serum HCG assay and pelvic ultrasonography with colour Doppler flow measurement. Most cases of choriocarcinoma follow a hydatidiform molar pregnancy, although it may also occur after either spontaneous abortion or normal-term pregnancy. If choriocarcinoma follows a molar pregnancy, molecular analysis reveals that the tumour DNA is entirely androgenetic, being derived from the father, with the loss of all maternal alleles. In contrast, post-term choriocarcinoma has a biparental genotype. Nonetheless, all cases of choriocarcinoma include paternal DNA sequences that are absent from the patient's genome and may be used to confirm the diagnosis genetically if necessary.

Treatment

Gestational trophoblastic disease was the first cancer to be cured by chemotherapy alone in the early 1960s. A scoring scheme has been devised that determines the risk of developing drug resistance to methotrexate, and women at low risk can be successfully treated with single-agent methotrexate, with very high success rates and very few long-term sequelae. Women at higher risk of resistance require combination chemotherapy schedules, which, although still highly successful, run a small risk of second malignancy. Serum HCG acts as the ideal tumour marker in this disease. HCG can be used to screen women following a molar pregnancy, to identify persistent trophoblastic disease that requires chemotherapy. Serum HCG can be used as a diagnostic investigation and in some circumstances obviates the need for a tissue diagnosis. Serum HCG levels form part of the prognostic scoring index and can be used to follow treatment: to determine the effectiveness of treatment and to detect remission or chemoresistance. Finally, HCG can be used in follow-up to identify relapse.

Prognosis

The prognosis of gestational trophoblastic tumours is excellent, with the rare exceptions of placental site histological subtype. The cure rates exceed 95%, and much of the current focus of clinical research is aimed at minimizing the long-term side effects of any treatment rather than attempts to increase the cure rates.

Chapter 20

Cervical cancer

Epidemiology and pathogenesis

Cancer of the cervix is thought to affect over one-third of a million women worldwide and represents 10% of all female cancers. Eighty percent of all cases of cervical cancer occur in the developing world. The incidence in the UK, as in many developed countries, is decreasing. In 2007, 2800 women were diagnosed and 941 women died of cervical cancer in the UK. In the UK, cervical cancer is the seventh most common of all female cancers, representing 2.5% of all cancer cases.

Invasive cervical cancer is believed to be the final stage in a continuum that starts with cervical infection by high-risk genotypes of human papillomavirus (HPV) and progresses via cervical intraepithelial neoplasia (CIN) to invasive cancer. CIN is a cytological diagnosis and is divided into three grades (CIN1–3). The histological equivalent of CIN is the squamous intraepithelial lesion (SIL), which is divided into low-grade SIL (LGSIL) that is similar to CIN1, and high-grade SIL (HGSIL) analogous to CIN2 and CIN3.

The decline in incidence of cervical cancer is associated with the development of the screening programmes, which began in 1964. Screening is based upon cervical smear assessment, and the current recommendation is for three-yearly screening. Four and a half million women are screened annually in the UK, and there has been a decline of 40% in the age-specific incidence over the last 20 years. Mortality has also decreased, falling from 11.2 deaths per 100000 women in 1950 to 2.4 in 2007. Screening is currently a subjective process, which, although well regulated, may be subject to human error. The accuracy of screening is likely to improve with the integration of molecular biological approaches to the process such as screening for the HPV genome.

Cervical cancer is associated with smoking, promiscuity, low socioeconomic status, the use of oral contraceptives, genital warts, herpes simplex virus 2 infection and, most particularly, infection with HPV 16 and 18. The average age of women with cervical cancer ranges from 35 to 44 years.

Presentation

Women with cervical cancer may present to their doctors with inter-menstrual bleeding, post-coital bleeding or painful intercourse. There may frequently be a vaginal discharge that can be bloody or offensive or symptoms suggestive of a urinary infection such as urinary frequency or urgency. When the cancer has spread, common symptoms include back pain due to enlarged abdominal lymph nodes or referred pain in the legs due to involvement of the nerve plexuses of the pelvis. These symptoms may be accompanied by loss of

Lecture Notes: Oncology, 2nd edition. By M. Bower and J. Waxman. Published 2010 by Blackwell Publishing Ltd.

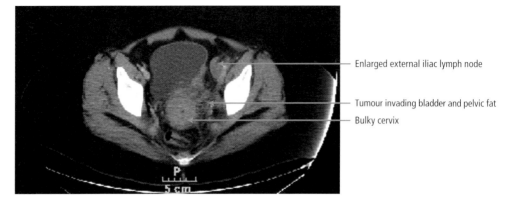

Enlarged external iliac lymph node

Tumour invading bladder and pelvic fat

Bulky cervix

Figure 20.1 Cervical cancer with extensive, locally infiltrating tumour. This CT scan of a 65-year-old woman who had never had a cervical smear shows a bulky cervix with loss of the normal fat plane that separates it from the bladder. There is extension of the invasive cervical cancer into the posterolateral bladder wall anteriorly and into the pelvic fat laterally. There is also an enlarged left external iliac lymph node. The staging was therefore T4N1M0 (IVA).

weight. The examination should include an assessment of the patient's general state of health together with palpation of the abdomen and a vaginal assessment. This may confirm the presence of a discharge and reveal a cervical mass (Figure 20.1).

Outpatient diagnosis

The GP should refer the patient to a gynaecologist who will repeat the examination, take smears from the cervix for cytological examination and then organize admission for examination under anaesthesia and cervical biopsy. Colposcopy should be performed as an outpatient procedure prior to admission. This technique allows direct visualization of the cervix with properly directed biopsies. After these assessments have been performed and a histological diagnosis has been obtained, staging investigations should be organized. These should include a full blood count, profile, chest X-ray and a CT or magnetic resonance scan of the abdomen and pelvis.

Staging and grading

Carcinoma of the cervix is staged as a result of these findings as follows:
- Stage 0: carcinoma *in situ*. Intraepithelial carcinoma grades 1–3

- Stage 1A: microscopic disease confined to the cervix
- Stage 1B: disease confined to the cervix and greater than stage 1A
- Stage 2A: carcinoma extending beyond the cervix without parametrial involvement
- Stage 2B: parametrial involvement
- Stage 3A: extension to the pelvic side wall
- Stage 3B: extension to the pelvic wall with hydronephrosis or a non-functioning kidney
- Stage 4A: extension beyond the true pelvis to adjacent organs
- Stage 4B: spread to distant organs.

Sixty-six percent of cervical cancers are squamous cell tumours. These are graded as G1, G2 or G3 tumours, according to their microscopic appearance: G1 tumours are well differentiated, G2 tumours moderately and G3 tumours poorly differentiated. Fifteen percent are adenocarcinomas, and these are also graded G1–3. Other rarer tumours include small cell cancers and lymphomas. Carcinomas *in situ* are graded I–III and abbreviated to CIN or CGIN, depending on whether squamous or adenocarcinoma cells are present.

Treatment

The treatment of cervical cancer depends upon the stage of disease. Stage 0 carcinoma of the cervix should be treated by cone biopsy or by surgical excision. Stage 1A disease can sometimes be managed by cone biopsy or local excision but usually by hysterectomy. Stage 1B and 2A cervical cancer is usually treated by either radical hysterectomy with pelvic lymphadenectomy or by pelvic irradiation. Both methods are equally effective in the long-term control of the disease. Stage 2B and 3 carcinoma of the cervix should be treated by pelvic radiotherapy and stage 4 carcinoma with chemotherapy.

Patients treated with pelvic radiotherapy with curative intent are frequently prescribed additional concurrent adjuvant chemotherapy. Typically, patients will be treated with weekly courses of single-agent cisplatin. Chemoradiation has been subjected to a number of randomized trials, and it has been concluded that concomitant chemoradiation appears to improve overall survival and progression-free survival in locally advanced cervical cancer. Progressive or metastatic cervical carcinoma is treated with combination chemotherapy usually using a PMB regimen that contains cisplatin, methotrexate and bleomycin.

Carcinoma *in situ*

As a result of treatment, virtually 100% of patients with CIN disease are cured. Approximately 0.05–0.3% of treated women subsequently develop invasive carcinoma. If CIN is left untreated, then over a 30-year follow-up period, 10–40% of patients will develop invasive cancer. The evidence for this is based on data from a single study carried out in New Zealand of untreated patients with CIN, by a clinician who apparently was convinced that CIN did not progress.

Prognosis

Approximately 5% of patients treated for stage 1A carcinoma of the cervix will progress to develop advanced disease. 65 to 85% of all patients with stage 1B and 2A carcinoma of the cervix survive five years after treatment by a radical hysterectomy or radiation. The chance for a cure is smaller in stage 2B disease, and the expectation is that approximately 50–65% survive with radiotherapy

alone. About 40–60% of patients with stage 3A disease, and 25–45% of patients with stage 3B disease, survive five years and are treated with radiotherapy and frequently with chemotherapy.

These statistics are relevant to patients with squamous cancers or adenocarcinomas. Variant histologies, such as small cell carcinomas, are associated with a poor prognosis, with the expectation that, even at an early stage, survival is less than 5% at 5 years.

Patients with stage 4 cervical cancer do very poorly. In this situation, it is very unlikely that a cure will be achieved. Chemotherapy is the treatment of first choice. A number of agents have activity in the order of 15% and their combination is accompanied by some synergy of effect. The most commonly applied treatment programme involves the combination of cisplatin, methotrexate and bleomycin. About 30–40% of patients will respond to treatment, but durable cures are rare. Chemotherapy is associated with toxicity, and this includes nausea and vomiting, hair loss, infections and kidney failure. Because of the toxicities of treatment, an alternative approach is to palliate symptoms with pain killers alone.

Terminal care

In the terminal phases of illness, patients with cervical cancer may have a number of problems that prove difficult to manage. These include fistulae from the vagina to bladder and from the rectum to vagina or bladder, as a result of local progression of the tumour. Obstruction of kidney function may occur as a result of blockage of the ureters, either by enlarged lymph nodes or by tumour from the cervix growing within the pelvis, blocking the ureters. These situations can be treated surgically, in which case a colostomy or ileostomy may be formed, relieving bowel or ureteric obstruction, or radiologically by the passage of a stent to reverse obstructive damage to the kidneys.

New treatment

We hope that with the successful introduction of HPV vaccination and the institution of public health measures to eliminate smoking, there will be no need for treatment of cervical cancer in the future. In the developing world this utopian view may be a little optimistic. A number of vaccines have become available for the prevention of cervical cancer. It is estimated that there will be a significant reduction in cervical cancer rates, but only when 90% of all girls aged 11–12 years have been vaccinated for many years. New quadrivalent vaccines given to women who are seropositive for HPV lead to major increases in antibodies directed against HPV 16 or 18, and it may be that this initiative prevents the development of invasive cervical cancer in HPV seropositive patients.

Chapter 21

Endometrial cancer

Epidemiology and pathogenesis

The key to endometrial function lies in the effects of oestrogen and progesterone on the endometrium, enabling it to progress through the normal menstrual cycle and to prepare for embryo implantation. Oestrogen stimulates proliferation in the glands and stroma. Progesterone inhibits mitotic activity and stimulates secretion in the glands and decidualization of the stroma, where the cells acquire more cytoplasm. It is therefore perhaps not surprising that unopposed oestrogens will promote continuous mitotic activity, leading to cancers. Endometrial cancer is associated with elevated endogenous levels of free oestrogens due to falls in sex hormone-binding globulin or to increased aromatization and sulphation of androgens (androstenedione to oestrone). Thus, endometrial cancer is ten times more common in obese women due to peripheral conversion of androstenedione to oestrone by extraglandular aromatization in adipose tissue. Exogenous oestrogens also increase the risk of endometrial cancer. The use of unopposed oestrogens carries a 4–8-fold relative risk, especially in hormone replacement therapy, which is abrogated almost completely by combining progesterone with oestrogen. A great

deal of attention has been paid to the induction of endometrial cancer by tamoxifen and has led to the development of new selective oestrogen receptor modulators (SERMs), including raloxifene. Although the benefit of tamoxifen therapy for breast cancer outweighs the potential increase in endometrial cancer, the relative risk is six to seven-fold. Screening for endometrial cancer in women with breast cancer taking tamoxifen has no proven benefit, but abnormal bleeding should prompt rapid investigation. Endometrial cancer is a feature of hereditary Lynch type II non-polyposis colon cancer.

Endometrial cancer is the fifth most common cancer in women in England and Wales (see Table 18.1). It rarely develops before the menopause, and, since it causes abnormal vaginal bleeding, it can usually be diagnosed at an early stage.

Presentation

These tumours present in postmenopausal women as uterine bleeding. Postmenopausal bleeding is always abnormal and requires prompt investigation. Hysteroscopy, which allows visual inspection of the uterine lining, is often used for diagnosis and can detect abnormalities in 95–100% of cases. The probability of endometrial cancer among women with postmenopausal bleeding who do not use hormone replacement therapy (HRT) is 10%. If

Lecture Notes: Oncology, 2nd edition. By M. Bower and J. Waxman. Published 2010 by Blackwell Publishing Ltd.

the transvaginal ultrasound scan is normal, this probability falls to 1%, so ultrasound allows the majority of women to be quickly reassured. Outpatient endometrial biopsy methods are now as accurate as dilatation and curettage (D&C), which requires a general anaesthetic.

Treatment and prognosis

The optimum treatment for endometrial cancer depends on the stage and grade of the disease and on the risk of tumour in lymph nodes. When the cancer is confined to the inner third of the myometrium, the lymph nodes are likely to be clear and total hysterectomy is usually sufficient as treatment. This applies to about 90% of women with endometrial cancer, and their 5-year survival exceeds 70%. In women with tumour that extends beyond the inner half of the myometrium or with regional lymph node involvement, adjuvant pelvic radiotherapy is widely used. This has been shown to reduce the rate of local recurrence but may have long-term sequelae, including lymphoedema.

It would appear that endometrial cancer can be divided into two different classes of disease, with contrasting outlook. One group of endometrial cancer patients have tumours that are strongly hormone receptor positive and have an excellent prognosis, whilst a second variant develops in the elderly, has atypical histology, is poorly responsive to hormonal therapy and has a poor outlook. Endometrial cancer of typical histology expresses receptors for oestrogen, progesterone and gonadotrophin-releasing hormone. The expression of these receptors leads to opportunities for hormonal treatment.

Patients with endometrial cancer do respond to chemotherapy and the current standard is for the use of combination therapy with carboplatin and paclitaxel, and this is of particular use in the atypical histology patient. Nevertheless, hormonal therapy is of use in the treatment of endometrial carcinoma, and excellent palliation is seen with treatments such as progestogens.

New treatment

There appears to be little benefit from the use of new chemotherapy agents for patients with recurrent disease who have previously received chemotherapy. Response rates to investigational drugs, such as the exotically named ixabepilone, are in the order of 10%. In the situation of recurrent disease, chemotherapy should only be administered with palliative intent. As in so many tumour groups, there is interest in the possibility of an effect of tyrosine kinase inhibitors. Uterine carcinomas stain positively for epidermal growth factor receptor in up to 60% of cases, suggesting that this receptor could be targeted for treatment. The tumour suppressor gene, PTEN, and the oncogene, PIK3CA, are frequently mutated in endometrial carcinoma, suggesting again a target for therapy. The steroid sulphatase enzyme is involved in the hydrolysis of oestrone sulphate and dehydroepiandrosterone sulphate to oestrone and dehydroepiandrosterone, and this is an important step in the formation of oestrodial. Inhibitors of the steroid sulphatase enzyme have been developed and shown to be of value in breast cancer. It is likely that these inhibitors would also have potential activity in endometrial cancer.

Chapter 22

Ovarian cancer

Epidemiology and pathogenesis

Carcinoma of the ovary is a common tumour affecting nearly 6600 women annually and leading to the death of 4300 women each year in the UK. Ovarian cancer is the fourth most frequent cause of cancer death in women. The average age at which the disease occurs is approximately 65 years. By far the most common pathological subtype of ovarian cancer is epithelial, and this chapter concentrates virtually exclusively upon ovarian epithelial malignancy. There is a familial association between breast and ovarian cancer. This relates to germline mutations in the BRCA1 and BRCA2 genes, which are associated with a risk approaching 60% of developing ovarian cancer. In an analysis of benign, borderline and malignant ovarian cancers, somatic loss of heterozygosity for BRCA1 was demonstrated in none of the benign, in 15% of the borderline and in 66% of the malignant cancers. There is controversy as to other associated risk factors of the development of ovarian cancer. For example, long-term oestrogen replacement therapy may be associated with the development of these tumours, and in one prospective study of over 31 000 postmenopausal women, the increased risk of the development of ovarian cancer was 1.7-fold. As in many other tumours HER-2 overexpression is significantly associated with poorer survival pros-

pects. HER-2 expression occurs in a minority of tumours; that is, in approximately 20% of patients.

Because ovarian cancer patients generally present with late-stage tumours, attempts have been made to reduce this risk by population screening. One of the largest published studies involved the prospective screening of nearly 4000 women by annual ultrasound examination and measurement of the serum tumour marker CA-125. This led to the identification of approximately 350 women with abnormalities, and 330 of these proceeded to laparotomy. In this group, there were 30 patients with ovarian tumours, the majority of which were at an advanced stage; so it seems that the value of screening using current technologies is low. Future screening programmes may benefit from a more refined approach. One technique involves the use of surface-enhanced laser absorption and ionization protein mass spectra. This rather complicated terminology describes the simple process of the separation of proteomic spectra from sera by electrophoresis. A number of protein patterns were identified in women with ovarian cancer, leading to a specificity of almost 90% in the identification of ovarian cancer. This would seem to be of interest in the development of more accurate screening technologies, particularly if the protein identities could be targeted using a rapid diagnostic test. This approach, of course, assumes that ovarian cancer progresses by an orderly process according to early and late stage. This is by no means clear, however, and there is genetic evidence that early- and late-

Lecture Notes: Oncology, 2nd edition. By M. Bower and J. Waxman. Published 2010 by Blackwell Publishing Ltd.

Omental cake of metastatic ovarian cancer

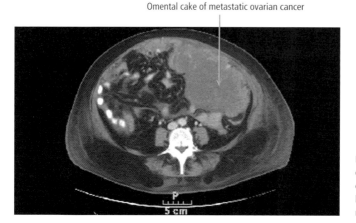

Figure 22.1 CT scan showing an omental cake of metastatic ovarian cancer deposits anteriorly with a large lobulated mass that extends from the midline to the left flank.

stage ovarian cancers may be different diseases that do not progress from one to the other.

Presentation

Patients with ovarian cancer usually present to their GPs with non-specific abdominal symptoms such as abdominal discomfort and swelling. There may be associated urinary frequency, alteration of bowel habit, tenesmus, colicky abdominal pain or postmenopausal bleeding. Patients with disseminated disease may have loss of appetite and weight. Early repletion is another common finding in the history. A patient with these symptoms should be examined by her GP, and if there is abdominal swelling or a pelvic mass, the patient should be referred on to a specialist gynaecologist for his or her views as to the patient's management. It is unfortunately the nature of ovarian cancer to present late, and almost 70% of patients have advanced disease at diagnosis. Patients with early-stage, localized tumours are often diagnosed as a result of the investigation of another medical condition.

The specialist should see the patient in outpatients and take a full clinical history and examine the patient. The examination should include a pelvic assessment. If the patient is thought clinically to have ovarian cancer, the investigations organized should include a full blood count, routine biochemistry, chest X-ray, a pelvic ultrasound and an abdominal and pelvic CT scan,

Lobulated heterogeneous ovarian cancer mass extending from the pelvis

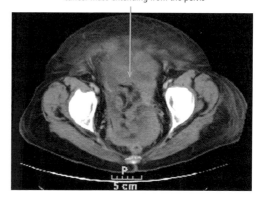

Figure 22.2 Ovarian cancer: pelvic mass. The CT scan shows a huge, lobulated, heterogenous pelvic mass that extends anteriorly. This mass was due to epithelial ovarian cancer.

together with measurement of serum levels of CA-125 (Figures 22.1–22.3 and see Plate 22.1). Ovarian cancer secretes CA-125, which is a glycoprotein. Approximately 80% of patients with advanced ovarian cancer have elevated CA-125 levels. Raised CA-125 levels may also occur in patients with almost any gynaecological, pancreatic, breast, colon, lung or hepatocellular tumour. CA-125 levels are elevated in a number of benign conditions including endometriosis, pancreatitis, pelvic inflammatory disease and peritonitis. Changing levels may be used to monitor treatment. If the tumour is operable, the patient should then be booked for a laparotomy. Surgery should be under-

Extensive mass of para-aortic lymph nodes

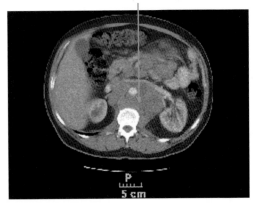

Figure 22.3 Lymph node metastases from ovarian cancer.

taken in specialist centres by a surgical gynaecological oncologist. At operation, the abdominal contents are examined and, where possible, tumour debulking should be undertaken. This should include removal of the omentum, ovaries, fallopian tubes and uterus, with excision of all visible peritoneal deposits. The aim of surgery is to remove as much tumour as possible, optimally reducing the maximum diameter of any tumour deposit to 1 cm or less.

Staging and grading

Ninety-five percent of ovarian cancers are epithelial tumours. The classification of tumours is as in Table 22.1.

An attempt should be made to stage the patient's tumour. The staging used is the FIGO classification, which is as follows:
- Stage 1: growth limited to the ovaries
- Stage 1A: one ovary, no malignant ascites
- Stage 1B: both ovaries, no malignant ascites
- Stage 1C: tumour on ovarian surface or capsular rupture or ascites positive for malignant cell
- Stage 2: growth involving one or both ovaries with pelvic extension
- Stage 3: growth involving one or both ovaries with peritoneal implants or superficial liver metastases or abdominopelvic lymph node involvement
- Stage 4: tumour metastazing to liver parenchyma, pleura or other visceral metastatic sites.

Table 22.1 Pathological classification of ovarian tumours.

A. Epithelial	Serous
	Mucinous
	Endometrioid
	Clear cell
	Brenner
	Mixed
	Undifferentiated
	Unclassified
B. Sex cord/stromal	Granulosa
	Androblastoma
	Gynandroblastoma
	Unclassified
C. Lipid cell	
D. Gonadoblastoma	
E. Soft tissue	
F. Germ cell	Dysgerminoma
	Endodermal sinus
	Embryonal
	Polyembryonal
	Teratoma
	Mixed
G. Unclassifiable	
H. Metastatic	

Treatment

Treatment is defined by the FIGO staging system. If the tumour is confined to one ovary, the gynaecological oncologist may choose to observe the patient after definitive surgery. For stage 1A and 1B ovarian cancer, patients derive no benefit from adjuvant chemotherapy, and studies suggest that all patients with more advanced stages can be offered chemotherapy with benefit. Most specialists would agree that stage 1A or 1B well differentiated tumours can be observed, but adjuvant chemotherapy is increasingly offered to most patients with grade 2 and upwards disease irrespective of stage, and stage 1C and upwards irrespective of grade. Patients with early-stage ovarian cancer are usually offered single-agent carboplatin as adjuvant chemotherapy. Ovarian cancer is chemosensitive, and there is a long history of the use of chemical agents in the treatment of this condition. The discovery of responsiveness to single-agent treatments led to the use of combination chemotherapy programmes. Intensive treatment using multiple drug regimens was advocated throughout the 1970s and early 1980s.

For patients with advanced ovarian cancer it was thought during the early 1990s that single-agent therapy carboplatin was just as effective as combination treatments in terms of overall survival, although it was thought that there might be a minor advantage in terms of initial response rates and response duration to combination programmes. In the late 1990s, fashions changed again and treatment involved the use of combination therapy. There was evidence from randomized studies that combination therapy with cisplatin and paclitaxel had the highest response rates and in two high-profile studies showed superiority over another platinum-based regimen in terms of disease-free result and overall survival. In this century, treatment recommendations have come full cycle, and in the results of the ICON 3 study, a large trial conducted in the UK and Italy, single-agent carboplatin was not shown to be inferior to carboplatin and paclitaxel together. Ovarian cancer is, however, a highly heterogenous condition of many entities, and current advice from the National Institute for Health and Clinical Excellence (NICE) is that the patient and oncologist should discuss whether better benefit might be obtained from single-agent carboplatin or carboplatin and paclitaxel on a case-by-case basis.

Non-epithelial ovarian cancer is treated initially, where possible, by surgery. The procedures may range from oophorectomy to extensive tumour debulking. In relapse, or where a patient has presented with gross metastatic disease, treatment may involve similar chemotherapy programmes to those used for testicular cancer. Occasional responses are seen to hormonal therapy, using luteinizing hormone-releasing hormone (LHRH) agonists for those patients with ovarian malignancies secreting sex steroids.

Prognosis

Localized ovarian cancer constitutes 24% of all presenting patients. Patients with stage 1A and 1B ovarian cancer have an excellent outlook, with a 95% chance of survival. The survival of patients with stage 1C disease with ovarian cyst rupture is variably reported and depends on tumour grade. In one series, just 63% of patients survived five years. Approximately 60–80% of patients with advanced ovarian cancer respond to suitable chemotherapy. The median survival for this group of patients is 2.5 years, with less than 30% of patients surviving for five years.

New treatment

At present the main 'new' treatment for ovarian cancer consists of new lines of chemotherapy. Agents such as pemetrexed, gemcitabine, topotecan, oxaliplatin and ixabepilone have been shown to be effective. Chemotherapy resistance is one of the major features of patients with end-stage ovarian cancer, and this may be due to clonal evolution with gains of chromosomal material on the chromosomes 1 and 17 and losses at chromosome 3.

However, the explosion of targeted biotherapies informed by the results of the Human Genome Project is beginning to find its way into ovarian cancer clinical trials. The main targets under consideration currently are the epidermal growth factor (EGF) receptor's tyrosine kinase intracellular domain and its extracellular ligand-binding component, the vascular endothelial growth factor (VEGF) and its receptor, and the IGF/PI3 kinase pathway. Treatments are being developed from an understanding of platinum resistance, which may take its origin from BRCA1 mutant states and MSH4 suppressed states, which may respectively mediate platinum sensitivity and resistance.

Other targets for the modern therapy of ovarian cancer include small molecular weight inhibitors ('nibs') and monoclonal antibodies ('mabs'), and treatment with these agents has in some senses undergone a renaissance. The early antibody studies, with radioisotope-labelled antibodies directed against the human milk fat globulin given intraperitoneally as an adjuvant to systemic chemotherapy, produced some exciting, but non-reproducible, survival data. The development of new antibodies that are relatively specific to ovarian cancer is now offering real promise.

Chapter 23

Head and neck cancers

To the oncologist, the head and neck comprises six regions: the nasopharynx (the area behind the nose and pharynx), the oral cavity (including the lips, floor of the mouth, tongue, cheeks, gums and hard palate), the oropharynx (the base of the tongue, the tonsillar region, the soft palate and pharyngeal walls), the hypopharynx (the lower throat), the larynx (including the vocal cords and both supraglottis and subglottis) and the nasal cavity (the ethmoid and maxillary sinuses and the parotid, submandibular and minor salivary glands) (Figure 23.1). Although lymphomas, sarcomas, melanomas and other tumours may affect these regions, the term 'head and neck cancers' generally refer to squamous tumours, which make up 90% of cancers at these sites. Cancers of the nasopharynx include not only squamous cancers but also non-keratinizing transitional cell cancers and undifferentiated lymphoepitheliomas. The latter are the most common, and, unlike most other head and neck cancers, they frequently spread to distant sites. Tumours of the salivary glands are the most heterogeneous group of tumours of any tissue in the body, with almost 40 histological types of salivary gland tumours. Salivary gland tumours are more often benign than malignant. Sigmund Freud succumbed to cancer of the head and neck in 1939, attributed to smoking.

Epidemiology and pathogenesis

Head and neck cancers comprise 5% of all cancers in the UK and account for 2.5% of cancer deaths. They are twice as common in men as women and generally occur in those over 50 years old. The sites in order of frequency are: the larynx, oral cavity, pharynx and salivary glands. Over 90% are squamous carcinomas. Cancer of the head and neck is often preventable, and, if diagnosed early, is usually curable. Patients, however, often have advanced disease at the time of diagnosis. This is incurable or requires aggressive treatment, which leaves them functionally disabled. The optimum management of these tumours requires a multidisciplinary approach, including oncologists, otorhinolaryngologists, oromaxillofacial surgeons and plastic surgeons, along with clinical nurse specialists, speech and language therapists, dieticians and prosthetics technicians.

The incidence of head and neck cancers varies geographically, as does the most common anatomical site of these cancers. Smoking, high alcohol intake and poor oral hygiene are well-established risk factors for the development of head and neck tumours. In addition, Epstein–Barr virus is implicated in the aetiology of nasopharyngeal carcinoma in southern China, betel nut chewing in oral cancer in Asia, and wood dust inhalation by furniture makers, who may contract nasal cavity adenocarcinomas. In the UK, the incidence and mortality are greater in deprived populations, most notably for carcinoma of the tongue.

Lecture Notes: Oncology, 2nd edition. By M. Bower and J. Waxman. Published 2010 by Blackwell Publishing Ltd.

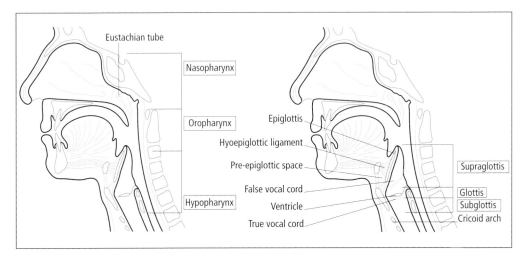

Figure 23.1 The head and neck.

Primary prevention by smoking cessation and alcohol abstention are the most effective methods of reducing the risk of head and neck cancers. Increasing awareness of head and neck cancers may encourage earlier referral and diagnosis at a stage when the cancer is still curable. In this respect, dentists play an important role in examining the oral mucosa. Retinoids may reduce the risk of both recurrence and second primary tumours in patients following primary therapy. Moreover, they may reduce malignant transformation in precancerous conditions such as leukoplakia.

Students who are concerned about biodiversity or just simply fans of the Looney Tunes cartoon character Taz may be concerned to learn that the carnivorous marsupial the Tasmanian devil has become an endangered species because of a head and neck tumour that threatens the survival of the whole species. Devil facial tumour disease is a parasitic tumour allograft transmitted between individual devils. The tumours are all derived from the same original cells. Transmissible cancer is extremely rare. The only other well-described example is canine transmissible venereal tumour in dogs, where again it is the actual cancer cells themselves that are spread from animal to animal rather than transmission of an infection that causes the cancer. Occasional similar cancer transmission has been described in humans. For

example, organ transplant recipients very rarely develop cancers that are shown genetically to derive from the donor. Transplacental transmission of malignancy has also been described with spread of melanoma from mother to child.

Clinical presentation

Most head and neck tumours present as malignant ulcers with raised indurated edges on a surface mucosa. Oral tumours present as non-healing ulcers with ipsilateral otalgia. Oropharyngeal tumours present with dysphagia, pain and otalgia. Hypopharyngeal tumours present with dysphagia, odynophagia, referred otalgia and neck nodes. Laryngeal cancers present with persistent hoarseness, pain, otalgia, dyspnoea and stridor. Nasopharyngeal cancers present with a bloody nasal discharge, nasal obstruction, conductive deafness, atypical facial pain, diplopia, hoarseness and Horner's syndrome. Nasal and sinus tumours present with a bloody discharge or obstruction. Salivary gland tumours present as painless swellings or facial nerve palsies. Cervical lymph node enlargement as the presenting feature is not uncommon, particularly when the primary tumour lies in certain hidden sites, such as the base of the tongue, supraglottis and nasopharynx. Systemic metastases are uncommon at presentation

Table 23.1 Indications for urgent referral for suspected head and neck cancer.

Hoarseness persisting for >6 weeks
Ulceration of oral mucosa persisting for >3 weeks
Oral swellings persisting for >3 weeks
All red or red-and-white patches on the oral mucosa
Dysphagia persisting for >3 weeks
Unilateral nasal obstruction, particularly when associated with purulent discharge
Unexplained tooth mobility not associated with periodontal disease
Unresolved neck masses for >3 weeks
Cranial neuropathies
Orbital masses

(10%). Synchronous or metachronous tumours of the upper aerodigestive tract occur in 10–15% of patients.

A number of criteria for urgent referral have been established (Table 23.1). Diagnostic surgical resection of cervical nodes, without first determining the site of the primary tumour, may compromise subsequent therapy, increases the morbidity and worsens the outcome.

Treatment

The approach to managing these tumours varies according to their site, but in general the primary site and potential for cervical lymph node metastases should be considered. Small early stage 1 and 2 tumours, where there are no regional lymph node metastases, should be treated with surgery or radiotherapy, with 60–69% cure rates. The decision between surgery and radiotherapy is often determined by the anatomical site and the long-term morbidity. Function is generally better after radiotherapy but requires daily attendance for four to six weeks, whilst surgical treatment is quicker, but patients need to be fit for anaesthesia.

More advanced tumours are usually managed surgically, providing that the tumour is resectable. This is followed by adjuvant radiotherapy if the margins are insufficient, or if there is extranodal spread, multiple lymph node involvement or poorly differentiated histology. The resection of large tumours may leave sizeable defects, requiring myocutaneous flaps. Inoperable or recurrent disease may be treated with combinations of chemotherapy and radiotherapy, but outcomes generally remain poor, and in many cases of advanced disease symptomatic palliation is a more valued approach.

If cervical lymph node metastases are present, surgical resection is recommended, and, recently, more limited and selective neck dissection has been advocated. This preserves function, especially in relation to the accessory nerve, which, if sacrificed, usually gives rise to a stiff and painful shoulder. A scoring index can be used to predict the likelihood of metastasis to cervical lymph nodes. If the expected incidence of lymph node involvement exceeds 20%, neck dissection is usually recommended.

The addition of chemotherapy to radiotherapy, the use of hyperfractionated radiotherapy as well as intensity-modulated radiotherapy have all improved the delivery of radiotherapy for patients with advanced head and neck tumours, resulting in modest improvements in survival and declines in morbidity. The addition of the monoclonal antibody cetuximab, which targets epidermal growth factor receptor (EGFR), to radiotherapy has been shown to double survival in advanced head and neck cancer, especially tumours of the oropharynx. However, this widely quoted landmark phase III trial did not use cisplatin chemoradiotherapy, the gold standard therapy, as the control arm. Recurrent or metastatic tumour may be palliated with further surgery or radiotherapy to aid local control, and systemic chemotherapy has a response rate of around 30%. Second malignancies are frequent in patients who have been successfully treated for head and neck tumours, with an annual rate of 3%, and all patients should be encouraged to give up smoking and drinking to lower this risk. In addition, a number of studies have addressed the role of retinoids and β-carotene as secondary prophylaxis, but none have proved to have any significant effect.

Quality of life issues are especially important in head and neck cancers, given the anatomical site of the disease and the consequences of treatment, which can affect facial appearance, speech, swallowing and breathing. These cancers have enormous sociopsychological impact and may result in physical disability. These concerns must be addressed sympathetically with patients. Rehabilitation following treatment for head and neck cancers needs input from many professionals, particularly speech and language therapists, dieticians and prosthetics technicians. Rehabilitation, furthermore, requires enormous patience and effort on behalf of the patient. For example, 40% of patients will achieve communication by oesophageal speech following total laryngectomy.

Prognosis

Five-year survival rates for patients with head and neck tumours are listed in Table 23.2.

Salivary gland tumours

Salivary gland tumours represent around 5% of all head and neck cancers and affect both genders equally. They are most common in the sixth and seventh decades of life. Over half of the tumours are benign, and 80% originate in the parotid gland. Approximately 25% of parotid tumours, 40% of submandibular tumours and over 90% of sublingual gland tumours are malignant. Histologically, the most common benign tumour is the pleomorphic adenoma, and the most common malignant tumour is the mucoepidermoid carcinoma. Most patients present with painless swelling of the parotid, submandibular or sublingual glands.

Table 23.2 Five-year survival rates for head and neck tumours.

Tumour	5-year survival
Larynx	68%
Larynx (glottic)	85%
Larynx (supraglottic)	55%
Oral cavity	54%
Oropharynx	45%
Nasopharynx	45%
Hypopharynx	25%
Salivary glands	60%

Facial numbness or weakness due to cranial nerve involvement usually indicates malignancy and is an ominous sign. Pleomorphic adenomas, although not malignant, often recur if not completely excised, and a small proportion may become malignant if left untreated. Early-stage, low-grade malignant salivary gland tumours are usually curable by surgical resection alone. The prognosis is best for parotid tumours, then submandibular tumours; the least favourable sites are the sublingual and minor salivary glands. Larger or high-grade tumours require postoperative radiotherapy. Complications of surgical treatment for parotid neoplasms include facial nerve palsy and Frey's syndrome. Frey's syndrome is gustatory flushing and sweating of the ipsilateral forehead because the sympathetic nerve fibers to the sweat glands of the scalp and parasympathetic fibers to the parotid gland have reconnected wrongly after the auriculotemporal branch of the trigeminal nerve has been severed in surgery; instead of salivating the patient sweats.

New treatment

Conventional radiotherapy is delivered by photons or occasionally electron beams (β-radiation) for superficial tumours. However, particle beam radiotherapy uses hadrons (colour charge neutral collections of quarks bound by the strong nuclear force) usually protons, neutrons or positive ions. Proton beam therapy is the most commonly used of these techniques but is only available in one institution in the UK currently. The theoretical advantage of proton beam radiotherapy is that the higher mass of protons results in less scatter and a more concentrated delivery of energy to the tumour and greater sparing of normal adjacent tissues. Proton beam therapy offers promise in the management of head and neck cancers as well as other tumours located in anatomically challenging sites such as intraocular melanoma and retinoblastoma. In recent times it has been suggested that antiprotons (a fermion formed of two anti-up quarks and one anti-down quark) and pi-mesons (formed of an up and an anti-down quark) could be used as particle beam radiotherapy (Box 23.1).

Box 23.1: A brief lesson in fundamental particles

According to the standard model of quantum theory, the universe is made up of fermions (quarks and leptons) and bosons (force carriers). There are three sets of quark pairs and three sets of lepton pairs and for every particle there is a corresponding antiparticle, denoted by a bar over the symbol. Quarks are named after a quote in James Joyce's *Finnegan's Wake* 'Three quarks for Muster Mark!' and they carry three types of colour charge (which have nothing to do with visible colours). Quarks do not exist in isolation but are confined in colour charge neutral hadrons. Two types of hadrons exist, mesons that are formed from a combination of a quark and an antiquark, and baryons that are formed of three quarks. Protons are baryons formed of three quarks (uud) that carry a net +1 electrical charge, whilst neutrons are baryons with no net electrical charge (udd), and pi-mesons are formed by a quark (u) and an antiquark ($[\bar{d}]$) and carry a +1 electrical charge.

Four forces or interactions are known, strong force, weak force, electromagnetic force and gravitational force. The force carriers or bosons for all but gravity have been identified. The strong nuclear force (also known as the colour charge) that holds protons and neutrons together in atomic nuclei is mediated by gluons exchanging colour charges with quarks. The weak nuclear force is responsible for lepton decay and β-radiation and is mediated by W^+, W^- and Z bosons. The electromagnetic force is, of course, mediated by photons whilst the force carrier particle for gravity has not been observed but nevertheless has been named graviton.

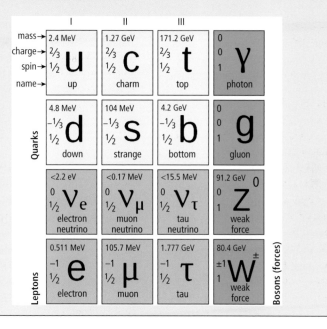

Chapter 24

Endocrine cancers

Endocrine cancers are a group of tumours whose clinical manifestations seem to delight old-fashioned physicians almost as much as they are concerned for the patients with these cancers. In particular, the products that they secrete give rise to many unusual syndromes. The majority of endocrine tumours are rare, with an incidence of 0.5 per million of population per annum. But others are more common, such as carcinoid tumours, which have a reported incidence of 1.5 per 10^5 of people per annum. These tumours are frequently listed as occurring in the context of multiple endocrine neoplasia (MEN). MENs are due to gene mutations. The MEN 1 gene is encoded at chromosome 11q13. The gene product is called, imaginatively, menin and encodes a nuclear protein that partners with JunD, NF-κB and many other proteins. The function of menin is, however, not known, and is lost in MEN 1. Mutations in MEN 2 lead to changes in the RET proto-oncogene.

The RET gene encodes a receptor tyrosine kinase and mutations at different sites within the RET gene are associated with MEN type 2A and type 2B, Hirschsprung's disease (congenital aganglionic megacolon) and medullary thyroid carcinoma. This one-gene source of multiple diseases is of course a blow to traditional paradigms of genetic disease but should perhaps be seen in the context of the shrinking genome. The number of genes postulated for the human genome has steadily fallen from the early days of the Human Genome Project, when it was speculated that 50 000–75 000 genes were present in the human genome, to the present 'post-genomic' era, when estimates have decreased to 25 000 genes only.

The MEN syndromes are described in Table 24.1.

Thyroid cancer, adrenal cancers and carcinoid tumours are discussed in detail in the following three chapters.

Lecture Notes: Oncology, 2nd edition. By M. Bower and J. Waxman. Published 2010 by Blackwell Publishing Ltd.

Table 24.1 Features of multiple endocrine neoplasia syndromes.

	MEN 1 (Werner's syndrome)	MEN 2A (Sipple's syndrome)	MEN 2B (also known as MEN 3)
Components	Parathyroid hyperplasia or adenoma (90%)	Medullary thyroid cancer (100%)	Mucosal neuromas (100%)
	Pancreatic islets adenoma, carcinoma or more rarely diffuse hyperplasia (80%)	Phaeochromocytoma (50%)	Medullary thyroid cancer (90%)
	Pituitary anterior adenomas (65%)	Parathryoid hyperplasia or adenoma (40%)	Marfanoid habitus (65%)
	Adrenal cortex hyperplasia or adenoma (40%)		Phaeochromocytoma (45%)
Genetic locus	Chromosome 11q13	Chromosome 10q11	Chromosome 10q11
	Menin gene	RET gene	RET gene

Chapter 25

Thyroid cancer

Epidemiology and pathogenesis

Thyroid cancers are relatively uncommon malignancies. There were 1933 patients registered a year in the UK with this condition and 341 deaths reported in the last national statistics publication. There is a 3 to 1 ratio of women to men affected with thyroid malignancies. Radiation exposure is the most common predisposing factor to the development of thyroid cancer, and it was reported for many thousands of people across Europe following the Chernobyl disaster and in Japanese populations after the atomic bomb devastations.

Thyroid cancer includes a number of clinical entities, ranging from the classical papillary, follicular and anaplastic tumours to the atypic Hurthle and medullary cell carcinomas, as well as thyroid lymphoma. Mutations in BRAF(V599E) are seen in 40% of papillary carcinomas. Cyclin D1 overexpression is observed in approximately 50% of papillary carcinomas, while the transcription factor E2F1, which is part of the Rb oncogene signalling pathway, is upregulated in 80% of papillary and anaplastic thyroid carcinomas. Medullary thyroid carcinoma is associated with multiple endocrine neoplasia (MEN) types 2A and 2B (see Table 24.1). The RET gene encodes a transmembrane tyrosine kinase receptor. This gene is mutated in almost 100% of all MEN 2A patients and in 85% of patients with familial medullary thyroid carcinoma families.

Presentation

The most common presentation of thyroid malignancy is with a thyroid nodule or with cervical lymphadenopathy. Much less frequently, patients will present with features suggestive of advanced disease, such as vocal cord paralysis or with symptoms due to metastases.

Investigations

The diagnosis of a thyroid malignancy is made following routine investigations, which should include thyroid function, thyroid isotope scanning and thyroid ultrasound. Under ultrasound control, fine needle aspiration biopsy is used to obtain a cytological diagnosis and thereby define treatment. Other staging investigations should include CT scanning of the neck and thorax. Serum calcitonin levels are measured in patients with medullary thyroid carcinomas, while serum thyroglobulin can be used to monitor relapse in well differentiated carcinomas after thyroid ablation.

Lecture Notes: Oncology, 2nd edition. By M. Bower and J. Waxman. Published 2010 by Blackwell Publishing Ltd.

Treatment

After initial staging, patients with thyroid malignancies proceed to surgery. In the majority of patients with thyroid cancers, the surgical options are either subtotal thyroid resection, removing the lobe bearing the tumour together with the thyroid isthmus, or total thyroidectomy. Generally, partial thryoidectomy is only considered in those patients with low-risk tumours, for example those with a single focus of papillary carcinoma measuring less than 1 cm in diameter. There is no evidence that routine lymph node dissection has any added survival advantage. Subsequent to surgery, patients are treated with thyroid replacement, aiming to suppress thyroid-stimulating hormone (TSH) completely, which may be a driver for the development of recurrence.

When patients with thyroid tumours develop recurrent disease, further options for management may include surgery or radiation therapy. Surgery is the treatment of choice for patients with recurrent medullary carcinoma of the thyroid, which is relatively resistant to radiation therapy and chemotherapy. Radiation treatment is given both by using external beam radiotherapy and by treating with radioiodine, which localizes to thyroid tissue. Thyroid lymphomas are treated with standard lymphoma chemotherapy. Their prognosis is said to be poor, but this information is based upon limited clinical studies and may not be true. These data, however, do lead most clinicians to recommend that chemotherapy is followed by adjuvant radiotherapy to the thyroid.

Table 25.1 Five-year survival rates for thyroid cancers.

Tumour	5-year survival
Papillary thyroid cancer	80%
Follicular thyroid cancer	60%
Anaplastic thyroid cancer	10%
Medullary thyroid cancer	50%

Prognosis

Table 25.1 shows the five-year survival rates for thyroid tumours according to histological subtype.

New treatment

New treatments for thyroid cancers target the molecular changes seen in this tumour, and in particular it is possible that the RET oncogenes could be a target for treatment with small molecule tyrosine kinase inhibitors such as sorafenib and sunitinib. Laboratory work is showing that this group of compounds is effective in inhibiting kinase activity of RET/PTC3 and leads to reversion of the malignant characteristics of transformed thyroid cell lines. Sunitinib also causes a dose-related inhibition of growth of rat thyroid cells. Supporting this theoretical basis for activity is very limited clinical trial work, which shows a response rate of up to 30%.

Chapter 26

Adrenal cancers

Epidemiology of adrenal cortical cancers

Adrenal cortical cancers are likely to occur with an incidence of approximately one per million of population per annum. Adrenal cortical cancers are derived from the adrenal cortex and may be secretory. The major adrenal hormone products of these tumours include androgens, aldosterone and cortisol. Serum levels of these hormones may be elevated, and 24-hour urinary cortisol secretion may be increased.

Presentation of adrenal cortical cancers

Patients with adrenal cortical cancers generally present with non-specific symptoms, such as weight loss and general fatigue, or specific symptoms relating to their anatomical position, which include abdominal or loin pain. Adrenal cortical cancers may also produce symptoms related to the hormones that they secrete. Women may be virilized by the excessive production of androgenic hormones. Occasionally, adrenal cortical cancers are picked up as a result of an abdominal ultrasound or CT scan carried out for another reason.

Investigations of adrenal cortical cancers

[The patient with a suspected diagnosis of adrenal cortical cancer will generally be investigated in an endocrinological or surgical outpatient setting where routine blood testing together with specific endocrinological investigations will be arranged. These will include measurement of the adrenal androgens, diurnal cortisol production, adrenocorticotrophic hormone (ACTH) levels, 24-hour urinary cortisol levels, plain X-rays and CT scans of the abdomen, pelvis and chest (Figure 26.1).

Initial treatment of adrenal cortical cancers

Once staging investigations have been completed, the patient with a suspected diagnosis of an adrenal cortical cancer should be referred on to a specialist endocrine surgeon. The patient will proceed to laparotomy, and an attempt is made to resect the tumour. Surgery is complex, and there may be a major morbidity and mortality associated with the procedure. There is no clinical advantage to any adjuvant treatment.

Treatment of metastatic or locally advanced adrenal cortical cancer

The secretory symptoms of adrenal cortical tumours are unpleasant. Secretory symptoms are

Lecture Notes: Oncology, 2nd edition. By M. Bower and J. Waxman. Published 2010 by Blackwell Publishing Ltd.

Right adrenal phaeochromocytoma

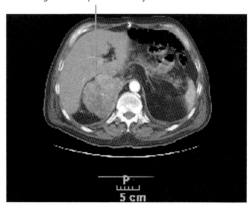

5 cm

Figure 26.1 Adrenal tumour. This CT scan was performed on a 28-year-old man with hypertension and shows a lobulated heterogeneous right adrenal mass which was due to phaeochromocytoma.

most unpleasant in women because of a virilization caused by androgenic steroid production. These symptoms may include acne, hirsutism, change in habitus and increased libido. Attempts are made to block the production of hormones by an adrenal cortical cancer, using blocking agents such as metyrapone and ketoconazole, which inhibit steroidogenesis. Treatment may be given using OPDD, which is also called 'Mitotane'. Mitotane is a selective adrenal poison that is structurally related to the chlorinated insecticide DDT. DDT is a cheap insecticide developed in the 1940s that has cumulative toxicity in mammals. It is estimated that DDT saved 500 million people globally from malaria. In 1962, however, Rachel Carson published *The Silent Spring*, in which she attributed the declining song-bird population to widespread DDT use, and there since have been calls to ban DDT globally. The alternative insecticides are far more expensive, however, as they remain subject to patents owned by the pharmaceutical industry. Patients with adrenal cortical cancers are also pre-

scribed chemotherapy. Approximately 40% of patients will respond and the most effective agents include doxorubicin and cisplatin.

The secretory symptoms of adrenal carcinoma can be controlled with octreotide. This agent has no effect on survival and does not lead to reductions in tumour bulk.

Prognosis of adrenal cortical cancers

The outlook for the majority of patients with adrenal cortical cancers is very poor, except in the patient with localized, small bulk disease. For this group of patients, the expectation is for a 70% chance of complete cure following surgery. For patients with bulky tumours, the expectation is for a median survival of one year. Patients with metastatic tumours survive a median period of four months.

Adrenal medullary tumours

These uncommon tumours occurring in association with multiple endocrine neoplasia are a rare cause of hypertension. Phaeochromocytomas of the adrenal medulla produce their effects by the secretion of catecholamines, resulting in intermittent, episodic or sustained hypertension, anxiety, tremor, palpitations, sweating, flushing, headaches, gastrointestinal disturbances and polyuria. Twenty-four-hour urinary collection for urinary free catecholamines (epinephrine, norepinephrine and dopamine) is now the most widely employed diagnostic test, although some centres also measure catecholamine metabolites such as metanephrines and vanillylmandelic acid (VMA). The treatment is surgical and the results of treatment generally excellent. Metastatic phaeochromocytoma may be treated with ^{131}I-MIBG (meta-iodobenzyl guanidine), a catecholamine precursor, which may also be used to image the tumour.

Chapter 27

Carcinoid tumours

Carcinoid tumours are neuroendocrine tumours that may arise in numerous anatomical sites, particularly the gastrointestinal tract and lungs (Table 27.1). Much of their medical notoriety derives from their secretion of vasoactive compounds that give rise to the carcinoid syndrome. This usually follows the development of liver metastases, when first pass metabolism of these products is bypassed. Carcinoid tumours are much more common than previously recognized but the true incidence is not clearly known.

Presentation

Patients with carcinoid tumours may be asymptomatic or may present with symptoms due to the secretory products of their tumour, if there is significant metastatic disease. These metabolic products cause diarrhoea, flushing and occasionally bronchospasm. These symptoms are so specific that there is little difficulty in making a diagnosis, which is often achieved in general practice.

Investigations

The presence of symptoms is likely to indicate that the patient with a carcinoid tumour has metastatic

disease. The examination of such a patient should be confined to establishing the extent of disease and obtaining a histological diagnosis. The investigations that are required include a blood count, liver function test, chest X-ray and a CT scan of the chest and abdomen (Figure 27.1). Twenty-four-hour urinary 5HIAA (5-hydroxyindole-acetic acid) levels should be measured. This is because 5HIAA is the excretory product of the metabolites produced by carcinoids and results from the breakdown of 5HT (5-hydroxytryptamine or serotonin). There has been interest in the use of chromagranin A as a serum marker for carcinoid. This is a neurosecretory product that is of value because we can monitor carcinoid using this as a blood test, rather than having to carry out 24-hour urinary collections to measure 5HIAA.

Treatment

Pharmacological control

These agents act to block the synthesis, release and peripheral blockade of circulating tumour products. The list of drugs used in the treatment of carcinoid symptoms include inhibitors of 5HT synthesis such as parachlorphenylalanine, peripheral 5HT antagonists such as cyproheptadine, antihistamines, and inhibitors of 5HT release such as somatostatin and its long-acting analogues. The most frequently used somatostatin analogue is

Lecture Notes: Oncology, 2nd edition. By M. Bower and J. Waxman. Published 2010 by Blackwell Publishing Ltd.

Table 27.1 Comparison of carcinoid tumours by site of origin.

	Foregut	Midgut	Hindgut
Site	Respiratory tract, pancreas, stomach, proximal duodenum	Jejunum, ileum, appendix, Meckle's diverticulum, ascending colon	Transverse and descending colon, rectum
Tumour products	Low 5HTP, multihormones*	High 5HTP, multihormones*	Rarely 5HTP, multihormones*
Blood	5HTP, histamine, multihormones,* occasionally ACTH	5HT, multihormones,* rarely ACTH	Rarely 5HT or ACTH
Urine	5HTP, 5HT, 5HIAA, histamine	5HT, 5HIAA	Negative
Carcinoid syndrome	Occurs but is atypical	Occurs frequently with metastases	Rarely occurs
Metastasizes to bone	Common	Rare	Common

*Multihormones include tachykinins (substance P, substance K, neuropeptide K), neurotensin, PYY, enkephalin, insulin, glucagon, glicentin, VIP, somatostatin, pancreatic polypeptide, ACTH and α-subunit of human chorionic gonadotrophin. ACTH, adrenocorticotrophic hormone; 5HIAA, 5-hydroxyindole-acetic acid; 5HT, 5-hydroxytryptamine (serotonin); 5HTP, 5-hydroxytryptophan.

octreotide, and this leads to a relief of symptoms in 80% of patients for a median duration of 10 months.

Cytokines

Interferon has been used to treat patients with metastatic carcinoid tumours. Symptom relief will occur in between 50% and 60% of patients. Less than 5% of patients, however, achieve any significant tumour regression. Treatment with interferon is associated with significant side effects, which may include flu-like symptoms; for this reason, it is not generally given.

Complications of carcinoid hormone production

Carcinoid heart disease develops in patients with 5HT-producing neuroendocrine tumours. It is due to the formation of fibrous plaques within the heart, causing valvular dysfunction. Classically, the valves affected are right-sided. Right-sided heart failure due to valve disease is treated surgically by valve replacement. In view of the underlining excellent prognosis for carcinoid tumours, this condition is actively treated. Carcinoid tumours also lead, because of their secreted prod-

ucts, to fibrosis at other sites, such as in the retroperitoneum, where it may lead to small bowel obstruction.

Embolization

When metastatic disease in the liver is extensive, hepatic artery embolization may be considered. This involves selective cannulation of the artery with injection of embolic material. This will lead to sustained symptom relief in the majority of patients. There may be significant side effects from embolization, and so this procedure is not entered into without due consideration of the benefits. In some clinical series, mortality rates are 3–5%.

Prognosis

The prognosis for patients with metastatic carcinoid tumour is relatively good in comparison to that for most metastastic tumours. Patients with metastatic carcinoid tumour commonly survive a considerable time and the expectation, even in the presence of liver disease, is that approximately 36% of patients will survive five years and 20% for 10 years. In the absence of metastases and following resection of the primary, the outlook is excellent. Carcinoid tumours of different primary sites

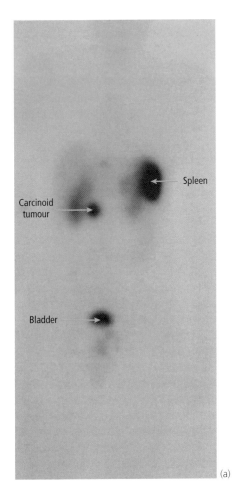

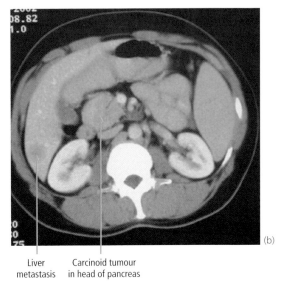

(b)

Liver   Carcinoid tumour
metastasis   in head of pancreas

Figure 27.1 (a) Indium-113-labelled somatostatin scan demonstrating a focus of carcinoid tumour in the pancreas as well as normal tracer uptake in the spleen and bladder. (b) Matched CT scan showing a tumour in the head of the pancreas and liver metastases.

(a)

are thought to have different outlooks, but this is very much debated.

New treatment

Carcinoid tumours highly express epidermal growth factor receptor (EGFR) but not ErbB. There is a potential therefore to treat this group of patients with EGFR inhibitors such as cetuximab or erlotinib. Neuroendocrine tumours express vascular endothelial growth factor (VEGF) and its receptor (VEGFR). Sunitinib, an agent that targets the tyrosine kinases of VEGF and VEGFR, has some minimal efficacy with up to 15% of patients improving and 70% having stable disease with treatment.

Chapter 28

Pituitary tumours

Pituitary tumours are common, and the most common are prolactinomas with an incidence of up to one in 3000 of the population per annum. Pituitary tumours arise from the anterior lobe and produce their effects by uncontrolled production of specific hormones, by destruction of normal pituitary tissues leading to hypopituitarism, or by compressing adjacent structures such as the optic chiasm, hypothalamus and bony structures (Table 28.1). Secretory tumours produce syndromes that cause gross clinical signs and symptoms. The local symptoms include headaches and visual field loss. The systemic symptoms produced depend upon the secreted product and range from acromegaly to pituitary Cushing's.

Treatment options include blocking agents, such as bromocriptine, neurosurgery and radiotherapy. The mainstay of therapy, however, is surgery,

Table 28.1 Comparison of clinical features of pituitary tumours.

Tumour	Percent of tumours	Morphology	Endocrine features	Neurological features
Prolactin-secreting adenoma	40%	Macroadenoma	Amenorrhoea, galactorrhoea, hypopituitarism in men	Headache, visual field defects
Non-secretory adenoma	20%	Macroadenoma	Hypopituitarism	Headache, visual field defects
Growth hormone-secreting adenoma	20%	Macroadenoma	Gigantism in children, acromegaly in adults	Headache, visual field defects
Corticotropin-secreting adenoma	15%	Microadenoma	Cushing's disease	Usually none
Gonadotropin-secreting adenoma	5%	Macroadenoma	Panhypopituitarism	Headache, visual field defects
Thyrotropin-secreting adenoma	<1%	Microadenoma	Hyperthyroidism	Usually none

Lecture Notes: Oncology, 2nd edition. By M. Bower and J. Waxman. Published 2010 by Blackwell Publishing Ltd.

which is important in establishing the histological diagnosis, in decompressing the optic chiasm and in relieving obstructive hydrocephalus, as well as in completely excising the tumour. A transfrontal approach is required for large tumours with extra-sellar extension, while a trans-sphenoidal approach is safer and tolerated better for smaller tumours. Radiotherapy may be used as the primary treatment for intrasellar tumours and as an adjunct to surgery for larger tumours. The outlook is generally excellent.

There are no classical oncogene mutations in pituitary tumours. However, there are clues to the development of this group of malignancies that come from dysregulation of the inhibitory components of the β-catenin pathway, and the relationship of this pathway to the cadherins. Both the Akt and MAPK pathways appear to be overexpressed in many pituitary tumours, and this causes an inhibition of the inhibitors of the cell cycle. This is equivalent to snapping the brake cable as you are bicycling down a steep hill.

Chapter 29

Parathyroid cancers

Parathyroid carcinomas are extremely rare, with an annual incidence of 0.5–1 per million of the population. Parathyroid cancers secrete parathormone, and for this reason the majority of patients present with hypercalcaemia. The hypercalcaemia is usually gross and, rather oddly, patients may be asymptomatic, with a calcium level that would normally be associated with death in the acute situation. The reason for this is that this condition generally has a long natural history and may have been present for many years prior to diagnosis. Calcium levels in excess of 4 mmol/l are frequently reported and the patient's cellular processes will have adapted to this level of hypercalcaemia. The primary treatment for this condition is surgical. The outlook for patients with metastatic disease is awful.

Lecture Notes: Oncology, 2nd edition. By M. Bower and J. Waxman. Published 2010 by Blackwell Publishing Ltd.

Chapter 30

Thoracic cancers

Table 30.1 Lung cancer registration data for southeast England from Thames in 2001 and five-year survival rates.

	Percentage of registrations		Rank of registrations		Lifetime risk of cancer		Change in ASR, 1997–2006		5-year survival
	Male	Female	Male	Female	Male	Female	Male	Female	
Lung cancer	15%	11%	2nd	3rd	1 in 13	1 in 23	−21%	+5%	6%
Mesothelioma	1%	0.2%	16th	>20th			+25%	+61%	8%

ASR, age-standardized rate.

In a celebrated television documentary *Death in the West*, produced in 1976 by Thames Television, the vice president of Philip Morris attempted to dismiss established links between tobacco and cancer. During the interview he said: 'Too much of anything can kill you. Too much apple sauce can kill you.' And: 'If there were something harmful in tobacco smoke, we could remove it'. Despite numerous court cases since, the tobacco industry continues to target the young and encourage smoking. It took until 1999 for the Royal Family to withdraw its royal warrant from the tobacco multi-national Gallaher, which entitled them to display 'By Appointment' on packs of Benson & Hedges cigarettes. This was despite the death of the last

Table 30.2 Five-year survival rates for lung cancer and mesothelioma.

Tumour	5-year survival
Non-small cell lung cancer	8%
Small cell lung cancer	5%
Mesothelioma	5%

three kings from tobacco-related disease, including King George VI, who died of lung cancer.

Thoracic cancers include primary lung cancers and mesotheliomas, although a number of other cancers may occur in the thorax: particularly haematological cancers. Primary lung cancer has recently been pushed into second place in the ranking order of cancer registration in men (Table 30.1) and has a very poor overall survival rate (Table 30.2).

Lecture Notes: Oncology, 2nd edition. By M. Bower and J. Waxman. Published 2010 by Blackwell Publishing Ltd.

Chapter 31

Lung cancer

Epidemiology and pathogenesis

Carcinoma of the bronchus is the second most common tumour of men and the second most common cancer of women. The overall prospects for survival are poor: only between 5% and 8% of patients survive five years from diagnosis. Currently in the UK, there are approximately 39 000 men and women registered annually with carcinoma of the bronchus: 22 300 men and 16 600 women. The latest survival figures indicate that 34 500 of these people will die from their tumour.

The most important cause of carcinoma of the bronchus is smoking, and the incidence of lung cancer is directly related to the number of cigarettes smoked. Although the overall incidence of smoking is decreasing in the UK at a rate of a little under 1% per annum, there has been an increase in women smokers and in young smokers, and this bodes poorly for the future.

There are other risk factors for developing lung cancer. These include exposure to asbestos and heavy metals, such as nickel, and fibrotic disease of the lung. Air pollution is a significant factor in the development of lung cancers, and it is often said that living in London has the equivalent effect on lung cancer incidence to smoking five cigarettes a

day. Similarly, proximity to industrial pollution has a significant impact upon mortality rates.

As with so many other tumour groups, there is significant interest in the molecular biology of lung cancer. Amongst the first observations of the molecular changes in lung cancer were mutations in the Ras family of oncogenes, which have guanosine triphosphatase (GTPase) activity and are important as second messengers linking events between the cell membrane and nucleus. The history of the molecular biology of lung cancer reads almost like a contemporaneous commentary on the development of our understanding of the molecular biology of cancer, and the next to be discovered were mutations in the tumour suppressor genes Rb and p53 present in at least 80% of all small cell lung cancers. Loss of heterozygosity of a number of chromosomes has been observed in small cell lung cancer. These include chromosomes 3, 9, 12, 13 and 17. The changes in chromosome 17 involve the c-erb-B2 oncogene and this has led to the development of new therapeutic approaches to the management of lung cancer.

More recently, observations of abnormal DNA methylation of the cyclin D2 gene has been described in approximately 60% of small cell cancer lines. The cyclin D2 gene has a primary function in cell cycle regulation and has recently been brought to the general public's attention because of the awards of the 2001 Nobel Prizes to the scientists involved in this discovery who

Lecture Notes: Oncology, 2nd edition. By M. Bower and J. Waxman. Published 2010 by Blackwell Publishing Ltd.

included Sir Paul Nurse. Sir Paul Nurse according to *The Sun* is 'the David Beckham of science'. He later became the director of CRUK (Cancer Research UK) but that did not stop him saying that Margaret Thatcher did 'a good job of ruining British science'.

Presentation

Patients with carcinoma of the bronchus generally present with a cough or haemoptysis. This may be associated with weight loss and symptoms of metastatic cancer, such as bone pain (Figure 31.1) or jaundice. Patients with chest symptoms suggestive of a diagnosis of carcinoma of the bronchus are generally referred promptly by general practitioners to a specialist chest physician. One of the concerns of oncologists in the 1990s was the lack of referral on from specialist chest physicians to oncologists, with patients regarded somewhat as property and their treatment proprietarily. One of the major changes that we have seen in this current decade has come about as a result of the central promotion of the philosophy of the multidisciplinary team. As a result, there is multispecialty input into the management of lung cancer patients and it is the view of these authors that the care of lung cancer patients has generally improved throughout the country.

The signs of carcinoma of the bronchus are many and of particular interest is the observation of clubbing of the fingers occurring in non-small cell carcinoma of the bronchus. The aetiology of finger clubbing, which is associated with hypertrophic osteoarthropathy and polyarthralgias, has been postulated as including the secretion of parathormone (PTH) by tumours and also, more recently, the ectopic secretion of platelet-derived growth factor (see Figures 45.2 and 45.3). Other clinical abnormalities may include Horner's syndrome (Figure 31.2) or hoarseness, which are pointers to inoperability as a result of nerve entrapment by the tumour, and dysphagia which comes as a result of mediastinal nodal enlargement. Paraneoplastic syndromes are commonly associated with lung cancer, particularly the small cell carcinoma variant. These include cutaneous syndromes of dermatomyositis and acanthosis nigricans, the neurological complications of peripheral neuropathy and the Eaton–Lambert syndrome. The endocrine features of ectopic PTH, adrenocorticotrophic hormone (ACTH) and antidiuretic hormone (ADH) secretion are all spectacular in their presentations.

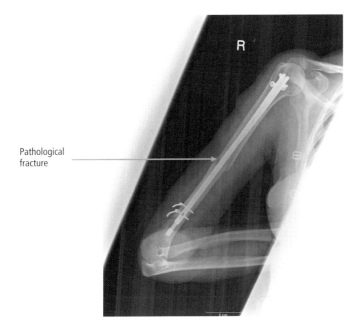

Figure 31.1 Pathological fracture of the mid-humerus in a patient with metastatic non-small cell lung cancer. The fracture has been pinned with an intramedullary nail.

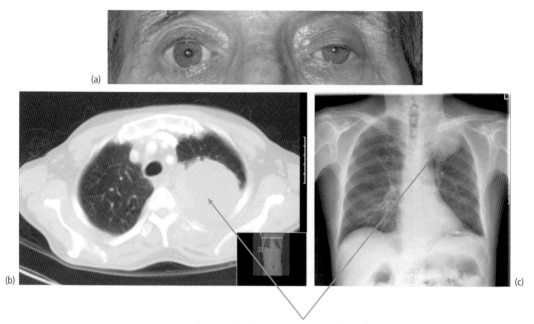

Non-small cell lung cancer at apex of left lung (Pancoast tumour)

Figure 31.2 (a) Unilateral ptosis and miosis (constricted pupil). The other features of Horner's syndrome are enophthalmos (sunken eye) and anhidrosis (no sweating). It is due to loss of sympathetic innervation due in this case to a Pancoast tumour of the left lung apex affecting the T1 nerve root (b, c) (also associated with ipsilateral wasting of the small muscles of the hand). Horner (1831–1886) was a Swiss ophthalmologist; Pancoast (1875–1939) was an American radiologist.

Investigations should include a full blood count, liver function tests, chest X-ray (Figure 31.3) and sputum cytology. Bronchoscopy is organized and should proceed within a few days (Plate 31.1). Biopsies and washings are then obtained and examined microscopically. By these means, a histological diagnosis will be achieved. Diagnosis may not be achieved in the context of peripheral lesions and if this is the case, then needle biopsies under CT scanning or fluoroscopic imaging should be arranged. (See also Figures 2.6, 45.1, 45.3, 46.1 and 46.5 and Plate 46.1.)

Pathology

There are a number of different variants of carcinoma of the bronchus, and these histological classifications are important in that they define the patient's further treatment. The main histological variants are squamous cell carcinoma, small cell carcinoma, adenocarcinoma and large cell carcinoma. For treatment purposes, tumours are described as either being small or non-small cell cancers. These constitute 95% of primary lung neoplasms. Squamous cell carcinoma accounts for approximately 40% of lung cancers, with adenocarcinoma accounting for 30% and small cell carcinoma for 25% of all lung tumours. Approximately 10% of lung cancers are of mixed histology. Rarer variants include carcinoid tumours, lymphomas and hamartomas.

Staging and grading

Lung cancer staging is usually by the TNM classification. Staging should include a CT scan of the chest and abdomen, a radioisotope bone scan, a liver ultrasound and ideally a positron emission tomography (PET) scan. Although not carried out routinely, examination of the bone marrow by aspiration and trephine in small cell lung cancer shows the presence of metastases in 95% of patients. Pulmonary function tests to assess vital capacity are essential, both to assess operability,

183

Right upper lobe
primary lung cancer

Ipsilateral hilar
lymphadenopathy

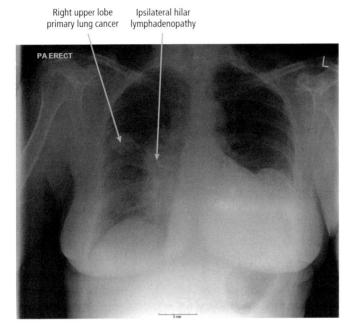

Figure 31.3 Chest X-ray of a 67-year-old woman with T2N2M0 small cell lung cancer showing a right upper lobe primary lesion with extensive ipsilateral and contralateral hilar lymphadenopathy.

and to ensure that the patient is not left with profound breathlessness following lung resection.

Treatment

Treatment of non-small cell lung cancer

Non-small cell lung cancer may be treated with either surgery or with radiation treatment. Surgery is only possible for patients with limited stage disease; that is, T1N0M0 and T2N0M0 disease, and a small number with T2N1M0 tumours. There is increasing surgical enthusiasm for operating on more extensive tumours, and it is not uncommon to find patients with T3 disease proceeding to surgery. The results of this approach are poor, however.

The UK falls below the European average in terms of the number of people proceeding to surgery because of issues of resource availability in terms of scans and surgeons. Surgery has a significant morbidity and mortality, and operability depends upon lung function prior to resection, together with cardiac status and the presence of other major illnesses. It is estimated that approximately 30% of patients with non-small cell carcinoma of the lung have operable tumours. The five-year survival for this group of patients is variably quoted at between 5% and 40%. A review of 2675 patients gave a five-year survival of 30%. There is a subgroup variation in survival, depending upon pathological staging and histology. For example, if those operable patients with adenocarcinoma are considered, the expectation for survival ranges between 38% and 79% and averages 65% at five years. If, on the other hand, operable patients under 40 years of age are considered, survival rises to 70%.

Radical radiotherapy, that is, radiotherapy given with curative intent, is considered for those patients who have inoperable disease by virtue of a poor medical state rather than spread of the cancer. Five-year survival figures of 6% were reported in a review of 1487 patients. Conventionally, patients receive 6000 cGy over a six-week period. More rapid treatment regimens are used, particularly in the north of England, and similar survival figures are found.

For the majority of patients with more advanced cancer, palliative radiotherapy is the only treatment option. This is given to patients who have symptoms as a result of their disease, which might include haemoptyses, breathlessness or chest pain.

Radiotherapy is given according to various prescriptions; some radiotherapists advise a single dose of 1000–1500 cGy, others 3000 cGy in 10 fractions over two weeks. Radiotherapy, too, has side effects, and these include tiredness, oesophagitis and skin changes.

There is a limited place for chemotherapy in this condition. Response rates for the most active regimens are in the range of 15–25%. The median survival of responding patients is six to seven months, offering only minor though statistically significant survival advantage over palliative therapy. Combination therapy using regimens such as MIC (mitomycin C, ifosfamide and cisplatin) is considered to be too toxic in view of the low response rates. Single-agent therapy using agents such as vinorelbine or platinum-based doublets have a role in the fitter patient, and may be used as primary neoadjuvant therapy in rendering operable the surgically inoperable patient and as adjuvant therapy following surgery.

Treatment of small cell lung cancer

Small cell lung cancer is an entirely different disease from non-small cell lung cancer. It is very rare for patients to have localized small cell lung cancer, and approximately 95% of patients with small cell lung cancer have metastatic disease at presentation.

The most important modality of treatment for small cell lung cancer is chemotherapy. The current chemotherapy programme of first choice is etoposide and cisplatin. Approximately 80% of patients have an initial response to chemotherapy with this and similar programmes, and this generally includes a complete remission rate of up to 60% of patients. However, the great majority of small cell lung cancers will recur after chemotherapy. Untreated, the median survival is three months. With treatment, 10–20% of patients will survive for two years and 5% for five years.

Treatment of paraneoplastic syndromes

Small cell lung cancer is associated with many paraneoplastic syndromes, due to secretion by the tumour of specific growth factors and hormones. One of the commonest is hyponatraemia, due to inappropriate secretion of ADH. This is treated by water restriction or tetracyclines. Steroids are prescribed in high dose for the treatment of polymyositis, Eaton–Lambert syndrome and the peripheral neuropathies associated with small cell lung cancer. Ectopic ACTH secretion may require high-dose therapy with adrenal enzyme-blocking drugs such as metyrapone and ketoconazole. Unfortunately, these two agents have toxicity in the dosages used and may make the patient feel awful. In this context, adrenalectomy may be rarely required.

New treatment

One of the most exciting developments of recent times has been that of specific therapies aimed at the molecular abnormalities expressed by cancer cells. The observation of aberrant epidermal growth factor receptor (EGFR) expression in non-small cell lung cancer has led to the hope that agents directed against this receptor may provide a therapeutic advance. The most interest recently has been around the use of gefitinib (Iressa) and erlotinib (Tarceva), which are EGFR tyrosine kinase inhibitors. There is some evidence of activity in non-small cell lung cancer, with disease stability being the best outcome. Women, non-smokers and patients with adenocarcinoma or bronchoalveolar carcinoma histologies are more likely to respond. These agents are used with a degree of optimism in patients with bronchioalveolar carcinomas and adenocarcinomas, with response rates of up to 30%. Response rates are highest in those patients with EGFR mutations reaching up to 80%. The proteasome inhibitor, bortezomib, has some efficacy in non-small cell carcinoma, but the best hope for this agent in terms of outcome is for stable disease. Future investigations of these agents hinge around their combination with cytotoxic chemotherapy and radiotherapy. Side effects are reported, the most common of which is an erythematous skin reaction, and the occurrence of this rash seems to be associated with tumour responsiveness.

Chapter 32

Mesothelioma

Epidemiology and pathogenesis

The incidence of mesothelioma has been steadily increasing, and it is estimated that the lifetime risk is around 0.5–1%. This tumour was originally described by occupational health doctors working in the asbestos factories in the East End of London around the time of the end of the First World War. It would appear, however, that this information was suppressed, and it was not until the 1960s that the association between mesothelioma and asbestos exposure was clearly publicized.

The development of mesothelioma is generally related to asbestos exposure, but this is not always the case. The risk of mesothelioma is not related to the amount of exposure. It may not only occur in the asbestos worker but also in family members exposed to the fibres of asbestos brought home in their spouse's, father's or mother's clothes. There are no specific chromosomal changes associated with the development of mesothelioma, but there are a host of abnormalities that may occur, which are entirely non-specific. Different asbestos fibres have different properties and carcinogenicity. The most carcinogenic fibres tend to be the needle-shaped blue (crocidolite) and brown (amosite)

asbestos rather than the commoner corkscrew-shaped white asbestos (chrysotile) (Table 32.1).

Presentation

Mesothelial tumours take their origins in the pleura or peritoneum. Patients with mesothelioma characteristically present with pleural effusions or ascites.

Investigations

The diagnosis of mesothelioma may be suspected from a chest X-ray (Figure 32.1), where a patient may have pleural thickening and an effusion. CT scanning will show the extent of the pleural or peritoneal tumour. The next step in the investigatory process is to carry out a pleural or peritoneal biopsy. Multiple biopsies are usually required to make the diagnosis.

Possibly the most important aspect of the care of patients with mesothelioma is to ensure that the appropriate compensatory mechanisms are put in place. In the UK, industrial compensation is usually arranged for patients by their union officers and involves an examination of the tumour by a pathology panel. It is enormously important for the patient and his or her family that the clinician signposts this process.

Often a pleural biopsy may not be sufficient to obtain diagnostic material, in which case

Lecture Notes: Oncology, 2nd edition. By M. Bower and J. Waxman. Published 2010 by Blackwell Publishing Ltd.

Table 32.1 Types of asbestos and cancer risk.

Type	Colour	Morphology	Usage	Cancer risk	Location of mining
Crocidolite	Blue	Amphibole needles	10%	+++	South Africa, Australia
Chrysotile	White	Serpentine corkscrew	85%	+	Canada
Amosite	Brown	Amphibole needles	5%	++	South Africa

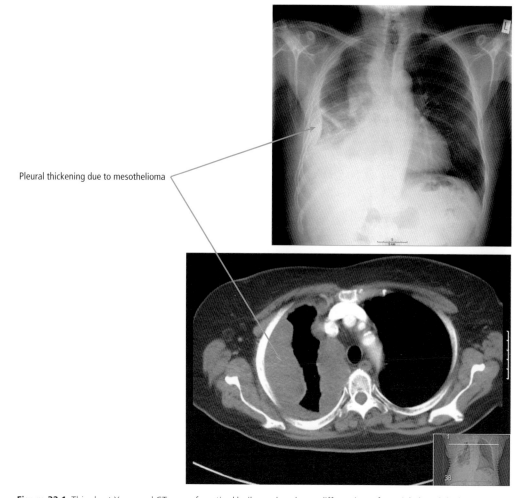

Pleural thickening due to mesothelioma

Figure 32.1 This chest X-ray and CT scan of a retired boiler-maker shows diffuse circumferential pleural thickening of the right hemithorax, extending to the mediastinal pleura. In addition there is substantial volume loss of the right hemithorax. The appearances are due to mesothelioma.

video-assisted thoracic screening may be required. Recurrent effusions are a dramatic problem for patients, and the intervention of a thoracic surgeon may be required to strip the pleura and provide an effective pleurodesis.

Treatment

Unfortunately, the majority of patients with mesothelioma present with incurable disease. Treatment options are limited. Chemotherapy is generally ineffective, with response rates in the order of less than 10% although newer combinations of cisplatinum and permetrexed offer promise. Radiation therapy may be helpful in controlling pain and is often given to pleural biopsy track sites to prevent the tumour growing down these channels. Multiple pleurodeses are often required, with installation into the pleural cavities of materials such as talc, tetracycline and bleomycin. There have been times when cytokine treatment was thought to be effective, with interferon being given into the thoracic cavity. This has, however, not proven to be a successful treatment option.

Prognosis

Unfortunately, the outlook for patients with mesothelioma is poor, with survival for patients with advanced disease ranging between 6 and 18 months.

New treatment

Recently, responses have been reported for pemetrexed, a dihydrofolate reductase inhibitor, and reductase. This is likely to become the standard. A 2009 analysis of survival in mesothelioma patients assessed 523 patients and defined prognosis according to four risk groups, but for all these groups the median progression-free survival ranged from 2.1 to 5.3 months, an indication of how poorly responsive to chemotherapy mesothelioma is.

Mesothelioma patients have high circulating levels of vascular endothelial growth factor (VEGF), and mesothelioma tissue stains strongly positively for VEGF receptor 3. For this reason patients with mesothelioma have been treated with antibodies to VEGF, such as bevacizumab, and with angiogenesis inhibitors, such as thalidomide. Bevacizumab, a recombinant monoclonal antibody to VEGF, has not been effective but agents such as thalidomide have led to disease stabilization in patients with progressive mesothelioma. Approximately 25% of patients have stable disease for a period of more than six months as a result of treatment with thalidomide. Sorafenib, a multikinase inhibitor of VEGF receptor and platelet-derived growth factor receptors, has led to responses in heavily pretreated patients.

Mesothelioma is an awful tumour to have and there is limited hope for new therapeutic strategies. The one true hope that exists is in the reduction of risk to workers, which is little compensation for those currently suffering as a result of the global epidemic.

Chapter 33

Haematological cancers

Louis Leakey found possibly the oldest hominid malignant tumour in 1932 in the remains of either a *Homo erectus* or an *Australopithecus*. This tumour was suggestive of a Burkitt's lymphoma, although that nomenclature was certainly not in use then. The leukaemias, lymphomas and myeloma are amongst the success stories in cancer treatment, with major advances in the second half of the 20th century. Cancer chemotherapy started with the treatment of these malignancies in the 1940s, following the demonstration by Alfred Gilman and Louis Goodman at Yale of lymphoma regression in mice with nitrogen mustard and their treatment of

the first patient in 1944. Shortly afterwards, Sidney Farber at Harvard began to use folate antagonists in children with acute leukaemia, and in 1947 he reported temporary remissions with aminopterin. Since that era, when childhood acute leukaemia was universally fatal, the long-term remission rate has risen to over 80%. Perhaps because of this success, medical oncologists and haematologists often fight over the management of haematological malignancies in the UK.

The leukaemias, lymphomas and myeloma are discussed in more detail in the following four chapters.

Lecture Notes: Oncology, 2nd edition. By M. Bower and J. Waxman. Published 2010 by Blackwell Publishing Ltd.

Chapter 34

The leukaemias

Epidemiology and pathogenesis

Leukaemias are relatively common with a preponderance of men affected. In the UK, the Office of National Statistics recently registered 4229 male and 3008 female leukaemia patients, with 2492 male and 1858 female deaths annually. The leukaemias are described generally as either acute or chronic. The main variants are lymphoid and myeloid leukaemia, which account for almost 95% of leukaemia. Acute lymphoid leukaemia is marginally more common than acute myeloid leukaemia (AML). Acute lymphoblastic leukaemia (ALL) is far more common in childhood than AML, and in adults approximately 80% of all the acute leukaemias are myeloid. Patients with Down's syndrome are at increased risk of leukaemia, as are patients with certain other conditions with a chromosomal basis, such as Klinefelter's syndrome, Fanconi's syndrome and ataxia telangiectasia.

The biology of leukaemia has been studied intensively over the last 20 years. With this investigation, the idea of a monoclonal origin of leukaemias has developed. The leukaemic clone is thought to have a survival advantage over normal haematological cells. One of the first leukaemias to be characterized at a molecular level was chronic myeloid

leukaemia (CML), where there is a fusion between chromosomes 9 and 22 that juxtaposes the BCR and ABL genes, which is observed cytogenetically as the 'Philadelphia' chromosome. This molecular abnormality may be seen in other haematological cells, such as platelet and red cell precursors. The protein product of a fusion gene may have aberrant function. For example, the BCR-ABL protein is thought to provide protection from chemotherapy drugs by interfering with apoptosis.

Other hybrid genes of interest occur in the leukaemias. For example, acute promyelocytic leukaemias (APMLs) are characterized by a translocation between chromosomes 15 and 17. The resultant fusion gene is formed between part of the PML gene and the retinoic acid alpha receptor gene, RARA. This hybrid gene interacts with chromosomal histone deacetylase complexes. Treatment with retinoic acid leads to dissociation of this complex and a transient remission of the leukaemia. Some examples of the fusion genes seen in leukaemia are described in Table 34.1.

Point mutations and gene deletions are also seen in leukaemias involving oncogenes such as p53 and RAS. P53 mutations are seen in ALL and blast crisis of CML, and N-RAS and c-KIT mutations are found in AML. It should be noted that the predominant molecular change in leukaemia is chromosomal translocation. This is in contrast with solid tumours, where the predominant changes are gene deletions and amplifications.

Lecture Notes: Oncology, 2nd edition. By M. Bower and J. Waxman. Published 2010 by Blackwell Publishing Ltd.

Table 34.1 Chromosomal abnormalities and their products.

Abnormalities	Disease	Fusion gene
Altered transcription regulators		
t(12;21)	ALL	*TEL/AML1*
t(8;21)	AML	*AML1/ETO*
t(15;17)	APML	*PML/RARA*
Activated kinases		
t(9:22)	CML, ALL	*BCR/ABL*
t(5;12)	CMML	*TEL/PDGFRB*

Table 34.2 The FAB classification of acute leukaemia.

M0	Acute myeloid leukaemia with minimal evidence of differentiation
M1	Acute myeloid leukaemia without maturation
M2	Acute myeloid leukaemia with maturation
M3	Acute promyelocytic leukaemia
M4	Acute myelomonocytic leukaemia
M5	Acute monocytic leukaemia
M6	Acute erythroleukaemia
M7	Acute megakaryoblastic leukaemia
L1	Small, monomorphic
L2	Large heterogeneous
L3	Large homogeneous (Burkitt)

Although there is a greater understanding of the molecular biology of leukaemia, the reason for the genetic changes observed is not known. The exceptions are those rare leukaemias that occur in the context of exposure to radiation or as secondary events following chemotherapy. Such secondary leukaemias are commonly associated with chromosome 5 and 7 abnormalities (see Figure 3.11).

Presentation

The presentation of patients with acute leukaemia is remarkable in its dramatic onset. It is usual to obtain a history that dates back only a few days, with features of anaemia, thrombocytopenia and leucopenia, although some people date their symptoms back for much longer periods. Chronic leukaemia may be diagnosed as an incidental finding, for example when a blood count is performed as part of a routine screen for another medical problem. Patients with chronic leukaemia may have abdominal discomfort due to splenomegaly or present with anaemia or lymphadenopathy. Such presentations generally tend to be insidious; this is particularly the case for chronic lymphocytic leukaemia (CLL). The situation is a little different for CML, which progresses from a chronic to an accelerated to a blast phase. The diagnosis can be made at any point in this clinical course.

Investigations and classification

The diagnosis of acute leukaemia is made by an examination of the peripheral blood and bone marrow (see Plates 34.1–34.3). In ALL, a lumbar puncture will be performed in order to investigate the possibility of CNS infiltration. Two common cytochemical stains are used to distinguish between acute myeloid and acute lymphoblastic leukaemias. These are the Sudan black, which is usually positive in AML and negative in ALL, and the periodic acid–Schiff (PAS) test, which is usually positive in ALL and negative in AML. The PAS stain is outmoded and has been largely replaced by immunophenotyping.

The classification of acute leukaemias usually follows the French–American–British (FAB) classification, which essentially describes the degree of differentiation and maturation. The myelogenous leukaemias are described as M1 to M7, and acute leukaemias as L1 to L3 (Table 34.2).

Immunophenotyping is also carried out in suspected acute lymphoblastic leukaemias, where the presence of B- and T-cell markers is sought out. More than 70% of adult acute lymphocytic leukaemias are of B-cell origin. Following immunophenotyping, cytogenic and molecular analysis is carried out in order to define chromosomal and molecular abnormalities, which provide prognostic information. Cytogenetic analysis is useful in the diagnosis of CML but may not be particularly helpful in CLL.

The 8;21 translocation in AML is associated with a good prognosis and occurs in about 8% of patients. The inversion or reciprocal translocation t(16;16) of chromosome 16 is associated with the M4 phenotype and again confers a favourable

Table 34.3 Chronic lymphocytic leukaemias.

B cell	T cell
B-cell chronic lymphocytic leukaemia/small lymphocytic lymphoma	T-cell chronic lymphocytic leukaemia (large granular lymphocytic leukaemia)
B-cell prolymphocytic leukaemia	T-cell prolymphocytic leukaemia
Hairy-cell leukaemia and variant	Adult T-cell leukaemia/lymphoma
Splenic marginal zone lymphoma, including splenic lymphoma with villous lymphocytes	Leukaemic phase of mycosis fungoides/Sézary syndrome
Leukaemic phase of mantle cell lymphoma	
Leukaemic phase of follicular lymphoma	
Leukaemic phase of lymphoplasmacytoid lymphoma	

response. Translocation with an 11q23 breakpoint is a poor prognostic feature. The presence of the Philadelphia chromosome is found in about 5% of childhood and 25% of adult ALL, and is thought to perhaps indicate transformation from a chronic myeloid leukaemia phase: this is an adverse prognostic feature. Chronic lymphocytic leukaemia (Table 34.3 and see Plates 34.4–34.6) is a tumour of B-cell origin in 95% of patients.

Cytogenetic changes are described in up to 80% of patients with CLL. Although there is no particular pattern that emerges to characterize this leukaemia, five or six abnormalities are usually observed. Trisomy 12, for example, the most common cytogenetic abnormality, is found in just one-third of patients. Patients with CLL are classified using a number of different systems, most of which are helpful in describing survival related to lymphocytosis, lymph node involvement and the presence or absence of anaemia or thrombocytopenia.

Treatment

The management of acute leukaemia is complex. It requires psychological support of the individual and of the family, and active and urgent treatment, particularly for the acute leukaemias. Initial treatment involves attempts to stabilize the patient by transfusion of red cells and platelets, combined with treatment of infection by antibiotics to limit the complications that may occur with the initiation of chemotherapy. These mainly revolve around the tumour lysis syndrome. Rehydration is required, and the patient is started on allopurinol to prevent the metabolic abnormalities that are described in detail in Chapter 46 of this book.

The chemotherapy that is given to patients with leukaemia has evolved as a result of many clinical trials over very many years, involving the Medical Research Council (MRC) in the UK, and the Cancer and Leukaemia Group B in the USA. The mainstay of induction chemotherapy in adult has been the use of daunorubicin and cytosine arabinoside given in a daily schedule, the dosage and duration of which is varied and repeated upon recovery of haematological parameters.

During treatment, patients require supportive therapies with blood products such as platelets and red cells. Platelet support is given to keep platelet counts above 10×10^9/l, which limits the risk of spontaneous haemorrhage. There is a risk of immunization against platelets, which may require human leucocyte antigen (HLA) matched transfusions rather than random donor platelet transfusion. Patients are of course at risk from neutropenic sepsis, which is treated with intravenous antibiotics. Prolonged neutropenia may be associated with fungal infection. In the context of persistent fever, particularly following transplantation, antifungal therapy is instituted. CT scanning may be appropriate in order to diagnose *Aspergillus* pneumonia. There is little evidence to suggest that any prophylactic antifungal treatment is of value, but randomized studies have shown that prophylaxis with antibiotics such as co-trimoxazole reduces the risk of *Pneumocystis* infection.

With recovery of the marrow, a further bone marrow examination is carried out. The majority of patients will have entered complete remission just before the second course of chemotherapy. Generally, four to six cycles of treatment are given in all, and this may be followed by post-remission treatment using an allogenic autologous stem cell transplant. These approaches are used in younger patients who have entered their first remission. Approximately 50–55% of patients who receive a transplant will be cured, but there is no evidence of better survival after transplantation in the good-prognosis patients.

The management of patients in transplant programmes is, of course, highly specialized, and medical training is focused on the recognition of the problems associated with profound and prolonged immunosuppression. The management of transplant patients has completely changed in recent years, because of the availability of recombinant growth factors. The use of granulocyte colony-stimulating factor (G-CSF) in transplant programmes has reduced the period of profound neutropenia such that the average duration of stay on a transplant ward has decreased from 28 to 17 days.

The management of chronic phase CML has evolved over the years from the use of single-agent alkylating agents, such as busulfan and hydroxyurea, to the use of interferon alpha and then allogeneic stem cell transplantation. Real hopes of cure came with the application of transplant programmes to CML. In the last few years, the introduction of imatinib (Glevec), a novel compound that acts to inhibit the tyrosine kinase activity of the BCR-ABL oncoprotein, has been most encouraging. Between 80% and 90% of patients respond to imatinib. In about half of these responding patients, a cytogenic response is also seen. There have been no serious adverse side effects from treatment with this agent, which offers a dramatic improvement over conventional therapy. Unfortunately, late relapses do occur, although at present we do not know the median duration of response.

CLL may be an entirely indolent disease with an excellent prognosis, and for many patients treatment may not be necessary. Therapy, when it is required, is similar to treatment given for low-grade lymphoma, with single-agent chlorambucil, steroids and occasionally combination therapy, all being helpful.

Treatment of recurrent disease

Although 50% of patients with good-prognosis acute leukaemia survive, the majority of patients still die. Relapse generally occurs within the first two years. Patients are usually re-treated with chemotherapy, with a 50% chance of re-entering remission and a 10% chance of cure. It is usual in these situations to use a different induction drug regimen, which is frequently more intensive, with a greater risk of treatment complications and death. Recurrence in chronic leukaemia may require stem cell transplantation, but this is not the practice for CLL.

Leukaemia in young children

Acute lymphocytic leukaemia is the commonest childhood leukaemia. Overall, the prospects for cure are very good, with a chance in excess of 80% of a sustained remission. The treatment of acute childhood leukaemia owes a great debt to the MRC-organized trials, which have examined issues such as the duration of therapy both for induction and maintenance, the need for cranial irradiation to prevent central nervous system relapse and the value of the individual drugs within the treatment programmes. Because of the high likelihood of a cure, recent clinical trials have concentrated on trying to moderate the side effects of treatment, and these are particularly important in limiting neurological toxicity, such as the effects upon intelligence, personality and pituitary function, and the effects on growth and fertility.

New treatment

In many ways, the future is 'here and now' for leukaemia. The treatment of CML has recently been transformed by the development of imatinib. Imatinib binds to the BCR-ABL protein, inhibiting its kinase activity and effectively controlling disease driven by this kinase. Remissions in CML are seen with clearance of the Philadelphia chromosome, as shown by cytogenetic analysis. Imatinib resistance emerges as a consequence of mutations in the kinase domains of BCR-ABL and new inhibitors including dasatinib and nilotinib, which are more potent, may overcome imatinib resistance. In other leukaemias where there is a major genetic base, such as those arising in the context of Fanconi's anaemia, haematopoietic stem cells using target effectors may offer hope for cure. Haematological malignancies offer a solid chance for targeted delivery of molecular therapies, with the possibility that naked DNA strategies or interfering mRNA therapeutic approaches may reach their target and help us cure leukaemia.

One of the major complications of transplantation is the development of graft versus host disease (GVHD), which is associated with a significant morbidity and mortality rate. New drugs to suppress GVHD have been developed over the last decade including sirolimus, tacrolimus and mycophenolate. Sirolimus, also known as rapamycin, was first discovered as a product of the bacterium *Streptomyces hygroscopicus* in a soil sample from Rapa Nui, one of the Easter Islands. Both sirolimus and tacrolimus inhibit mTOR (mammalian target of rapamycin), which is a cellular protein kinase that acts as a common step in many signal transduction pathways.

There have been major advances in cytogenetics and molecular biology, and these have been applied to leukaemia and are a significant aid to diagnosis, and define prognosis. One of the challenges in this area is in defining new markers for AML, where 50% of patients lack a characteristic cytogenetic signature.

Chapter 35

Hodgkin's disease

Epidemiology and pathogenesis

Hodgkin's disease is a relatively uncommon tumour, affecting approximately 1600 people each year in UK. Currently, there are about 310 deaths annually, including, in 2002, the original Albus Dumbledore actor Richard Harris. More men than women present with Hodgkin's disease, and there is a bimodal age distribution with peaks in the third and seventh decades. Little is known of the risk factors for the development of Hodgkin's disease, although there are minor associations with Down's syndrome and smoking. Geographical clustering has been noted, and there have been a few familial cases of Hodgkin's disease. Hodgkin's disease is also associated with sarcoidosis. The Epstein–Barr virus (EBV) genome is found incorporated within Reed–Sternberg cells, but we do not know for certain whether this virus is a causal agent for Hodgkin's disease. The Reed–Sternberg cell is pathognomonic for the diagnosis of Hodgkin's lymphoma and is thought to originate from lymphocytes affected by EBV. In HIV there is a tenfold increase in Hodgkin's disease. There is significant interest in the origins of the Reed–Sternberg cells, which are large cells with multinucleated or bilobed nuclei that according to histopathologists look like owl's eyes (Figure 35.1). Reed–Sternberg cells have a specific immunophenotype, express-ing CD15 and CD30, but not expressing CD20 or CD45. Immunoglobulin gene expression is mutated within Reed–Sternberg cells, and there are functional rearrangements that lead to abnormal immune function. This leads to defective apoptosis, prolonged B-cell survival and, ultimately, to the development of Hodgkin's disease. EBV proteins remain present in about 40% of Reed–Sternberg cells and there is a three-fold increased risk of Hodgkin's disease following infectious mononucleosis (glandular fever). This possibly suggests that EBV is a future target for immunotherapy.

Presentation

The presentation of Hodgkin's disease is usually with enlarged lymph nodes. This is generally painless and may be accompanied by constitutional symptoms that include profound sweating, sufficient to drench bedclothes, fevers greater than 38°C and weight loss exceeding 10% of body mass. These constitutional symptoms are prognostically important. There are other non-specific symptoms relating to the presentation of Hodgkin's disease, including alcohol-related pain and skin itching.

Investigations

In clinic, a careful history should be obtained and an examination made. Investigations will be organized which include a full blood count and erythrocyte sedimentation rate (ESR), liver and

Lecture Notes: Oncology, 2nd edition. By M. Bower and J. Waxman. Published 2010 by Blackwell Publishing Ltd.

RS cell

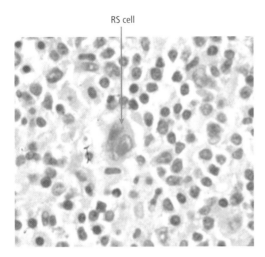

Figure 35.1 Histopathological sample demonstrating a Reed–Sternberg cell (a large binucleated cell with prominent nucleoli surrounded by a clear space or lacunae) diagnostic of Hodgkin's disease.

Mediastinal mass

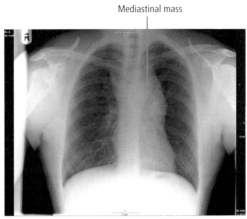

Figure 35.2 Hodgkin's disease with a mediastinal mass. This chest X-ray of a 20-year-old male student shows infilling of the aortopulmonary window and a wide left paratracheal stripe due to mediastinal lymph node enlargement from Hodgkin's disease.

renal function tests, a chest X-ray, CT scan of the chest and abdomen, bone marrow aspiration and trephine biopsy. The patient will be reviewed in outpatients with the results of these tests. Admission will then be organized for a biopsy of the lymph glands. The purpose of these investigations is to define the clinical stage of the disease and the purpose of the biopsy to make a histological diagnosis. The examination of bone marrow is commonly undertaken in the investigation of patients with Hodgkin's disease. Less than 5% of men and women with Hodgkin's disease have bone marrow involvement, however, and this is generally only present in patients with advanced tumours of stages greater than IIB. There are strong arguments against carrying out this assessment except in advanced-stage patients.

The investigation of Hodgkin's disease is a recapitulation of the history of imaging in the UK. Plain X-rays (Figure 35.2) remain helpful, but approaches such as lymphography have been replaced by CT and magnetic resonance imaging (MRI). There are significant errors in the accuracy of both CT and MRI in defining hepatic and splenic involvement, with an error rate of up to 60% in the specificity for indicating involvement by lymphoma. Staging laparotomy has long been aban-

doned as an investigative tool, and the saga of the downside to staging diagnostic splenectomy continues to this day. It includes an ever-enlarging list of infection susceptibilities for which antibiotic therapy and immunization are recommended.

Pathology

Four different histological variants of Hodgkin's disease are described: nodular sclerosing, mixed cellularity, lymphocyte-predominant and lymphocyte-depleted Hodgkin's disease. Nodular sclerosing Hodgkin's disease is subclassified as grade I or II. Lymphocyte-predominant Hodgkin's disease is rare, constituting less than 5% of all histological phenotypes. The nodular sclerosing variant occurs in about 70% of all cases and is even more common in Hodgkin's disease affecting young women. The mixed cellularity variant is commonly associated with HIV-related malignancy and will often be diagnosed in infradiaphragmatic presentations of Hodgkin's disease.

Staging

The results of the staging investigations will help the clinician to determine the clinical stage of the Hodgkin's disease, and this in turn defines treatment. In stage I Hodgkin's disease, one lymph node or two contiguous lymph node groups are affected. In stage II disease, two non-contiguous lymph node groups on the same side of the diaphragm are affected. In stage III Hodgkin's disease, lymph node groups on both sides of the diaphragm are affected. In stage IV disease, there is extranodal spread to the liver, lung or bone but rarely to other sites.

The tumour is further classified as A or B. 'A' defines a lack of constitutional symptoms and 'B' indicates the presence of the constitutional symptoms of Hodgkin's disease. Finally, the staging is defined by use of the subscript 'S', which indicates splenic involvement, or 'E', which defines extension to involve extranodal tissue in direct apposition to an enlarged lymph node group.

Treatment and side effects

The purpose of staging is to define treatment groups. The current recommendations for treatment are as follows: stage I and IIA Hodgkin's disease is generally treated with radiation. The exceptions are where there is bulky lymphadenopathy or constitutional symptoms. In these instances, chemotherapy may be the preferred option. Stage IIB–IV disease is usually treated with combination chemotherapy.

Radiation

Radiation treatment is generally given according to two well-defined treatment plans. Lymphadenopathy above the diaphragm is treated with mantle radiation which includes the lymph node groups in the neck, axillae and chest to a total dosage of 3500 cGy given over a period of four to six weeks. Infradiaphragmatic radiation is generally given in the inverted Y distribution that includes the para-aortic and iliac nodal groups. Treatment is given to a total dosage of 3500 cGy over a four to six-week period.

Mantle radiotherapy may be complicated by radiation pneumonitis, which is characterized by a period of breathlessness and fever and responds to

steroids. It is invariably accompanied by loss of saliva production and oesophagitis. Infradiaphragmatic radiotherapy may be complicated by some minor bowel disturbance but generally is well tolerated. Radiation is usually avoided in children and adolescents as it may lead to gross growth disturbance. Infradiaphragmatic radiation may cause sterility. In patients with good-prognosis disease the radiation fields may be reduced to lower toxicity. Thus extended field or mini-mantle treatments may be prescribed in order to reduce radiotherapy toxicity.

Chemotherapy

Combination chemotherapy for Hodgkin's disease was introduced in the mid-1960s. The original treatment regimen, which has the acronym MOPP, combined mustine, vincristine (Oncovin), prednisone and procarbazine. These drugs are given intravenously and orally for two weeks and repeated every four weeks. Six cycles are administered. Treatment is associated with acute nausea and vomiting, sterility in 90% of males and 50% of females, and the development of second tumours in approximately 5% of patients.

Chemotherapy treatments have been modified over the years in order to reduce side effects. Six is a 'magic number' in oncology, and it is possible that four cycles of therapy are as effective as six cycles. The most frequently used current programme is called ABVD which combines adriamycin, bleomycin, vinblastine and dacarbazine. These drugs cause neither sterility nor second malignancies and are of obvious advantage in a disease where there is a high expectation of cure. Randomized trials have shown an equivalence of ABVD to standard therapy with MOPP and to hybrid therapies.

Haemopoietic stem cell transplantation

High-dosage chemotherapy with either bone marrow transplantation or peripheral blood stem cell support is a relatively new and toxic treatment for drug-resistant Hodgkin's disease. The most commonly applied current programme in the UK uses 'mini-BEAM' or BEAM chemotherapy. Treatment is accompanied by either peripheral blood stem cell or bone marrow transplantation. Morbidity is high, and in certain groups, such as those pretreated with mediastinal radiotherapy, mortality reaches up to 30%. Long-term remissions occur in up to 40% of patients. The rationale for first-line treatment with high-dose chemotherapy and bone marrow product support is absent. There are no randomized trials comparing such treatment programmes with conventional approaches for first-line treatment of Hodgkin's disease.

Prognosis

The results of treatment of Hodgkin's disease are considered to be one of the miracles of modern oncology, in that approximately 90% of patients with small-volume, early-stage disease are curable with radiation and between 40% and 60% of patients with advanced disease are curable with chemotherapy. A poorer prognosis results from the presence of bulk disease, constitutional symptoms or poor-prognosis histology. The patient who is 'cured' as a result of treatment is unfortunately at risk from late relapse; this may occur 15–30 years after diagnosis. This risk of a late relapse is small and largely confined to lymphocyte-predominant Hodgkin's disease.

Complications of chemotherapy

Hodgkin's disease is a tumour with significant cure rates, occurring in young people with an expectation of prolonged survival. This leads to a significant onus for providing a therapy that is without major long-term toxicity. Conventional chemotherapy and radiotherapy for Hodgkin's disease using alkylating agents is associated with the development of second tumours. The incidence of second tumours reaches approximately 5%, with staggering increases in the rates of acute leukaemias and lymphomas. The leukaemias present early, two to four years after the completion of chemotherapy. The solid tumours, such as breast, colorectal and lung cancer, occur late, sometimes 15–20 years after diagnosis. Sterility is also an important consequence of treatment with any alkylating agent-containing regimen, reaching up to 80% in males and 50% in females.

New treatment

The most important prospect for Hodgkin's disease remains the development of immunization programmes for EBV. EBV antigens are present in up to 40% of patients with Hodgkin's disease, and it is thought that this herpes virus might be a significant cause for the development of this 'B-cell' malignancy. Vaccination strategies have been developed, and it is hoped that these may lead to the elimination of a proportion of cases of Hodgkin's lymphoma. Other attempts have been made to develop cytotoxic lymphocyte-based immunotherapy for Hodgkin's disease. They have, however, not been successful, because of the facility of EBV to use multiple strategies to avoid detection. Attempts at immunotherapy have included downregulation of immunodominant antigens, together with cytokine secretion.

Combination chemotherapy regimens using hybrid treatment programmes have been investigated for the treatment of advanced Hodgkin's disease for the reason that, in this group of patients, a significant proportion of patients remain incurable. Although some studies have shown a small advantage to such hybrid regimens, the treatment carries the disadvantage of increased long-term toxicity from the alkylating agent-containing regimens. A recent trial of 850 patients which compared ABVD with MOPP/ABVD has shown an identical complete remission and failure-free survival rate.

Where there is predominant CD20 expression, there are prospects for treatment with immunotherapy directed to this surface antigen, such as rituximab, which in a recent study has shown a response rate of 86% in a small group of patients.

Chapter 36

Non-Hodgkin's lymphoma

Epidemiology and pathogenesis

Non-Hodgkin's lymphoma is relatively common. In the UK there are just over 4500 deaths each year and 10 500 patients presenting with this condition. There have been many descriptions of the pathological classification of this disease. Rather than achieving clarity, however, most have tended to confuse the situation further because of their complexity. In terms of clinical practice, the most significant divisions are into high- and low-grade lymphoma.

High-grade lymphoma is much more common than low-grade lymphoma. About 1000 people with low-grade lymphoma present each year. Slightly more men are affected than women. Lymphomas arise from lymphoid organs or lymphatic tissue associated with other systems that contain lymphatic tissue. The latter, the so-called 'extranodal lymphomas', constitute up to 30% of all non-Hodgkin's lymphoma.

There have been extraordinary advances in the molecular biology of lymphoma, and from this we have begun to understand some of the aetiological features involved in this condition. It is thought that Epstein–Barr virus infection is linked to the development of African Burkitt's lymphoma,

certain other B-cell lymphomas, HIV-associated lymphomas and almost all lymphomas associated with the immunosuppression consequent to the transplantation of heart, kidneys and lung.

The human T-cell leukaemia lymphoma virus type 1 (HTLV-1) causes adult T-cell lymphoma and leukaemia and both are endemic in the Caribbean and Japan. Other viruses associated with the development of lymphoma include hepatitis C and human herpesvirus 8 (HHV-8). *Helicobacter* infection in the stomach leads to a proliferation of gastric lymphoid tissue and the development of low-grade mucosa-associated tumours. Such tumours may respond to *H. pylori* eradication treatment, but unfortunately they may evolve into classical lymphoma despite eradication.

Presentation

Patients present with nodal enlargement which may be accompanied by constitutional symptoms including weight loss, sweating and fever. These symptoms – where weight loss is in excess of 10% of pre-morbid weight, sweating is sufficient to drench night clothes, and fever exceeds 38°C – are described as 'B' symptoms. 'B' symptoms are less common in high-grade lymphoma than low-grade malignancies. Patients with such symptoms should be referred to specialist centres where the chance for survival and the quality of survival are significantly better than in peripheral non-

Lecture Notes: Oncology, 2nd edition. By M. Bower and J. Waxman. Published 2010 by Blackwell Publishing Ltd.

specialist centres. The care of patients with lymphoma should be by oncologists or haematologists, depending upon the specialist interests of the clinicians.

Staging and grading

In outpatients, a careful history is obtained from the patient who is then examined. The investigations organized should include a blood count, renal and hepatic function tests, chest X-ray, bone marrow aspiration and trephine, and CT scan of the abdomen and chest (Figures 36.1–36.4). These investigations are done in order to define the extent of the disease. From these investigations the clinical staging is obtained. This is defined as follows:

• Stage I: disease confined to one lymph node or two contiguous lymph node groups
• Stage II: disease on one side of the diaphragm in lymph node groups that are separate
• Stage III: disease on both sides of the diaphragm
• Stage IV: extranodal spread of the lymphoma.

Preliminary investigations having been organized, the patient should then proceed to a lymph node biopsy. Lymph node biopsies used to be required to describe the architectural arrangement of the tumour. In modern times, they are no longer

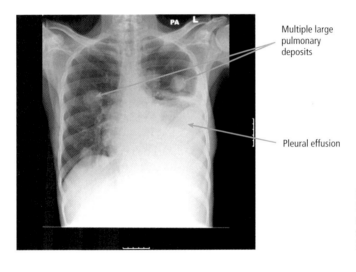

Multiple large pulmonary deposits

Pleural effusion

Figure 36.1 Chest radiograph showing multiple large pulmonary nodules and a left sided pleural effusion due to diffuse large B-cell non-Hodgkin's lymphoma.

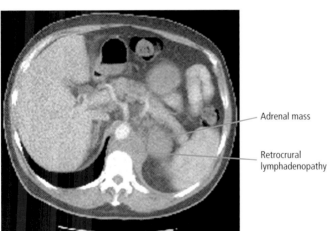

Adrenal mass

Retrocrural lymphadenopathy

Figure 36.2 CT scan showing extensive left retrocrural adenopathy and a left adrenal mass due to high-grade B-cell non-Hodgkin's lymphoma.

Extradural mass displacing and compressing spinal cord

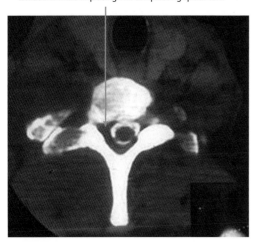

Figure 36.3 Spinal cord deviation and compression at T1 vertebra by an extradural mass of high grade non-Hodgkin's lymphoma.

Liver   Spleen

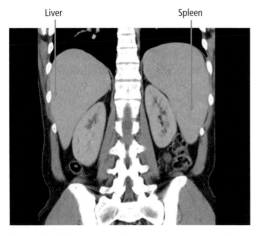

Figure 36.4 CT scan showing hepatosplenomegally due to follicular non-Hodgkin's lymphoma.

always considered to be necessary. Sufficient material can often be obtained from core needle biopsies to define the pathological diagnosis. There are many classification systems for non-Hodgkin's lymphoma, which include the WHO classification (Table 36.1), the Kiel classification, the Working Formulation and the Revised European and American Lymphoma Classification (REAL).

For the purposes of defining treatment, the most practical classification, however, is to describe the tumour as being low or high grade. A low-grade tumour tends to have a follicular nature and to contain relatively inactive cells. A high-grade tumour contains cells that have a high index of mitotic activity and there is no follicular structure to the lymph node. An intermediate-grade tumour, which generally behaves clinically like a high-grade tumour, has some of the features of both high- and low-grade tumours. There are variant lymphomas, such as mantle cell and Burkitt's lymphomas, which are clinical entities with poor prognosis.

Many modern techniques have been applied to the pathological diagnosis of lymphoma. Immunophenotyping using monoclonal antibodies is the most helpful, firstly, in initially distinguishing between a lymphoma or a carcinoma by using antibodies to the leukocyte common antigen (CD45), and secondly, in defining the lymphoma by using antibodies that are specific for B or T lymphocytes, such as CD20 or CD4, CD2 and CD3. T-cell receptor and immunoglobulin gene rearrangements are also carried out, and are helpful in describing tumour clonality. Fluorescent *in situ* hybridization is also useful. This is because of the observed cytogenetic abnormalities that are relatively specific for non-Hodgkin's lymphoma. Some of these are outlined in Table 36.2.

Treatment

Low-grade non-Hodgkin's lymphoma

Low-grade tumours are generally disseminated at diagnosis. If they are localized, that is stage I, small bulk, peripheral and without B symptoms, the treatment should be radiotherapy. For stage II–IV disease, treatment is with chemotherapy with oral alkylating agents such as chlorambucil or with an intravenous chemotherapy programme known as CVP which uses cyclophosphamide, vincristine and prednisone. Chlorambucil has very little early toxicity but at high total dosages causes sterility, secondary myelodysplasia (MDS) and acute myeloid leukaemia (AML). CVP leads to hair loss, but apart from this it is without significant morbidity. Both regimens may be associated with marrow toxicity which results in admissions with neutropenic

Table 36.1 World Health Organization (WHO) classification of lymphomas. (More common lymphomas are shown in italics.)

B-cell neoplasms	T-cell and NK-cell neoplasms
Precursor B-cell neoplasms	**Precursor T-cell neoplasms**
B-lymphoblastic leukaemia/lymphoma	T-lymphoblastic leukaemia/lymphoma
Mature B-cell neoplasms	**Mature T-cell and NK-cell neoplasms**
B-cell chronic lymphocytic leukaemia/small lymphocytic lymphoma	T-cell prolymphocytic leukaemia/lymphoma
B-cell prolymphocytic leukaemia	T-cell large granular cell lymphocytic leukaemia
Lymphoplasmacytic lymphoma	NK-cell leukaemia
Splenic marginal zone B-cell lymphoma	Adult T-cell leukaemia/lymphoma (± villous lymphocytes)
Hairy cell leukaemia	Extranodal NK-/T-cell lymphoma, nasal type
Plasma cell myeloma/plasmacytoma	Enteropathic-type intestinal T-cell lymphoma
Extranodal marginal zone lymphoma	Hepatosplenic γ/δ T-cell lymphoma
(of MALT type)	Subcutaneous panniculitis-like T-cell lymphoma
Nodal marginal zone lymphoma	Mycosis fungoides/Sézary syndrome
Follicular lymphoma	Primary cutaneous anaplastic large cell lymphoma
Mantle cell lymphoma	Peripheral T-cell lymphoma, not otherwise
Diffuse large B-cell lymphoma	characterized
Subtypes: mediastinal (thymic),	Angioimmunoblastic T-cell lymphoma
intravascular, primary effusion lymphoma	Systemic anaplastic large cell lymphoma
Burkitt's lymphoma/Burkitt's cell leukaemia	
MALT, mucosa-associated lymphoid tissue.	

sepsis or with thrombocytopenic bleeding. The monoclonal antibody rituximab that targets CD20 is frequently added to these cytotoxic agents.

Patients with stage I non-Hodgkin's lymphoma have a 70–95% chance of cure with radiotherapy. The patient with disseminated low-grade lymphoma is not cured by treatment. Although 85% of patients achieve a complete response to therapy, this response is transient. After a median period of 18 months, the patient relapses and requires re-treatment. The average patient has four such episodes of response and relapse. Finally after a median period of 7.5 years, there is transformation to high-grade lymphoma.

High-grade and intermediate-grade non-Hodgkin's lymphoma

Paradoxically, high-grade and intermediate-grade lymphomas are more likely to be confined to one lymph node group than low-grade tumours and are curable. Stage I disease may be treated with radiotherapy. Some clinicians will then proceed to treat with adjuvant chemotherapy. Patients with small bulk stage I non-Hodgkin's lymphoma have a 95% chance of cure with radiation, and this chance is only minimally improved with chemotherapy. If the stage I disease is bulky, chemotherapy alone may be given. Treatment is with the R-CHOP regimen, and there is little evidence that more complex regimens add to the chance of cure. Of all patients, 70–80% enter remission, which is sustained in about 40–60% of cases. CHOP consists of cyclophosphamide, doxorubicin (hydroxydaunorubicin), vincristine (oncovin) and prednisolone and was introduced in the 1970s. It has remained the gold standard therapy for many high-grade lymphomas ever since with the addition of rituximab for CD20-expressing lymphomas in the 1990s. In 1993 a pivotal trial compared CHOP with several newer chemotherapy regimens with less memorable but more exotic names (e.g. m-BACOD, ProMACE-CytaBOM, MACOP-B); CHOP emerged as the regimen with the least toxicity but similar efficacy.

Table 36.2 Recurrent chromosomal translocations in non-Hodgkin's lymphoma subtypes, resulting in oncogene dysregulation.

Histology	Translocation	Alteration of gene function	Mechanism/features of translocation	Frequency
Follicular lymphoma	t(14;18)(q32;21)	Upregulation of BCL2 (inhibitor of apoptosis)	BCL2 relocates to IgH locus. Error in physiological IgH rearrangement. Seen rarely in normal B cells	80%
Burkitt's lymphoma	t(8;14)(q24;q32); t(2;8)(p12;q24); t(8;22)(q24;q11)	Upregulation of c-MYC (transcription factor for cell cycle progression/proliferation)	c-myc relocates to IgH locus or to one of the light chain gene loci	100%
Mantle cell lymphoma	t(11;14)(q13;q32)	Upregulation of cyclin D1 (G1 cyclin)	Cyclin D1 relocates to IgH	>90%
Diffuse large B-cell lymphoma*	t(3;14)(q27;32) and several others involving 3q27	Deregulation of BCL6 (zinc finger transcription factor)	BCL6 relocates to IgH, IgL, IgK or one of many other non-Ig loci	30–40%
Extranodal marginal zone lymphoma (MALT)	t(11;18)(q21;q21)	Gene fusion of AP12 and MLT/MALT1 genes (AP12 is inhibitor of apoptosis)	Gene fusion	20–35%
Extranodal marginal zone lymphoma (MALT)	t(1;14)(q22;q32)	Deregulation of BCL10 (apoptosis regulatory protein)	BCL10 relocates to IgH locus	<5%
Lymphoplasmacytic lymphoma	t(9;14)(q13;q32)	Deregulation of PAX5 (paired homeobox transcription factor)	PAX5 relocates to IgH locus	50%
Anaplastic large cell lymphoma	t(2;5)(p23;q35) and others involving 2p23	Gene fusion of ALK (anaplastic lymphoma kinase, a receptor tyrosine kinase) and NPM (located at 5q35) or other gene malignant transforming capacity *in vitro* and *in vivo*	Gene fusion	ALK-NPM, 50% Others, 15%

*BCL2 (30%) and c-myc (10%) rearrangements are also frequently seen in diffuse large B-cell non-Hodgkin's lymphoma. Ig, immunoglobulin; MALT, mucosa-associated lymphoid tissue.

High-dose therapy

Patients with poor-prognosis lymphomas at presentation or with recurrent high-grade lymphomas may be considered for high-dose chemotherapy with auto- or allogeneic bone marrow or other stem cell support. These programmes may be linked with attempts to purge the marrow or peripheral blood stem cells of specific cell populations. Immunosuppression is required for patients receiving allografts. Prognosis depends on a number of risk factors. There is an associated mortality rate to these procedures that may exceed 10%.

New treatment

New agents have become available for the treatment of lymphoma. Amongst the most interesting are antibody treatments directed against B-cell antigens, such as rituximab. Rituximab is directed against CD20 and usually has very little toxicity apart from the possibility of a hypersensitivity response. It has been used mainly in the treatment of recurrent lymphoma. In more recent trials, however, rituximab has been prescribed as first-line therapy for patients with B-cell lymphomas. These trials have been successful, and rituximab in combination with chemotherapy is considered to be standard first-line treatment for patients with B-cell lymphomas. There are other anti-CD20, -CD40 and -CD8 antibody treatments, which show some promise and these have been combined with radioisotopes such as iodine-131. Vaccine trials using patient-specific immunization with immunoglobulin idiotype are also underway. There is new hope for lymphoma patients!

Chapter 37

Myeloma

Epidemiology and pathogenesis

Myeloma is a relatively common haematological malignancy affecting 3987 people each year in the UK, and leading to 2695 deaths per year. There is an equal sex distribution and an increasing incidence with age. The rate of myeloma is higher amongst black populations, and the disease is associated with industrial and radiation exposure.

Multiple myeloma is a B-cell neoplasm characterized by the proliferation of plasma cells that synthesize and secrete monoclonal immunoglobulins or fragments thereof. The molecular basis of the transformation that characterizes this tumour is not clearly known. Karyotypic abnormalities have been identified in up to 50% of myeloma patients, but there is no clear, unifying change that underlies this transformation. Several molecular events have been described. These involve 14q32 translocations, chromosome 13 deletion and fibroblast growth factor receptor 3 (FGFR3) activation. These abnormalities are seen in no more than 20% of all myeloma patients. The translocations that have been described mostly involve the switch rearrangements of the heavy chain locus with partner genes such as FGFR3. Mutations have been observed in tumour suppressor genes and abnormalities of expression in apoptosis-related genes

such as BCL-2. T cells secrete interleukin 6 (IL-6), which appears to be an essential growth factor for myeloma cells in culture. Excessive secretion of IL-6 occurs in myeloma and this may be a primary cause for the condition.

The destructive bone lesions that are seen in myeloma are thought to be due to dysregulation of the osteoprotegerin Rankl system. Rankl is the ligand for osteoprotegerin and is relaeased in myeloma by the malignant plasma cells and bone marrow stroma, leading to osteoclast activation and hence osteolysis. The osteolytic bone lesions of myeloma are best seen on plain X-rays rather than bone scans as they generally lack osteoblastic activity. They appear as punched-out lesions, including the classical 'pepper pot' appearance of the skull X-ray, and the bone breakdown releases calcium and may cause hypercalcaemia.

Presentation

Patients with myeloma often present in a dramatic fashion with significant bone pain due to the lytic lesions that characterize this disease (Figure 37.1). Vertebral collapse is often a feature of presentation, and this may lead to symptoms of cord compression. Patients with myeloma may present with symptoms of hypercalcaemia, which every medical student reading this chapter is able to describe. Hypercalcaemia can be one of the precipitating factors for renal failure commonly observed in myeloma. The other causes include amyloidosis

Lecture Notes: Oncology, 2nd edition. By M. Bower and J. Waxman. Published 2010 by Blackwell Publishing Ltd.

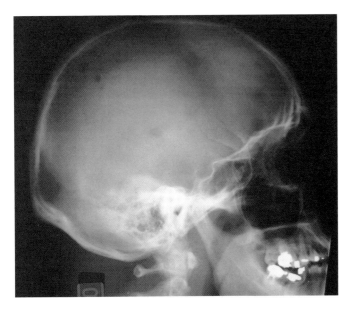

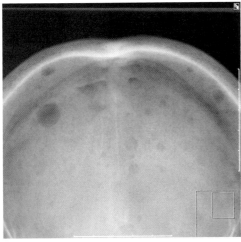

Figure 37.1 Skull radiograph of a 52-year-old man with multiple myeloma showing multiple, well-defined lucencies that are fairly uniform in size, unlike bone metastases which usually vary in size.

(AL amyloid containing immunoglobulin light chains), precipitation of Bence–Jones protein (urinary free light chain papprotein), direct infiltration and infection. An excess of immunoglobulin may cause the hyperviscosity syndrome, which is more common with an IgG myeloma than an IgM myeloma. This is explained by the fact that a far greater proportion of patients have IgG than have IgM myelomas, which represents just 0.5% of all myeloma cases.

The raised paraprotein levels may cause other problems, including peripheral neuropathy. Marrow infiltration with an excess of plasma cells leads to a decrease in numbers of other marrow constituents, causing anaemia, thrombocytopenia and neutropenia. This in turn has consequences for both the presentation and the clinical features of the disease as it evolves.

Investigations

The investigation of myeloma is relatively simple. It requires the examination of the peripheral blood, paraprotein levels, blood count, β_2-

microglobulin levels, renal function and calcium levels (see Plates 37.1 and 37.2), assessment of the bone marrow, examination of the urine for Bence–Jones protein urea and a skeletal survey. Bone scanning is of low diagnostic value in myeloma. Myeloma is staged, and the staging has prognostic value (Table 37.1). Two systems are used, that of Durie and Salmon and that of the Medical Research Council (MRC) (Tables 37.2 and 37.3).

Treatment

The initial treatment of myeloma requires stabilization of the patient and correction of renal function abnormalities and hypercalcaemia (Table 37.4). The patient is started on allopurinol and may require hydration or transfusion. Hypercalcaemia is treated with bisphosphonates, steroids and rehydration. Where there is significant bone pain, which is poorly responsive to opiates, radiotherapy may be required. A single fraction treatment will alleviate bone pain in approximately 80% of patients. Anaemia may require transfusion and significant hyperviscosity needs plasmaphoresis.

Chemotherapy for myeloma has a 50-year history, beginning with the use of alkylating agents such as melphalan and cyclosphosphamide. Nowadays, the initial treatment of multiple myeloma depends on the patient's age and co-morbidities. High-dose chemotherapy with hematopoietic stem cell transplantation has become the preferred treatment for patients under the age of 65. Prior to stem cell transplantation, these patients receive an initial course of induction chemotherapy. The

most common induction regimens used are thalidomide–dexamethasone, bortezomib-based regimens, and lenalidomide–dexamethasone. Unfortunately, many patients are older and frailer

Table 37.1 Diagnostic criteria for myeloma.

Major criteria	
I	Plasmacytoma or tissue biopsy
II	Bone marrow plasmacytosis >30%
III	Monoclonal (M) spike on electrophoresis:
	>35 g/l (IgG peaks)
	or>20 g/l (IgA peaks)
	*or*κ or λ light chain excretion >1.0 g/24 hours
Minor criteria	
	Distant metastases
a	Bone-marrow plasmacytosis 10–30%
b	M spike present but less than in major criteria
c	Lytic bone lesions
d	Normal immunoglobulin levels decreased:
	IgM < 0.05 g/l
	or IgA < 0.01 g/l
	or IgG < 0.60 g/l
	Diagnosis of myeloma requires a minimum of one major plus one minor criteria *or* three minor criteria
Diagnostic criteria for MGUS	
I	Monoclonal gammopathy
II	Bone marrow plasma cells <10%
III	Monoclonal (M) component level:
	IgG < 35 g/l
	or IgA < 20 g/l
	*or*κ or λ light chains <1.0 g/24 hours
IV	No overt bone lesions
V	No symptoms to suggest myeloma

MGUS, monoclonal gammapathy of uncertain significance.

Table 37.2 Durie and Salmon staging system for myeloma.

Cell mass category: Requirements:		High (stage III) One of A, B, C or D	Low (stage I) All of A, B, C and D	Intermediate (stage II)
Haemoglobin (pre-transfusion)	A	<85 g/dl%	>10 g/dl%	
Serum calcium	B	>12 mg%	Normal	Neither
M component	C	IgG >nbsp;7 g/dl%	<5 g/dl%	I or III
IgA >nbsp;5 g/dl%	<3 g/dl%			
Bence–Jones >12 g/day	<4 g/day			
Bone lesion on skeletal survey	D	Advanced lytic disease	None/solitary lesion	

Table 37.3 MRC staging system.

		Poor prognosis (stage III) A, C or B, C	Good prognosis (stage I) All of A, B, C and D	Intermediate (stage II) Not in I or III
Blood urea concentration	A	>10 mM/l	=8 mM/l	Not in I or III
Haemoglobin	B	=7.5 g/dl	>10.0 g/dl	Not in I or III
Performance status	C	Restricted activity	Minimal symptoms or asymptomatic	Not in I or III

Table 37.4 Southwest Oncology Group myeloma response criteria.

A. Responsive patients who satisfy all the following criteria are considered to have achieved definite objective improvement:

    1. A sustained decrease in the synthesis index of serum monoclonal protein to 25% or less of the pre-treatment value, and to less than 25 g/l on at least two measurements separated by 4 weeks. For IgA and Ig_3M proteins, the synthetic index is the same as the serum concentration. For IgG proteins of subclasses 1, 2 and 4, the synthetic index must be estimated using a nomogram

    2. A sustained decrease in 24-hour urine globulin to 10% or less of the pre-treatment value, and to less than 0.2 g/24 hours on at least two occasions separated by 4 weeks

    3. In all responsive patients the size and number of lytic skull lesions must not increase, and the serum calcium must remain normal. Correction of anaemia (haematocrit >27 vol%) and hypoalbuminaemia (>3.0 g/dl) is required if they are considered to be secondary to myeloma. With equivocal data (e.g. non-secretors or L-chain producers for whom the pre-treatment urine collection was lost), the following two points support the conclusion that an objective response has occurred

    4. Recalcification of lytic skull lesions

    5. Significant increments in depressed normal immunoglobulins (e.g. increments >200 mg/l IgM, >400 mg/l IgA, and >4000 mg/l IgG)

B. Improved patients show a decline in the serum M protein synthesis rate to less than 50%, but not less than 25%, of the pre-treatment value

C. Unresponsive patients fail to satisfy the criteria for responsive or improved patients

patients and here the standard of care has been chemotherapy with melphalan and prednisone. Bortezomib and lenalidomide are suitable treatments at relapse. Bortezomib inhibits proteosome, the cellular organelles that identify tagged proteins in the cytoplasm, and breaks them down. It is not quite clear how thalidomide and lenalidomide work but they seem to have both immunomodulatory and anti-angiogenic actions. Both are potent teratogens and it is essential that they are not prescribed to women who could become pregnant.

New treatment

Because myeloma is a clonal disease that expresses a unique surface immunoglobulin, it was thought possible that patients might mount an immune defense against these myeloma cells if they were somehow used as a vaccine. Myeloma cell/dendritic cell fusions have been examined as a vaccination strategy for multiple myeloma and have been found to induce myeloma-specific cell death. Similarly, antisense oligonucleotides have been shown to have some efficacy in patients with recurrent myeloma. *In vitro*, IL-6 causes the proliferation of myeloma cells, and a monoclonal antibody that blocks the IL-6 receptor is being used in trials as treatment for myeloma.

Chapter 38

Skin cancer

Cinema has wide-ranging influence on fashion trends and one of the most striking examples was the mid-20th century trend towards sun tanning. The fashion of the Victorian era was sun avoidance; the upper classes stayed pale in part to distinguish themselves from lower class workers who had to toil in the sun. Yet by the 1950s, the beach culture of southern California spread worldwide via the movies. The ill effects of chronic exposure to ultraviolet radiation on skin ageing are well demonstrated by Clint Eastwood. The carcinogenic effects of sunlight led to the removal of a basal cell carcinoma from the former actor, US President Ronald Reagan, whilst his eldest daughter Maureen Reagan died of melanoma.

The following two chapters discuss both non-melanoma skin tumours and melanomas.

Lecture Notes: Oncology, 2nd edition. By M. Bower and J. Waxman. Published 2010 by Blackwell Publishing Ltd.

Chapter 39

Non-melanoma skin tumours

Epidemiology and pathogenesis

Non-melanoma skin cancers probably comprise more than one-third of all cancers in the UK and have been described as a worldwide epidemic. The term includes two major types: basal cell carcinoma (BCC) and squamous cell carcinoma (SCC). Other less common non-melanoma skin cancers include Kaposi's sarcoma, cutaneous lymphoma and Merkel cell carcinoma. Despite their frequency, these tumours account for only 2% of cancer deaths.

BCC is four times more common than SCC. Sun damage is the major cause of both cancers, especially the ultraviolet B (UVB) spectrum (290–320 nm wavelength). The UV radiation produces DNA mutations, particularly thymidine dimers in the p53 tumour suppressor gene. The incidence of skin cancer rises with latitudes approaching the equator. Light-exposed areas of the body are the most frequent sites for tumours, and occupations with high sun exposure like farming have an increased incidence of BCC and SCC. Ozone absorbs UVB, and progressive destruction of the ozone layer by fluorinated hydrocarbons may lead to increased rates. Melanin absorbs UV light, and its lower levels in melanocytes of white people

accounts for the higher incidence of skin cancers in white people. The benefits of melanin in areas of high UV exposure are offset against the reduced production of vitamin D3, which requires UV light, so in regions of low sunlight, black people are prone to rickets. This delicately balanced system of biological geodiversity has been abused to justify some of the most inhumane behaviour. Genetic predispositions to skin cancers include xeroderma pigmentosum, Gorlin's basal cell naevus syndrome and familial melanoma syndromes. Patients with xeroderma pigmentosa are unable to repair the UV-induced DNA damage and develop both BCC and SCC under the age of 10 years old. Gorlin's basal cell naevus syndrome patients develop BCC in their teens and brain tumours later in life; it is caused by a mutation of a patched gene involved in the Hedgehog pathway signal transduction. The gene name *Hedgehog* was originally coined because mutations lead to spikes on *Drosophila* fruit flies. Humans have three homologues of the gene named after the two common varieties of hedgehogs, 'Indian' and 'Desert'. The third human gene was named *Sonic* after Sega's game character. Familial melanoma is caused by inherited mutations of the CDKN2 (p16) gene (chromosome 9p21) and of CDK4 (chromosome 12q13), both implicated in insensitivity to cell cycle checkpoints. Chemical carcinogens, including arsenic, are associated with SCC. Sir Percival Pott's description in 1775 of scrotal cancers in chimney sweeps

Lecture Notes: Oncology, 2nd edition. By M. Bower and J. Waxman. Published 2010 by Blackwell Publishing Ltd.

is thought to be due to industrial exposure to coal tar. Radiation is associated with an increased incidence of SCC, BCC and Bowen's disease (SCC *in situ*). Allogeneic organ transplant recipients are at greatly increased risk of SCC, with as many as 80% having SCC within 20 years of the graft. This may be related to the finding of genotypes five and eight of human papillomavirus in some skin SCC.

Presentation

BCC begins in the basal cell layer of the epidermis, usually develops on chronically sun-exposed areas of the skin, rarely metastasizes, and is usually slow growing. If left untreated, however, BCC may spread locally to the bone or other tissues beneath the skin. BCC starts as painless, translucent, pearly nodules with telangiectasia on sun-exposed skin. As they enlarge, they ulcerate and bleed and develop a rolled shiny edge sometimes referred to as a 'rodent ulcer' (see Plate 39.1). They may progress slowly over many months to years, but less than 0.1% metastasize to regional lymph nodes. They occur mostly on the face, especially the nose, nasolabial fold and inner canthus, usually in elderly people and are more common in men than in women.

SCC arises from more superficial layers of the epidermis and tends to be more aggressive. SCC can invade tissues beneath the skin and 1–2% spread to the lymph nodes. These cancers typically appear on sun-exposed areas of the body, such as the face, ears, neck, lips and backs of the hands (see Plate 39.2). Marjolin ulcers are SCCs arising in long-standing, benign ulcers, such as venous ulcers, or scars, such as old burns. SCCs are irregular, red hyperkeratotic tumours that ulcerate and crust. Unlike BCCs, SCCs grow more rapidly over months rather than years and occasionally bleed. Precursors to SCC include actinic keratosis and SCC *in situ*, which is also called Bowen's disease. SCC *in situ* is a full-thickness malignant transformation of the epidermis that, by definition, has not invaded the dermis.

Merkel cell carcinoma is a highly malignant tumour in the basal layer of the epidermis, most commonly found in elderly, white patients. It consists of rapidly growing, painless and shiny purple nodules that may occur anywhere on the body. These tumours are thought to arise from neuroendocrine cells and are positive for neuron-specific enolase staining. They resemble small cell lung cancer in their clinical course. In 2008, a polyomavirus (Merkel cell polyomavirus, MCV) was identified in most of these tumours and represents the first of a new class of human oncogenic viruses. Max Perutz, who won the Nobel Prize for his work on crystallography and who was Watson and Crick's PhD supervisor whilst they were discovering the structure of DNA, died of Merkel cell tumour. Distant metastases are common, and treatment is with combination chemotherapy, although relapses are frequent and the prognosis is poor. Other, rarer non-melanoma skin cancers include Kaposi's sarcoma, which usually starts within the dermis but can also develop in internal organs. This cancer, once extremely rare, has become more common due to its association with HIV/AIDS. It is caused by infection with an oncogenic herpesvirus, HHV8 (human herpesvirus 8). Primary cutaneous lymphoma or mycosis fungoides is a low-grade lymphoma that primarily affects the skin. Generally, it has a slow course and often remains confined to the skin, but progression of the tumour to a more aggressive, life-threatening stage is more likely the longer it has been present. Adnexal tumours, which start in the hair follicles or sweat glands, are extremely rare and usually benign.

Treatment

The goal of treatment for BCC and SCC is to eradicate local disease and achieve the best cosmetic appearance. For BCC, a complete skin examination is indicated because of the increased risk of actinic keratosis or cancers located at other skin sites in persons presenting with a suspicious lesion. For SCC, regional lymph nodes should also be examined. The main options include: (i) surgery, which offers a single brief procedure and histological confirmation of completeness of excision; (ii) curettage, which is suitable for small, nodular lesions of less than 1 cm and yields good cosmesis; and (iii) cryotherapy, which can be used for lesions of less than 2 cm but may leave an area of depigmentation, and radiotherapy. Mohs' micrographic surgery is a specialized form of excisional surgery that provides 100% microscopically controlled histological margins. The technique involves tumour excision, mapping of the removed tissue and immediate microscopic assessment of the surgical specimen. If occult tumour extension is detected microscopically, the process is repeated until a tumour-free margin is attained. Frederick Mohs developed this surgical approach whilst still a medical student and, according to at least one of our surgical colleagues, it is analogous to peeling rather than chopping a vegetable. Mohs' surgery is curative for 99% of primary BCCs and for 97% of primary SCCs, the highest documented cure rates. Radiotherapy has the advantages of no pain, no hospitalization and no keloids or contracture; it preserves uninvolved tissue and produces smaller defects. It does, however, require multiple visits and results in depigmentation and loss of hair follicles and sweat glands at the treated site. The decision between surgery and radiotherapy is based on size and site, histology, age of patient, recurrence rates and anticipated cosmetic results. Topical 5-fluorouracil chemotherapy may be used for actinic keratosis and small, superficial, non-invasive tumours. Side effects include progressive inflammation, erythema, erosions and contact dermatitis. Systemic chemotherapy is reserved for treating locally advanced and metastatic disease. The most widely used regimens include cisplatin in combination with 5-fluorouracil or doxorubicin.

Prevention remains the most important aspect of the management of skin cancers and requires campaigns to increase public awareness. Children should not get sunburnt, and white-skinned people should limit their total cumulative sun exposure. The public should be encouraged to look out for new skin lesions, and those that are not obviously benign should be seen and removed in their entirety for pathological examination within four weeks.

Prognosis

The prognosis of five-year survival for patients with non-melanoma skin tumours is given in Table 39.1.

Table 39.1 A prognosis of five-year survival for patients with non-melanoma skin tumours.

Tumour	5-year survival
Basal cell carcinoma	95–100%
Squamous cell carcinoma	92–99%

Chapter 40

Melanoma

Epidemiology and pathogenesis

Melanoma is a tumour of melanocytes: the pigmented cells of the skin. The incidence of melanoma has increased by a factor of 4 since 1971. More than 10 000 people were diagnosed with melanoma in the UK in 2006. The primary cause is thought to be an increase in exposure to sunlight. Risk factors for the development of melanoma, however, include being Caucasian and having dysplastic naevi or familial melanoma. It is encouraging to note that recently there has been a stabilization of the increase in melanoma incidence. One hopes that with all the publicity, the risks of exposure to sun are at last entering into the public consciousness.

Less than 10% of all melanoma cases constitute families with an inherited predisposition to melanoma. Mutations in two genes, CDKN2A and CDK4, have been shown to confer increased risk of melanoma, but these mutations only constitute about one-fifth of all familial cases. The melanocortin receptor gene, *MC1R*, influences skin pigmentation and polymorphisms in this gene are linked to an increased risk of melanoma. In other families, there is linkage around the 1p22 chromosomal region. Loss of the transcription factor AP-2 is also thought to have some tumour suppressor-like role in melanoma progression.

Presentation

Patients with malignant melanoma generally present with a history of a growing mole, which may bleed or itch (see Plates 40.1 and 40.2). Because of the public awareness of melanoma, generally there is quite rapid self-referral to GPs with these symptoms. Specialist referral to plastic surgery or dermatology is also quick, and many hospitals now offer walk-in skin lesion clinics. In clinic, the specialist will on initial examination seek to confirm the diagnosis. If there is no evidence for metastases, he will make arrangements to excise the primary lesion. This proceedure requires specialist surgery with wide excision of the surrounding normal tissue. The reasons for this are, firstly, concerns about the incidence of local recurrence following inadequate resection (see Plates 40.3 and 40.4) and, secondly, the need for good cosmesis. Although wide excision is practised, there is no evidence from a randomized trial that supports this practice.

Staging and grading

There are four main clinical descriptions of melanoma and these are the superficial spreading, nodular, lentigo maligna and acral lentiginous subtypes (Table 40.1).

Lecture Notes: Oncology, 2nd edition. By M. Bower and J. Waxman. Published 2010 by Blackwell Publishing Ltd.

Table 40.1 Clinicopathological features of four common forms of melanoma.

Type	Location	Age (median)	Gender and race	Edge	Colour	Frequency
Superficial spreading	All body surfaces, especially legs	56 years	White females	Palpable, irregular	Brown, black, grey or pink; central or halo depigmentation	50%
Nodular	All body surfaces	49 years	White males	Palpable	Uniform bluish black	30%
Lentigo maligna	Sun exposed, areas, especially head and neck	70 years	White females	Flat, irregular	Shades of brown or black, hypopigmentation	15%
Acral lentigenous	Palms, soles and mucous membranes	61 years	Black males	Palpable, irregular nodule	Black, irregularly coloured	5%

Following excision and confirmation of the diagnosis histologically, staging investigations, which should include CT scanning, should be performed. As a result of surgery and staging procedures, the clinical stage can be defined as follows:

• Stage 1a: localized melanoma less than 0.75 mm thick
• Stage 1b: localized melanoma 0.76–1.5 mm thick
• Stage 2a: localized melanoma 1.6–4 mm thick
• Stage 2b: localized melanoma greater than 4 mm thick
• Stage 3: limited nodal metastases involving only one regional lymph node group
• Stage 4: advanced regional metastases or distant metastases.

There are additional, widely practised staging systems, which are not included in this book. For prognostic purposes, however, pathological staging is significant and includes the Breslow thickness and Clark's levels:

• Clark's level I: melanoma confined to the epidermis
• Clark's level II: penetration into the papillary dermis
• Clark's level III: extension to the reticular dermis
• Clark's level IV: extension into the deep reticular dermis
• Clark's level V: invasion of the subcutaneous fat.

Breslow's staging system measures the vertical thickness of the primary tumour, grouping melanomas into 'Breslow's thickness', as less then 0.75 mm, 0.76–1.5 mm, 1.51–3.99 mm and greater than 4 mm.

Treatment

Adjuvant therapy

There have been many studies of the use of adjuvant immunotherapy in melanoma. Adjuvant immunotherapy using the interferons has led to some conflicting findings. Some studies have been positive and others not. In patients with poor-prognosis melanoma the consensus now is that treatment with adjuvant interferons may have a slight survival benefit. Cancer vaccines have been developed, enhancing antitumour immune responses, and in some recent studies prolonged survival has been reported. Treatment with adjuvant chemotherapy has largely been without any benefit at all and has produced remarkable levels of toxicities without any effect.

Management of local skin metastases and nodal disease

The treatment of this pattern of relapse is primarily surgical. Localized recurrence is excised and nodal metastases are managed by radical lymph node dissection. There are advocates of regional infusional programmes using cytotoxic chemotherapy, but the value of this is contentious. Radiotherapy may be used where localized disease is inoperable or as an adjuvant to surgery, reducing the bulk of disease prior to definitive surgery.

Treatment of metastatic melanoma

The outlook for patients with metastatic melanoma is poor. Patients generally have disease in multiple sites, and the median survival is approximately four to six months. Treatment depends upon the patient, on his or her fitness and on the disease site. Patients with multiple disease sites are treated with chemotherapy or biological therapies or a combination of the two. The most effective chemotherapeutic drugs are dacarbazine, the nitrosoureas and vindesine. The response rate to these compounds is in the range of 5–10%. Prolonged survival is very rare, and the consensus view is that there is no advantage to the combination of single agents. New chemotherapy agents are being developed for melanoma, and there is interest in the role of temozolomide.

It is clear that biological therapies are effective in melanoma. Within this group, the interferons lead to response rates of 10%. The median duration of a partial response is approximately four months, and of a complete response seven months. More recently, adoptive immunotherapy using interleukin 2 and LAK (lymphokine-activated killer) cells has been evaluated in melanoma. The high response rates initially reported have not been confirmed, and the true response rates are in the order of 10% with a median duration of 3 months. Very rarely, spontaneous regression of metastatic disease occurs.

Prognosis

The most important prognostic factor is clinical stage, as reported in a group of 4000 patients treated in America and Australia. Approximately 90% of stage 1 patients, 60% of stage 2 patients and 30% of stage 3 patients survive for 10 years. The survival of stage 4 patients depends upon the metastatic site. Median survival for patients with metastases in the skin is seven months, in the lung is one year, in the brain is five months, in the liver is two months and in bone is six months. The depth of tumour invasion is the most important prognostic factor for localized melanoma. This can be described according to Clark's stage and Breslow's thickness. Ten-year survival for a lesion less than 0.75 mm thick or for a Clark's level I melanoma is 90%, for a lesion 0.75–1.5 mm thick or Clark's level II is 80%, for a lesion 1.6–2.49 mm thick or Clark's level III is 60%, for a lesion 2.5–3.99 mm thick or Clark's level IV is 50%, and for a lesion greater than 4 mm or Clark's level V is approximately 30%.

Other important survival factors have been described from multifactorial analyses. They include the type of initial surgical management, pathological stage, ulceration, presence of satellite nodules, a peripheral anatomical location and, to a much lesser extent, the patient's sex, age and tumour diameter.

The American Joint Committee on Cancer, in a study involving 17 600 patients, has provided recent information on survival. This ranges from 90% survival at five years for early-stage disease to, as might be expected, the usual miserable outlook of only 5% survival at five years for metastatic disease.

New treatment

Angiogenesis inhibitors such as thalidomide are currently under evaluation and responses have been reported. Antitumour vaccination programmes have also been developed, based on the initial observation by Morton and others.

Chapter 41

Paediatric solid tumours

Epidemiology and pathogenesis

Cancer is a leading cause of death in children in England and Wales, second only to accidental injury. It is responsible for around 10% of deaths in childhood. Cancer in children is nonetheless relatively rare, affecting 1 in 600 children, and includes a different spectrum of cancers than adults. The solid tumours encountered in childhood are often embryonal in origin, and many are associated with an inherited predisposition. There are few areas of medicine that can rival the advances made in paediatric oncology in the second half of the 20th century. 7 in 10 children with cancer are now cured, compared with fewer than three in ten in 1962–1966. It is estimated that in 2000, 55 000 young adults in Britain aged 16–40 years were survivors of childhood cancer.

Many paediatric tumours are associated with recognized familial predispositions that are due to inherited mutations of tumour suppressor genes and therefore are inherited as autosomal dominant traits. Examples are hereditary retinoblastoma (mutations of the RB gene on chromosome 13q14) and familial Wilms' tumours (mutations of the WT1 gene on chromosome 11p13). In contrast, environmental oncogenic factors have been less

Lecture Notes: Oncology, 2nd edition. By M. Bower and J. Waxman. Published 2010 by Blackwell Publishing Ltd.

readily identified for paediatric solid tumours; one example, however, is the excess of papillary thyroid cancers in children following the nuclear explosion at Chernobyl (see Chapter 2).

After leukaemias, which account for 22% of childhood malignancies or 440 cases per year in the UK, central nervous system (CNS) tumours are the most common (20% or 330 cases), accounting for 2.5 in 100 000 persons under 18 years old, followed by lymphoma (non-Hodgkin's lymphoma, 8%; Hodgkin's lymphoma, 6%), neuroblastoma (8%), Wilms' tumour (6%) and bone tumours (6%).

Presentation and management of CNS tumours

Tumours in the CNS occur throughout childhood; the age distribution of paediatric CNS tumours is 15% between birth and two years old, 30% from two to five years old, 30% from 5 to 10 years old, and 25% from 11 to 18 years old. In contrast to adult brain tumours, most (60%) are infratentorial and 75% are midline, involving the cerebellum, midbrain, pons and medulla. The most common tumours, accounting for 45%, are astrocytomas of varying grades. They include optic nerve gliomas, which are usually well differentiated tumours. A further 20% are medulloblastomas, a small round cell tumour of childhood, of neuroectodermal origin. Medulloblastomas usually arise in the posterior fossa and may seed metastases in the neuraxis by dropping them down the subarachoid space into the spinal canal. Craniopharyngiomas make up 5–10% of CNS tumours of childhood and cause raised intracranial pressure, visual defects and pituitary dysfunction: usually reduced growth hormone, thyroid-stimulating hormone (TSH), antidiuretic hormone (ADH: diabetes insipidus) or luteinizing hormone/follicle-stimulating hormone (LH/FSH) abnormalities (precocious puberty or delayed secondary sexual characteristics). Suprasellar calcification is a characteristic X-ray finding. A further 1–2% are pineal region tumours that present with Perinaud's syndrome (failure of conjugate upward gaze). Histologically, most pineal tumours are extragonadal germ cell tumours (teratomas and germinomas). Naturally, the management of these children will be determined both by the histological diagnosis and the anatomical location of the tumour and frequently involves surgery, radiotherapy and (occasionally) chemotherapy. The overall five-year survival rates according to the histology are shown in Table 41.1.

Presentation and management of neuroblastoma

Neuroblastoma is the most common malignancy in infants and often is clinically apparent at birth. About 100 new cases of neuroblastoma are diagnosed each year in the UK. Tumours often have

amplification of the n-Myc oncogene on chromosome 1, either as small 'double minute' (DM) chromosomes, or as 'homogenously staining regions' (HSR). They may arise from any site along the craniospinal axis derived from neural crest. The sites include abdominal sites (55%) such as the adrenal medulla (33%), pelvis (25%), thorax (13%) and head and neck (7%). In the case of head and neck neuroblastoma, these occur most commonly in the sympathetic ganglion or olfactory bulb (the latter are more common in adults). The most common finding is a large, firm and irregular abdominal mass that crosses the midline. Tumours may present with non-specific symptoms such as weight loss, failure to thrive, fever and pallor of anaemia, especially if widespread metastases are present. 70% are disseminated at diagnosis via lymphatic and haematogenous spread. Metastases to bones of the skull are common, and orbital swelling is a frequent presentation. Paraneoplastic opsoclonus or myoclonus is a rare feature. These tumours have the highest spontaneous regression rate of any tumour, usually by maturation to ganglioneuroma. Plain abdominal X-ray may show calcification: this occurs in 70% of neuroblastoma and 15% of Wilms' tumours. Other diagnostic investigations include [131]-I-labelled MIBG (metaiodobenzyl guanidine) scan and urinary catecholamines including VMA (vanillylmandelic acid), serum NSE (neuron-specific enolase) and ferritin. Localized disease has a high cure rate with surgery and radiotherapy. On account of the high rate of disseminated disease at presentation, which is 70%, however, the overall five-year survival rate for neuroblastoma is 55%.

Presentation and management of Wilms' tumours

This highly malignant embryonal tumour of the kidney is the most common malignant lesion of the genitourinary tract in children. It was named after Dr Max Wilms, who first described it, and is also known as nephroblastoma. Most occur in children under five years old, and some are hereditary. Only about 75 children develop a Wilms' tumour each year in Britain. Wilms' tumours are associated

Table 41.1 The 5-year survival rates for paediatric CNS tumours.

Tumour	5-year survival
Any paediatric CNS tumours	56%
Low-grade glioma	80%
High-grade glioma	25%
Optic glioma	80%
Brainstem glioma	5–50%
Medulloblastoma	60%
Ependymoma	60%
Pineal germinoma	90%
Pineal teratoma	65%
Craniopharyngioma	90%

with congenital abnormalities including aniridia and the WAGR syndrome (Wilms' tumour, aniridia, gonadoblastoma and mental retardation), Denys–Drash syndrome (Wilms' tumour, male pseudohermaphroditism and diffuse glomerular disease) and Beckwith–Wiedemann syndrome (organomegaly, hemihypertrophy, increased incidence of Wilms' tumour, hepatoblastoma and adrenocortical tumours). Wilms' tumours present in usually healthy children as abdominal swellings with a smooth, firm, non-tender mass. A quarter have gross haematuria, and occasionally children present with hypertension, malaise or fever. Up to 20% have metastases at diagnosis; lungs are the most common site of metastases. The main stay of treatment is surgical resection with adjuvant radiotherapy to the tumour bed, reserved for children with a high risk of relapse. The five-year survival for Wilms' tumours now exceeds 80%, and one of the goals of more recent trials is to reduce the long-term morbidity of treatment.

Presentation and management of liver tumours

Fewer than 10 children in the UK develop liver tumours each year. Liver cancers are divided into hepatoblastoma (66%), which usually occurs before the age of three years, and hepatocellular cancers (33%), which occur at any age. Hepatoblastoma occurs as part of the Beckwith–Wiedemann syndrome and is also associated with familial adenomatous polyposis. Hepatoblastoma is the third most common intra-abdominal malignancy in young children – after neuroblastoma and Wilms' tumours. It most frequently affects the right lobe of the liver, and 10% have disseminated disease at presentation with regional lymph node involvement or lung metastases. Hepatocellular carcinoma is associated with hepatitis B and C infection, tyrosinaemia, biliary cirrhosis and α_1-antitrypsin deficiency. Surgical resection with or without neoadjuvant chemotherapy has dramatically improved the prognosis in hepatoblastoma, where the five-year overall survival is now 70%. In contrast, the prognosis for hepatocellular carcinoma in children is not greatly different from that for adults, with five-year overall survival rates of around 25%.

Presentation and management of retinoblastoma

Retinoblastoma most often occurs in children under five years old and in a third of cases is bilateral. There are about 40 new cases of retinoblastoma diagnosed each year in the UK. Up to 40% are hereditary due to germline mutations of the retinoblastoma (RB) gene, and these children frequently have bilateral retinoblastoma and present at a younger age. Hereditary retinoblastoma was the basis of Knudsen's two-hit model of tumour suppressor genes. These tumours present with whitening of the pupil, squint or secondary glaucoma. Retinoblastoma is usually confined to the orbit, and hence the cure rate with enucleation is high. Smaller tumours may be treated with localized cryotherapy, laser treatment or a radioactive iodine plaque stitched to the outer surface of the eye. Overall, 90% of children with retinoblastoma are cured. Hereditary retinoblastoma, however, is also associated with other malignancies, especially osteosarcoma, soft tissue sarcoma and melanoma. Genetic counselling is an integral part of therapy for retinoblastoma. All siblings should be examined periodically: DNA polymorphism analysis may identify relatives at high risk.

Presentation and management of bone tumours and sarcomas

Osteosarcoma

The incidence of bone tumours is highest during adolescence, although they only represent 3% of all childhood cancers. Only about 30 children develop these tumours each year in the UK. Most tumours occur in areas of rapid growth in the metaphysis near the growth plate, where cellular proliferation and remodelling are greatest during long bone growth. The most active growth plates are in the distal femur and proximal tibia. These are also the most common sites for primary bone cancers. Known risk factors include hereditary retinoblastoma, Li–Fraumeni syndrome and prior radiotherapy. Most primary bone tumours present as painful swellings which may cause stiffness and effusions in nearby joints. Occasionally, tumours present as pathological fractures. The radiological appearances are a lytic or sclerotic expansile lesion, associated with a wide transition zone, cortical destruction, a soft tissue mass, periosteal reaction and calcification. The clinical management of bone tumours requires a specialist multidisciplinary unit including orthopaedic surgeons, plastic surgeons and oncologists. Clinical management should happen in the context of an adolescent oncology unit, since the majority of patients fit into this age group, with all its special needs. Neoadjuvant chemotherapy plays an important role in localized osteosarcoma and Ewing's sarcoma to shrink the tumour and hopefully allow limb sparing surgery without increasing relapse rates. Postoperative adjuvant chemotherapy and radiotherapy are useful in some tumours. The five-year survival has steadily risen from under 20% in the late 1960s to over 60%.

Ewing's sarcoma

Ewing's sarcoma is named after Dr James Ewing, who described the tumour in the 1920s. Ewing's sarcoma is a childhood bone malignancy of uncertain cellular origin that is associated with the t(11;22) chromosomal translocation that juxtaposes the EWS and Fli-1 genes, resulting in a hybrid transcript from these two transcription factor genes. This same chromosomal translocation occurs in peripheral neuroectodermal tumours (PNETs) and Askin lung tumours, suggesting a possible common origin. PNETs are thought to arise from peripheral autonomic nervous system tissue and stain for NSE as well as S-100. Morphologically, all three tumours are small round blue cell tumours – a group that also includes embryonal rhabdomyosarcoma, non-Hodgkin's lymphoma, neuroblastoma and small cell lung cancer. About 30 children each year in the UK develop Ewing's sarcoma. It most frequently occurs in the teenage years. Ewing's sarcoma is very rare in African and Asian children and is not associated with familial

syndromes or prior radiotherapy. It usually starts in a bone at the diaphysis or, less frequently, the metaphysic – most commonly in one of the bones of the hips, upper arm or thigh, although it can also develop in soft tissue. The most common symptom is pain and swelling, but systemic symptoms such as pyrexia, weight loss and night sweats may also occur. X-rays usually demonstrate ill-defined medullary destruction, small areas of new bone formation, periosteal reaction and soft tissue expansion. Approximately a fifth of patients have metastases in their lungs or bones at presentation. Multimodality treatment including surgery, radiotherapy and chemotherapy is standard practice for Ewing's sarcoma, and the five-year survival rate is 55%.

Rhabdomyosarcoma

Rhabdomyosarcoma is the most common paediatric soft tissue sarcoma, although only 60 children are diagnosed with this tumour in the UK each year, and most are under 10 years old. Rhabdomyosarcoma may be divided into alveolar (25–30%), embryonal (50–60%) and pleomorphic (5%). The embryonal type occurs in the first decade, most often in the head and neck and genitourinary tract. The alveolar type occurs in adolescents, in the forearms and trunk. The pleomorphic type occurs in adults. Consistent chromosomal translocations have been found in a number of soft tissue sarcomas, both benign and malignant. These chromosomal rearrangements may be of help diagnostically; for example, 75% of alveolar rhabdomyosarcomas harbour the t(2:13)(q35:q14) chromosomal translocation that fuses the PAX3 gene and the FKHR (*forkhead*) gene. The consequence of many of these translocations is the transcription of chimeric mRNA, containing 5′ sequences of one gene and 3′ sequences from another gene, and translation to hybrid proteins. Many of the genes involved with these translocations are themselves transcription factors, and it is postulated that the consequence of these translocations is the aberrant expression of a number of downstream genes. Rhabdomyosarcomas present as masses that grow and may become hard and painful. Approximately 15% have metastases at presentation; most frequently in the lungs, bones and lymph nodes. Treatment involves both surgery and chemotherapy but is risk stratified, with radiotherapy reserved for those at higher risk of relapse in order to save those at low risk of recurrence from the late effects of radiotherapy. The five-year overall survival is 75%.

Langerhans' cell histiocytosis

Langerhans' cell histiocytosis (LCH), previously known as histiocytosis X, is not strictly a cancer but may behave in an aggressive fashion and is often treated by oncologists. About 30 children develop LCH in the UK each year; most of them are under two years old. LCH is a proliferation of epidermal histiocytes or Langerhans' cells, which are antigen-presenting dendritic cells named after Paul Langerhans, who first described them in 1868 when he was a 21-year-old medical student in Berlin. LCH comprises three overlapping syndromes: unifocal bone diease (solitary eosinophilic granuloma), multifocal disease of bone (Hand–Schüller–Christian disease) and multifocal, multisystem disease (Letterer–Siwe disease). Letterer–Siwe disease occurs mainly in boys under two years old; Hand–Schüller–Christian syndrome has a peak of onset in children aged 2–10 years; whilst solitary eosinophilic granuloma occurs in those aged 5–15 years. Solitary eosinophilic granuloma occurs at any site in bones, is usually asymptomatic and is frequently an incidental finding. Patients with Hand–Schüller–Christian syndrome often present with recurrent episodes of otitis media and mastoiditis or with polyuria and polydipsia due to diabetes insipidus. Letterer–Siwe disease presents with symptoms suggestive of a systemic infection or malignancy with a generalized skin eruption, anaemia and hepatosplenomegaly and other protean manifestations (Table 41.2). This eponymous classification of LCH has in part been abandoned, and a simpler classification into either restricted LCH (skin or bone lesions) or extensive LCH (visceral organ involvement) has been introduced. The diagnosis is confirmed histologically; the characteristic cytological features are

Table 41.2 Clinical manifestations of extensive Langerhans' cell histiocytosis.

System	Clinical manifestations
Systemic effects	Pyrexia, weight loss, fatigue
Bone	Painful swelling (skull (50%), femur (17%), ribs (8%), pelvis, vertebrae), associated soft tissue swelling (proptosis, mastoiditis and deafness, gums)
Skin	Scaly, erythematous, seborrhoea-like brown to red papules (behind the ears and in the axillary, inguinal and perineal areas) (50%)
Endocrine glands	Diabetes insipidus (20%) due to involvement of the hypothalamus or pituitary stalk
Bone marrow	Pancytopenia
Lymph nodes	Lymphadenopathy (30%)
Liver and spleen	Hepatosplenomegaly
Gastrointestinal tract	Failure to thrive, malabsorption, diarrhoea, vomiting (5–10%)
Lungs	Dyspnoea, honey-comb lungs, bullae, spontaneous pneumothorax, emphysema (20%)
Central nervous system	Progressive ataxia, dysarthria, intracranial hypertension, cranial nerve palsies (10%)

CD1a surface antigen expression and cytoplasmic Birbeck granules. Localized bone disease is treated surgically or, less frequently, with radiotherapy, whilst systemic disease requires chemotherapy with cladribine often with desmopressin for the management of the diabetes insipidus. Survival exceeds 95% in unifocal disease and 80% in multifocal bone disease, but is only 50% in patients with systemic multiorgan disease.

Complications of treatment

Although many of the delayed effects of chemotherapy and radiotherapy in children are similar to those in adults, the effects on developing organs also produce unique late side effects, particularly on the skeleton, brain and endocrine systems.

These delayed effects of multimodality therapy on the developing child are substantial and the late sequelae cause considerable morbidity in this group of patients where the long-term survival rates are high. Radiotherapy retards bone and cartilage growth, and causes intellectual impairment, gonadal toxicity, hypothalamic and thyroid dysfunction, as well as pneumonitis, nephrotoxicity and hepatotoxicity. Late consequences of chemo- therapy include infertility, anthracycline-related cardiotoxicity, bleomycin-related pulmonary fibrosis and platinum-related nephrotoxicity and neurotoxicity. Up to 5% of children cured of this cancer will develop a second malignancy as a consequence of an inherited cancer predisposition or the late sequelae of cancer treatment. Second malignancies occur most frequently following combined chemotherapy and radiotherapy.

Chapter 42

Bone cancers and sarcomas

Epidemiology and pathogenesis

Bone tumours are amongst the oldest cancers discovered in humans according to palaeopathological evidence. A Bronze Age woman with bone metastases in her skull has been dated to 1600–1900 BC, whilst Saxon bones from Standlake in Oxfordshire, UK, demonstrate features of osteosarcoma in a young adult warrior. St Peregrine, born in 1260 at Forlì, Italy, is the patron saint of cancer sufferers (the feast day is on 4 May). He was due for an amputation for a sarcoma of the leg, but the cancer was cured on the night prior to surgery, following a vision of Christ. He lived a further 20 years and was canonized in 1726. The presumed origins of primary bone tumours are shown in Table 42.1.

Sarcomas are tumours of the connective tissue, which supports the body and includes bone muscle, tendon, fat and synovial tissue. These tumours represent less than 1% of all malignancies. They have an incidence of approximately 1–2 per 100 000 per annum. There are no known associated aetiological factors, although sarcomas rarely occur as second malignancies in areas of the body that have been previously irradiated. The most common bone tumours are osteosarcoma (see Figure 2.12) and Ewing's sarcoma.

Ewing's sarcoma occurs in childhood and in early adult life. Molecular biology studies have shown the presence of a specific chromosomal translocation between chromosomes 22 and 11. This translocation is present in a group of small, round, blue cell tumours which include peripheral neuroectodermal tumours (PNETs), classic Ewing's and extraosseous Ewing's sarcoma; these are now grouped together for treatment purposes. In patients with this group of tumours there may be difficulty in obtaining a histopathological diagnosis. Modern advances in molecular biology have led to the identification of the EWS/FLI-1 translocation present in patients with Ewing's sarcoma. The presence of this translocation is identifiable by fluorescence *in situ* hybridization (FISH).

Osteosarcoma occurs in two groups of patients: firstly in adolescence or early adult life and secondly in old age, where osteosarcoma complicates Paget's disease. p53 mutations are commonly seen in osteosarcoma, as are mutations in the retinoblastoma gene.

Presentation

Most soft tissue sarcomas occur in the limbs, and patients present to their GPs with localized swelling. Patients with Ewing's tumours and sarcomas generally present with pain, and the diagnosis

Lecture Notes: Oncology, 2nd edition. By M. Bower and J. Waxman. Published 2010 by Blackwell Publishing Ltd.

usually comes as a result of the classic X-ray appearances of these tumours. Fractures are common and nerve palsies may be seen where there is a cranial presentation. Patients may also present with metastases. Because of the rarity of these tumours and the requirement for a multidisciplinary specialist approach, patients with a suspected diagnosis of sarcoma should be referred on to specialist centres, where results have been shown to be vastly superior to those achieved by peripheral clinics. These tumours are usually diagnosed after a significant delay.

Tables 42.2–42.4 list the clinical features of the different types of bone cancers and sarcomas, some of which are illustrated in Figures 42.1–42.4.

Investigations and management

In a patient where a diagnosis of soft tissue sarcoma is suspected, an initial biopsy should be carried out by the surgeon who is to perform definitive surgery. Fine needle aspiration cytology, core needle biopsy and incisional biopsies are all techniques that are considered by the surgeon and, for those patients with rare abdominal or thoracic soft tissue sarcomas, CT-guided biopsies may be required. After the pathological diagnosis has been established, definitive surgery can be planned. This requires a

Table 42.1 Origins of primary bone tumours.

Origin	Benign tumour	Malignant tumour
Cartilage	Enchondroma Osteochondroma Chondroblastoma	Chondrosarcoma
Bone	Osteoid osteoma Osteoblastoma	Osteosarcoma
Unknown origin	Giant cell tumour	Ewing's sarcoma Malignant fibrous histiocytoma

Table 42.2 Clinical features of cartilage-derived bone tumours.

	Enchondroma	Osteochondroma (exostosis)	Chondroblastoma	Chondrosarcoma
Age	10–50 years	10–20 years	5–20 years	30–60 years
Site	Hands, wrist Diaphysis	Knee, shoulder, pelvis Metaphysis	Knee, shoulder, ribs Epiphysis prior to fusion	Knee, shoulder, pelvis Metaphysis or diaphysis
X-ray	Well-defined lucency, thin sclerotic rim, calcification	Eccentric protrusion from bone, calcification	Well-defined lucency, thin sclerotic rim, calcification	Expansile lucency, sclerotic margin, cortical destruction, soft tissue mass
Notes	Ollier's disease = multiple enchondromas	1% transform to chondrosarcoma		

Table 42.3 Clinical features of osteoid-derived bone tumours.

	Osteoid osteoma	Osteoblastoma	Osteosarcoma
Age	10–30 years	10–20 years	10–25 years and >60 years
Site	Knee Diaphysis	Vertebra Metaphysis	Knee, shoulder, pelvis Metaphysis
X-ray	<1 cm central lucency, surrounding bone sclerosis, periosteal reaction	Well-defined lucency, sclerotic rim, cortex preserved, calcification	Lytic/sclerotic expansile lesion, wide transition zone, cortical destruction, soft tissue mass, periosteal reaction, calcification

Table 42.4 Clinical features of bone tumours of uncertain origins.

	Giant cell tumour	Ewing's sarcoma	Malignant fibrous histiocytoma
Age	20–40 years	5–15 years	10–20 years and >60 years
Site	Long bones, knee	Knee, shoulder, pelvis	Knee, pelvis, shoulder
	Epiphysis and metaphysis post closure	Diaphysis, less often metaphysis	Metaphysis
X-ray	Lucency with ill-defined endosteal margin, cortical destruction, soft tissue mass, eccentric expansion bone/lung metastases	Ill-defined medullary destruction, small areas of new bone formation, periosteal reaction, soft tissue expansion,	Cortical destruction, periosteal reaction, soft tissue mass

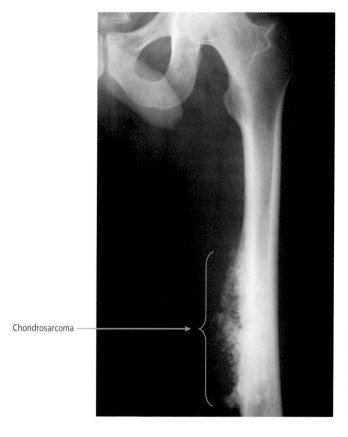

Chondrosarcoma

Figure 42.1 Femur chondrosarcoma showing an expansile lesion with sclerotic margin, cortical destruction and punctuate internal calcification and an associated soft tissue mass. These tumours are most common in middle age and occur around the knee, shoulder or pelvis.

multidisciplinary approach that takes place in the context of magnetic resonance (MR) staging of the local tumour and CT definition of the metastatic sites. The surgical approach requires the removal of the muscle compartment to include the fascia. This limits the risk of local relapse.

In those patients with Ewing's sarcoma and osteosarcoma, initial staging will include CT assessment of the chest, abdomen and pelvis, and MR imaging of the primary tumour site. The initial management option for Ewing's sarcoma includes the consideration of either primary surgery or

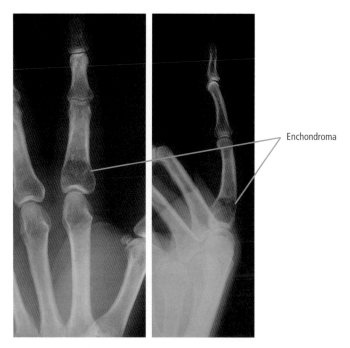

Figure 42.2 Enchondroma of the ring finger proximal phalynx showing well-defined lucency and a thin sclerotic rim with preserved cortex. These cartilage-derived tumours occur in 10–50-year-olds most frequently in the diaphyses of the hand or wrist. Multiple enchondromas occur in Ollier's disease, a non-hereditary condition that is associated with an increased risk of chondrosarcoma.

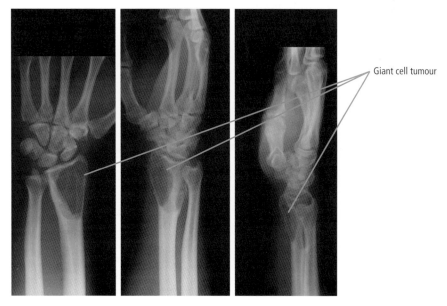

Figure 42.3 Giant cell tumour of the distal radius showing expansion and lucency with cortical destruction giving a multi-loculated appearance. These tumours occur most commonly in 20–40-year-olds in long bones at the epiphyses and metaphyses after closure.

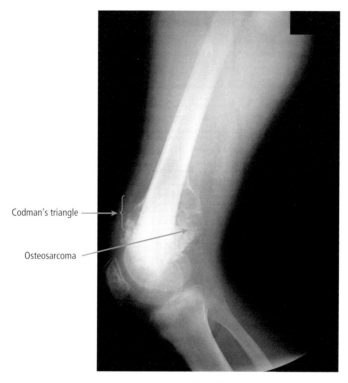

Codman's triangle

Osteosarcoma

Figure 42.4 Osteosarcoma of the distal femur showing an expansile soft tissue mass with internal calcification and cortical destruction. There is a marked periosteal reaction with lifting of the periosteum that is described as Codman's triangle, which is almost always due to an aggressive malignant bone tumour extending into adjacent soft tissues.

radiotherapy to control the local lesion. If the lesion is small and it is possible to have substantial resection margins, surgery is the best option with immediate endoprosthetic replacement. For the majority of patients, however, radiotherapy remains the most important treatment modality for the control of local disease.

Osteosarcomas are rare and for this reason also best managed in specialist centres. This is particularly important for teenage patients with sarcomas. For these patients, chemotherapy, radiation, surgery and counselling all have a significant role in management. Patients with osteosarcomas are generally managed well because of the excellent results achieved using multidisciplinary specialist approaches. In osteosarcoma, bone scanning as well as CT and MR scanning are essential in the initial work up of a patient. Biopsy of the tumour is required with the open approach preferred. Surgi-

cal advances have meant that bone tumours are managed much better than they were, with the aim of limb-sparing prosthetic surgery.

Pathology

The most helpful classification of soft tissue tumours is into tumours of fibrous tissue, fibrohistiocytic tumours, adipose tissue tumours including liposarcomas, tumours of muscle, tumours of blood vessels, tumours of lymph vessels, tumours of synovium, tumours of mesothelium, tumours of peripheral nerves, tumours of autonomic ganglia, tumours of paraganglionic structures, tumours of cartilage and bone-forming tissue, tumours of pleuripotential mesochyme, tumours of uncertain histogenesis and unclassified soft tissue tumours. This latter tumour group is extremely diverse, with at least 50 different subtypes.

These groups may in turn be divided into benign and malignant conditions. Benign tumours do not generally metastasize, and microscopic examination shows a low mitotic rate. Malignant tumours have a high mitotic rate and do tend to metastasize. Approximately one-third of tumours are low grade and two-thirds are high grade. Osteosarcomas are described as being of low, intermediate and high grade.

grade tumours, which by definition should not spread, should be treated by surgical excision alone. Local control should result in 85–100% recovery in these patients. The situation is different for those patients with high-grade tumours, and there is debate as to whether surgery alone, surgery combined with radiation, or surgery, radiation and chemotherapy in combination is the correct approach.

Treatment of soft tissue sarcomas

The clinical features of soft tissue sarcomas are listed in Table 42.5, along with the primary therapy.

Treatment of the primary tumour

There is considerable discussion as to the appropriate management of a soft tissue sarcoma. Low-

Surgery

There is little argument that surgery is necessary, and the operation of first choice should be one that allows a reasonably wide margin of normal tissue to be excised with the tumour. If a good procedure is carried out, such as muscle compartmental excision, the local failure rate is 7–18%. If less radical procedures such as excision biopsy are performed, then the local failure rate is approximately 50%. More radical procedures such as amputation have a

Table 42.5 Clinical features of soft tissue sarcomas.

Tumour	Age (years)	Commonest sites	Primary therapy	5-year survival
Fibrosarcoma	20–50	Thigh, arm, head and neck	Wide excision and adjuvant radiation	90% (well differentiated) 50% (poorly differentiated)
Liposarcoma	40–60	Thigh, head and neck (rarely arise from lipoma)	Wide excision and adjuvant radiation	66% (myxoid) 10% (pleomorphic)
Embryonal rhabdomyosarcoma	0–10	Head and neck, genitourinary (botyroid)	Neoadjuvant chemoradiation and surgery	40%
Alveolar rhabdomyosarcoma	10–20	Thigh	Neoadjuvant chemoradiation and surgery	60%
Pleomorphic rhabdomyosarcoma	40–70	Thigh, upper arm	Wide excision and adjuvant radiation	10%
Synovial sarcoma	20–40	Leg	Wide excision and adjuvant radiation	40%
Angiosarcoma	50–70	Skin, superficial soft tissues	Wide excision and adjuvant radiation	15%
Leiomyosarcoma	45–65	Retroperitoneal, uterine	Wide excision and adjuvant radiation	40%

lower local recurrence rate, of approximately 5%. Over the last decade, there has been a trend toward radical compartmental excision with limb-sparing procedures.

Adjuvant chemotherapy and radiation

After definitive surgery has been performed, the need for radiation and chemotherapy is assessed. Radiation is not given for low-grade tumours. In high-grade tumours, radiotherapy to the tumour bed has an advantage in terms of reduced local recurrence rates in extremity lesions where effective dosages can be given without risking vital structures. Local radiation has no effect upon the progression of distant metastases. Because patients with high-grade sarcomas are at great risk from the progression of their cancer to a metastatic state, adjuvant chemotherapy has been investigated in a number of trials. The original studies, which were non-randomized, showed an advantage to combination chemotherapy. This result has not held up, and the consensus view now is that adjuvant chemotherapy has no advantage in terms of five-year survival. This remains very much a subject for debate, however, and in many centres adjuvant chemotherapy is still administered.

Treatment of metastatic sarcoma

The treatment of metastatic soft tissue sarcoma requires the use of chemotherapy. The most effective single-agent treatments lead to responses in 15–35% of patients. Attempts are made to capitalize on this by the use of combination chemotherapy programmes. A slight increase in response rates has been found by some groups of clinicians. This supposed advantage is, however, much debated. Many cancer doctors would advocate the administration of single-agent chemotherapy to their patients simply because combination therapies maximize toxicities and do not provide a significant advantage.

Treatment of Ewing's sarcomas

For patients with Ewing's tumours, the last 20 or 30 years have seen a significant evolution of treatment protocols. One type of management generally consists of treatment with induction chemotherapy, followed by local treatment to the primary site with either surgery or radiotherapy or both. This will be followed by further consolidation chemotherapy.

Treatment of osteosarcomas

Similarly in sarcomas, primary chemotherapy to debulk the tumour is followed by surgery. Both chemotherapy and surgery are complex and highly specialized, requiring immense technical skill and input from many areas of medical and paramedical expertise. Patients with metastatic osteosarcoma can be cured, and, once more, surgery is enormously important. Surgical excision of pulmonary mestastases is considered and may be curative in a limited number of patients.

New treatment

Although there have been some developments in chemotherapy, it is not thought that chemotherapy will be the future for patients with sarcomas. Oncologists and their patients have been most encouraged by the development of imatinib (Glevec), which is an agent that inhibits the function of the BCR-ABL oncogene and of the KIT and platelet-derived growth factor (PDGF) tyrosine kinases. This agent is active in chronic myeloid leukaemia and is described in the leukaemia section of this book. It also has activity in gastrointestinal stromal sarcomas, which are rare sarcomas of the bowel. Patients who have gross metastatic disease have been seen to respond to this agent without any significant toxicity. This is clearly a wonderful development and may have a role in the management of bone tumours.

Chapter 43

Unknown primary cancer

Epidemiology and pathogenesis

For most patients who present with metastatic disease, routine examination and investigation will quickly disclose the underlying primary tumour. Occasionally, the primary tumour may be more elusive, and a number of clinical, histopathological and serological clues may help to establish the site. For 1–5% of patients, however, the primary site remains undisclosed because it is too small to be detected or has regressed. The usual histological diagnosis in these patients with an unknown primary site is adenocarcinoma or poorly differentiated carcinoma. The benefits of establishing the primary site include diagnosing treatable disease (Table 43.1), avoiding overtreating unresponsive disease and hence iatrogenic morbidity in resistant disease, preventing complications that relate to occult primary disease, such as bowel obstruction, and, finally, clarifying the prognosis. The methods commonly used to aid in the hunt for a primary site are described below.

Clinical sites of metastatic spread

Different tumours follow different patterns of metastatic spread. This may be related to chemokine

Lecture Notes: Oncology, 2nd edition. By M. Bower and J. Waxman. Published 2010 by Blackwell Publishing Ltd.

and chemokine receptor expression by tumours and stromal cells (see Part 1).

Brain and meningeal metastases

Up to 30% of solid tumours develop parenchymal brain metastases. Carcinomatous meningitis is less common. Carcinomatous meningitis presents with multiple, anatomically distant, cranial and spinal root neuropathies. The diagnosis may be confirmed by finding malignant cells in the cerebrospinal fluid. Treatment usually involves a combination of intrathecal chemotherapy and craniospinal radiotherapy. Carcinomatous meningitis most frequently occurs with leukaemias and lymphomas and occasionally with breast cancer. Parenchymal brain secondaries that may occur with any solid tumour are usually treated with whole-brain radiotherapy, although surgery may be considered for patients with solitary brain metastases and limited systemic disease (see Figure 15.2).

Bone metastases

Bone metastases are a major source of morbidity in patients with cancer and often have a prolonged course. Bone metastases cause pain, reduced mobility, pathological fractures, hypercalcaemia, myelosuppression and nerve compression syndromes. The tumours that commonly metastasize to bone are lung, breast, prostate, renal and thyroid tumours and sarcomas. Metastases usually occur in the axial skeleton, femur or humerus. If they are found elsewhere, then renal cancer and melanoma should be considered as possible primary tumour sites. Most bone metastases are lucent, lytic lesions; occasionally dense, sclerotic deposits are seen in prostate, breast, carcinoid tumours and Hodgkin's disease. The diagnosis of bone metastases is rarely complicated. The differential diagnosis is outlined in Table 43.2. (See also Figures 1.7, 16.1, 16.2 and 31.3.)

Lung metastases

The lungs are the second most common site for metastases via haematogenous spread. Tumours that commonly metastasize to the lung include lung, breast, renal, thyroid, sarcoma and germ cell tumours. Surgical resection of pulmonary metastases is occasionally undertaken where the primary site is controlled and the lungs are the sole site of metastasis. (See also Figures 2.7 and 17.1c.)

Liver metastases

Of all patients with liver metastases, 60% have a colorectal primary tumour, 25% have melanoma, 15% lung cancer and 5% breast cancer. Hepatic resection for patients with up to three metastases from colorectal cancer results in five-year survivals of 30% and is the best treatment available for selected patients.

Malignant effusions

Eighty percent of malignant pleural effusions are due to lung and breast cancer, lymphoma and

Table 43.1 Treatable unknown primary diagnoses.

Chemosensitive tumours	Hormone-sensitive tumours
Non-Hodgkin's lymphoma	Breast cancer
Germ cell tumours	Prostate cancer
Neuroendocrine tumours (including small cell lung cancer)	Endometrial cancer
Ovarian cancer	Thyroid cancer

Table 43.2 Differential diagnosis of bone metastases.

Diagnosis	Pain	Site	Age	X-ray	Bone scan, CT/MRI	Biochemistry
Metastases	Common	Axial skeleton	Any	Discrete lesions, pathological fracture, loss of vertebral pedicles	Soft tissue extension on MRI/CT	Raised ALP and Ca
Degenerative disease	Common	Limbs	Old	Symmetrical	Symmetrical uptake on bone scan	Normal
Osteoporosis	Painless (unless pathological fracture)	Vertebrae	Old (female)	Osteopenia	Normal bone scan/MRI	Normal
Paget's disease	Painless	Skull (often)	Old	Expanded sclerotic bones	Diffusely hot bone scan	Raised ALP and urinary hydroxyproline
Traumatic fracture	Always	Ribs	Any	Fracture	Intense linear uptake on bone scan	Normal

ALP, alkaline phosphatase; Ca, calcium; CT, computed tomography; MRI, magnetic resonance imaging.

leukaemia. Malignant pericardial effusion is rarer than pleural effusions; breast and lung cancer account for 75%. Metastases to the heart and pericardium are 40 times more common than primary tumours at these sites, but only 15% will develop tamponade. Malignant ascites is a common complication of ovarian, pancreatic, colorectal and gastric cancers and lymphoma. Measures for long-term control of malignant effusions include sclerosis with talc, bleomycin or tetracycline for pleural effusions, drainage by pericardial window for pericardial effusions and peritoneovenous shunts for malignant ascites (see Figure 46.6).

Clinical unknown primary syndromes

Five highly treatable subsets of unknown primary site have been identified, which have more favourable outcomes and require distinct management:
1. Women with isolated axillary lymphadenopathy (adenocarcinoma or undifferentiated carcinoma) usually have an occult breast primary and should be managed as stage II breast cancer. They have a similar prognosis (five-year survival is 70%).
2. Women with peritoneal carcinomatosis (often papillary carcinoma with elevated serum CA-125) should be managed as stage III ovarian cancer.
3. Men with extragonadal germ cell syndrome or atypical teratoma present with features reminiscent of gonadal germ cell tumours. They occur predominantly in young men with pulmonary or lymph node metastases. Germ cell tumour markers (α-fetoprotein (AFP) and human chorionic gonadotrophin (HCG)) may be detected in the serum and in tissue by immunocytochemistry. Cytogenetic analysis for isochromosome 12p (see Box 1.4) is positive in 90% of cases. Empirical chemotherapy with cisplatin-based combinations yield response rates of over 50% and up to 30% long-term survival.
4. Patients with neuroendocrine carcinoma of an unknown primary site overlap with extrapulmonary small cell carcinoma, anaplastic islet cell carcinoma, Merkel cell tumours and paragangliomas. Immunocytochemical staining for chromogranin, neuron-specific enolase, synapto-physin and epithelial antigens (cytokeratins and epithelial membrane antigen) are usually positive. Patients often present with bone metastases and diffuse liver involvement. These tumours are frequently responsive to platinum-based combination chemotherapy.
5. Patients with high cervical lymphadenopathy containing squamous cell carcinoma may have occult head and neck tumours of the nasopharynx, oropharynx or hypopharynx. Radical neck dissection followed by extended field radiotherapy that includes these possible primary sites may yield five-year survival rates of 30%. Adenocarcinoma in high cervical nodes and lower cervical adenopathy containing either histology, however, have a much worse prognosis and should not be treated in this aggressive fashion.

Unfortunately, the majority of unknown primary tumours do not fit into any of these subsets, and the response rates to chemotherapy are below 20%. These responses are usually of brief duration, with no impact on overall survival. The median survival is under 12 months. The exception to this rule is in the group of patients who are under 45 years old. In this group, treatment with BEP (bleomycin, etoposide and cisplatin) or a taxane combination is worthwhile. For this group of patients, 50% survive in excess of two years. Tumours from patients such as these do not have the characteristics of testicular cancer, that is, their tumours do not stain positively for HCG or AFP.

Histopathological characterization

The histopathological characterization of unknown primaries to establish their origin includes a number of techniques: light microscopy, immunocytochemical staining, immunophenotyping, electron microscopy, cytogenetics and molecular analysis. These are described in detail in Part 1.

Serological characterization

Tumour markers are proteins produced by cancers that are detectable in the blood of patients. Ideally, serum tumour markers should be quick and cheap

Table 43.3 The most common serum tumour markers and their uses.

Name	Natural occurrence	Tumour	Comments	Screening	Diagnosis	Prognosis	Follow-up
Carcino embryonic antigen (CEA)	Glycoprotein found in intestinal mucosa during embryonic and fetal life	Colorectal cancer (especially liver metastases), gastric, breast and lung cancer	Elevated in smokers' cirrhosis, chronic hepatitis, UC, Crohn's, pneumonia and TB (usually <10 ng/ml)	No	Yes	Yes	Yes
Alpha-fetoprotein (AFP)	Glycoprotein found in yolk sac and fetal liver	Germ cell tumours (GCTs) (80% non-seminomatous GCTs), hepatocellular cancer (50%), neural tube defects, Down's pregnancies	Role in screening in pregnancy not cancer Only prognostic for GCT not HCC Transient increase in liver diseases	No	Yes	Yes	Yes
Prostate-specific antigen (PSA)	Glycoprotein member of human kallikrein gene family. PSA is a serine protease that liquefies semen in excretory ducts of prostate	Prostate cancer (95%), also benign prostatic hypertrophy and prostatitis (usually <10 ng/ml)	Tissue specific but not tumour specific although a level of >10 ng/ml is 90% specific for cancer	*	Yes	No	Yes
Cancer antigen 125 (CA-125)	Differentiation antigen of coelomic epithelium (Muller's duct)	Ovarian epithelial cancer (75%), also gastrointestinal, lung and breast cancers	Raised in cirrhosis, chronic pancreatitis, autoimmune diseases and any cause of ascites	*	Yes	No	Yes
Human chorionic gondadotrophin (HCG)	Glycoprotein hormone, 14 kD α subunit and 24 kD β subunit from placental syncytiotrophoblasts	Choriocarcinoma (100%), hydatidiform moles (97%), non-seminomatous GCT (50–80%), seminoma (15%)	Screening post-hydatidiform mole for trophoblastic tumours, also used to follow pregnancies and diagnose ectopic pregnancies	Yes	Yes	Yes	Yes

Table 43.3 *Continued*

Name	Natural occurrence	Tumour	Comments	Screening	Diagnosis	Prognosis	Follow-up
Calcitonin	32 amino acid peptide from C cells of thyroid	Medullary cell carcinoma of thyroid	Screening test in MEN 2	Yes	Yes	Yes	Yes
Beta-2-microglobulin	Part of HLA common fragment present on surface of lymphocytes, macrophages and some epithelial cells	Non-Hodgkin's lymphoma, myeloma	Elevated in autoimmune disease, renal glomerular disease	No	No	Yes	Yes
Thyroglobulin	Matrix protein for thyroid hormone synthesis in normal thyroid follicles	Papillary and follicular thyroid cancer		No	Yes	No	Yes
Placental alkaline phosphatase (PLAP)	Isoenzyme of alkaline phosphatase	Seminoma and ovariandysgerminoma (50%)		No	Yes	No	Yes

* See Part 3.

HCC, hepatocellular carcinoma; HLA, human leucocyte antigen; TB, tuberculosis; UC, ulcerative colitis.

to measure, have high sensitivity (of more than 50%) and specificity (over 95%) and yield a high predictive value of positive (PPV) and negative (NPV) results. Under these circumstances, tumour markers may be used for population screening, diagnosis, as prognostic factors, for monitoring treatment, diagnosing remission and detecting relapse and for imaging metastases. A large number of serum tumour markers are available, and each may be valuable for any of screening, diagnosis, prognostication and monitoring treatment (Table 43.3).

Approach to investigation of metastatic disease to establish primary site

There is a worrying tendency to over-investigate patients with unknown primary cancer while at the same time ignoring their palliative care needs. So often the greater the eminence and number of consultants whose advice is sought, the larger the number of esoteric investigations ordered, and the less well the patient and their family are informed. Investigations should be restricted to those that will alter clinical management. It is estimated that in the absence of a localizing sympton, extensive radiological investigation leads to the identification of a primary site in less than 5% of all patients. The prognosis is generally poor, with a median survival of three to four months. Less than 25% of patients survive to one year, and less than 10% are alive after five years. The site of the primary is usually on the same side of the diaphragm as the metastases, and 75% of tumours are infradiaphragmatic; of the 25% that arise above the diaphragm, nearly all arise from the lung. Where identified, the most common primary sites, in order of frequency, are: lung, pancreas, liver, colorectal, stomach, kidney, prostate, ovary, breast, lymphoid and testis. A good performance status is the most important predictor of survival, while extensive weight loss and older age are adverse prognostic factors. With the exception of the five clinical syndromes listed above, treatment other than symptom palliation is rarely appropriate.

Chapter 44

Immunodeficiency and cancer

Hereditary or primary immunodeficiency

Primary immunodeficiencies are mainly single-gene inherited disorders that present in early childhood. They include nearly 100 syndromes, three-quarters of which have been characterized genetically. One important exception is common variable immunodeficiency (CVID), a complex, polygenic disease that is often first manifest in early adulthood. Classically, primary immunodeficiency disorders are classified into B-lymphocyte, T-lymphocyte, phagocytic cell and complement deficiencies. This classification is useful, as it helps us establish the clinical manifestations. For example, B-cell deficiencies usually present after the age of 6 months, when maternal antibodies are exhausted, and the most common pathogens are encapsulated bacteria (like *Streptococcus* and *Haemophillus*), fungi (such as *Giardia* and *Cryptosporidia*) and enteroviruses. In contrast, primary T-cell deficiencies usually present within the first 6 months of life, with opportunistic infections such as *Mycobacterium*, *Candida*, *Pneumocystis jiroveci* and cytomegalovirus. Both B-cell and T-cell primary immunodeficiency may be associated with an increased risk of malignancy (Table 44.1). An increased risk of cancer has not been found with complement deficiencies or phagocyte abnormalities.

Acquired or secondary immunodeficiency

Two forms of acquired immunodeficiency have dominated the last quarter of the 20th century and are responsible for the majority of cancers in the immunosuppressed. Both human immunodeficiency virus (HIV) and iatrogenic immunosuppression following allogenic transplantation are associated with cancers that are linked with oncogenic viruses. The first renal transplant was performed between identical twins by Joseph Murray at Boston's Brigham Hospital in 1953. The development of azathioprine by George Hitchins and Gertrude Elion 10 years later enabled successful allogeneic transplantation and began an era of transplantation medicine dependent upon iatrogenic immunosuppression. The allogeneic organ transplant recipients who received immunosuppressant therapy were found to be prone to post-transplantation lymphoproliferative diseases (PTLDs) and other tumours. The emergence of post-transplant tumours is widely quoted as evidence to support Burnet's immune surveillance theory that states that the immune system acts to remove abnormal clones of cells. In 1949, Frank Macfarlane Burnet described a theory of acquired

Lecture Notes: Oncology, 2nd edition. By M. Bower and J. Waxman. Published 2010 by Blackwell Publishing Ltd.

Table 44.1 Description of primary immunodeficiency syndromes.

Syndrome	Inheritance and incidence	Genetic defect	Immunological defect	Clinical manifestations	Cancer risk
B-cell/antibody deficiency					
X-linked (Bruton's) agammaglobulinemia (XLA)	X-linked recessive (1 in 200000 male live births)	Defect of btk Bruton's (B-cell progenitor tyrosine kinase) intracellular signalling path involved in pre-B cell development. Less often, the mutation is of the mu heavy chain gene	There are virtually no immunoglobulins present in the serum and the number of residual B lymphocytes in blood is very low	Recurrent pyogenic bacterial infections starting aged 6 months after maternal IgG is exhausted. Chronic sinusitis and bronchiectasis may follow	Small increased risk of lymphoma
Common variable immunodeficiency (CVID)	Polygenic, most common primary immunodeficiency (1 in 30000)		Characterized by variably decreased concentrations of all immunoglobulin classes	Recurrent bacterial infections of the respiratory tract. These disorders are also associated with autoimmune diseases (e.g. Crohn's)	Increased risk of lymphomas and digestive carcinomas
Selective IgA deficiency	(1 in 700 live births)	Mapped to chromosome 6p21	No secreted IgA but surface IgA present on B cells	Common mild onset in childhood. Sinusitis and recurrent lung infections	No increased risk
Hyper IgM syndrome (HIM)	X-linked (CD40 ligand = CD154; <1 in 1000000 male live births), autosomal recessive (CD40 or activation induced deaminase)	Three defects causing lack of isotype class switching from IgM to IgG, IgA and IgE	Excess IgM production but no IgG, IgA or IgE	Prone to opportunistic infections particularly *Pneumocystis carinii* and *Cryptosporidium parvum*. The latter may progress to sclerosing cholangitis and cirrhosis	Liver cancer in X-linked HIM
Hyper IgE syndrome (HIE)	Autosomal dominant	Gene not identified yet. Mapped to chromosome 4q	Elevated IgE, defective neutrophil chemotaxis, impaired lymphocyte response to *Candida* antigen	Recurrent bacterial skin and lung infections, chronic mucocutaneous candidiasis, craniofacial abnormalities, scoliosis and bone fractures	No increased risk

Disease	Genetics	Mechanism	Immune defect	Clinical features	Cancer risk
X-linked lymphoproliferative syndrome (XLPS; Duncan's syndrome)	X-linked signalling lymphocyte-activating molecule (SLAM)-associated protein (SAP) (<1 in 1 000 000 male live births)	SLAM activates cytotoxic T cells and this action is regulated by SAP	Overproduction of polyclonal CD8+ cytotoxic T cells in response to EBV infection	EBV-induced T-cell proliferation causes severe organ damage, progressive hypogammaglobulinaemia or	Increased risk of EBV-associated lymphomas
T-cell deficiency					
DiGeorge syndrome (thymic aplasia)	Most have deletions of 22q11; 1 in 3500 live births	The third and fourth branchial pouches fail to form properly	Moderate to severe lack of T cells	Tetany and cardiac malformations just after birth. Lack of T cells may lead to fungal, viral or other infection in infancy. Increased risk of autoimmune diseases (e.g. thyroiditis)	No increased risk
Severe combined immunodeficiency (SCID) syndromes	Nine genetic (8 autosomal recessive, 1 X-linked) defects of T-cell maturation; 1 in 30 000 live births	Genetic defects affect purine metabolism (e.g. adenosine deaminase), VDJ recombination (e.g. recombinase activating genes) and lymphocyte signalling (e.g. common γ chain of interleukin receptors)	A variety of profound deficiencies of both T-cell and B-cell function	Failure to thrive and repeated infections caused by opportunistic infections by 6 months old. Protracted diarrhoea and death by 2 years in the absence of treatment	None known

Table 44.1 *Continued*

Name of syndrome	Inheritance and incidence	Genetic defect	Immunological defect	Clinical manifestations	Cancer risk
DNA-repair defects (see Chapter 1)					
Ataxia telangiectasia (AT; Louis–Bar syndrome)	Autosomal recessive ataxia-telangiectasia mutated (ATM), a protein kinase that reacts to DNA damage and affects the accumulation of p53 (1 in 60 000 live births)	Chromosomal instability due to defective DNA repair may interfere with immunoglobulin and T-cell receptor gene rearrangement	Most have IgA deficiency. Other hypoimmunoglobulinaemia and T-cell function deficits occur	Progressive cerebellar ataxia, skin telangiectasia. Most die in third decade of respiratory infections or tumours	Increased risk of acute leukaemias and lymphomas
Nijmegen breakage syndrome	Autosomal recessive	Chromosomal instability due to defective DNA repair may interfere with immunoglobulin and T-cell receptor gene rearrangement	Lymphopenia	As for AT but in addition have progressive microcephaly ('bird-like face')	Increased risk of acute leukaemias and lymphomas
Other					
Wiskott–Aldrich syndrome	X-linked recessive	Defective gene for WASP (Wiskott–Aldrich syndrome protein) involved in cytoskeleton reorganization following activation of platelets and T cells	Low IgM and raised IgE levels	Thrombocytopenia, eczema and increased autoimmune diseases (including vasculitis). Usually die by age 10 years	Increased risk of EBV-associated lymphomas

immunological tolerance, proposing that lymphocytes that were able to respond to self-antigens were deleted in prenatal life. This hypothesis was confirmed experimentally by Peter Medawar who shared the Nobel Prize with Burnet in 1960. Peter Medawar also wrote several wonderful books and collections of essays and I would encourage anyone who is thinking of doing scientific research to read *Advice to a Young Scientist*. In the 1960s, however, in a *volte face* that signalled a paradigm shift, Burnet began to champion the view that a major function of the immune system is to eliminate malignant cells. This was based upon evidence that animals can be immunized against syngeneic transplantable tumours. This theory of immune surveillance led to the identification of tumour antigens and of immunotherapy strategies to treat tumours.

Tumours in allograft recipients

The risk of cancer following an organ transplant varies with both the organ that has been transplanted and the type of cancer. The greatest risks numerically are with heart and heart–lung transplants, which often require a more aggressive regimen of immunosuppression to prevent graft rejection. In addition to PTLD that is caused by the Epstein–Barr virus (EBV), the risks of Kaposi's sarcoma (caused by Kaposi sarcoma herpesvirus (KSHV)), cervical cancer (caused by human papillomavirus (HPV)) and non-melanoma skin cancers are most dramatically increased. In the case of PTLD and post-transplantation Kaposi's sarcoma, reducing the immunosuppression may cause regression of the tumours – but this of course increases the risk of graft rejection.

Tumours in HIV patients

Studies by the World Health Organization (WHO) estimated that by December 2007, over 25 million people had died of acquired immune deficiency syndrome (AIDS) and 33 million people are living with the virus. The number of people newly infected with HIV worldwide is approximately 2.5 million per year. Along with opportunistic infections, tumours are a major feature of HIV infection. The most frequent tumours in this population are Kaposi's sarcoma (KS), non-Hodgkin's lymphoma and cervical cancer, and these three are AIDS-defining illnesses. The management of cancer in the immunodeficient host requires careful attention to the balance between antitumour effects and the toxicity associated. Combination antiretroviral treatment has both dramatically reduced the incidence of opportunistic infections and prolonged the survival of people with HIV infection. In addition, this highly active antiretroviral therapy (HAART) has reduced the incidence of AIDS-defining malignancies and improved their prognosis. Less than five million of the estimated 33 million people infected with HIV worldwide, however, are receiving HAART, as the majority of affected people live in developing countries. In addition, even in the established market economies with access to medical treatment, many individuals remain undiagnosed and consequently do not receive HAART.

Tumours in primary immunodeficiency

The cancers that occur with primary immunodeficiency syndromes are rare, and as a consequence treatment protocols and outcome data are scarce. Most patients succumb to infections, and these continue to pose a major threat to life during treatment of associated tumours.

Management of immunodeficiency-associated malignancies

The incidence of congenital immunodeficiency-associated tumours is sufficiently low for there to be little consensus upon their clinical management. In contrast, the incidence of both PTLD and KS has risen dramatically in recent years with the spread of the HIV pandemic and the marked increase in transplant surgery. The management of PTLD relies upon enhanced immunity against EBV by reducing immunosuppression and infusing

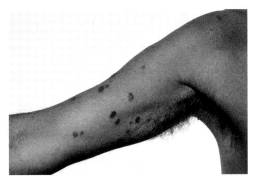

Figure 44.1 Multiple pigmented Kaposi sarcoma skin lesion in a man with HIV infection. Following antiretroviral therapy alone there was a marked regression of these lesions.

cytotoxic T lymphocytes against EBV. In addition, antiviral agents, low-dose chemotherapy and anti-CD20 monoclonal antibodies may be useful. The introduction of HAART has reduced the incidence of HIV-associated KS in established market economies where this treatment is available. Moreover, early-stage KS may be successfully treated with HAART alone, leading to regression of KS (Figure 44.1). Visceral KS is usually treated with systemic liposomal anthracycline chemotherapy with concomitant HAART. Other tumours that arise in immunodeficient individuals are generally treated along conventional lines, with extra attention to the risk of infectious complications of therapy.

Part 3

The Practice of Oncology

Chapter 45

Paraneoplastic complications of cancer

Paraneoplastic complications of malignancy are remote effects of cancer that arise without local spread. Most of these paraneoplastic syndromes arise due to secretion by tumours of hormones, cytokines and growth factors. Paraneoplastic syndromes also arise when normal cells secrete products in response to the presence of tumour cells. For example, antibodies produced in this fashion are responsible for many paraneoplastic neurological syndromes including cerebellar degeneration, Lambert–Eaton myasthenic syndrome and paraneoplastic retinopathy. Paraneoplastic neurological complications always appear on the list of differential diagnoses. However, just as viewers of *House MD* will know that 'it's not lupus', it is rarely paraneoplastic either.

Paraneoplastic endocrine complications

Cushing's syndrome

Cushing's syndrome is a clinical disorder resulting from prolonged exposure to excess glucocorticoids and should not be confused with Cushing's disease which refers exclusively to those cases that arise

due to an adrenocorticotrophic hormone (ACTH) secreting pituitary adenoma (Table 45.1). Clinically overt Cushing's syndrome caused by ectopic secretion of ACTH by non-endocrine-derived tumours is rare. Approximately 20% of cases of Cushing's syndrome are caused by ectopic ACTH secretion by a tumour that is frequently occult at presentation. For this reason the differential diagnosis between pituitary adenoma and ectopic ACTH is important clinically but biochemical overlap often makes this difficult. More than half the cases of ectopic ACTH syndrome are due to small cell lung cancer, with carcinoid tumours and neural crest tumours (phaeochromocytoma, neuroblastoma, medullary cell carcinoma of the thyroid) accounting for a further 15%. The typical presentation is of a middle-aged smoker with features of severe hypercortisolism and hypokalaemic metabolic alkalosis. Patients have muscle weakness or atrophy, oedema, hypertension, mental changes, glucose intolerance and weight loss. When ectopic ACTH production arises from a more benign tumour (e.g. bronchial carcinoid or thymoma), the other classic features of Cushing's syndrome may be present including truncal obesity, moon facies and cutaneous striae (Figure 45.1).

The diagnosis of Cushing's syndrome may be confirmed by elevated urinary free cortisol, loss of diurnal variation of plasma cortisol and failure of

Lecture Notes: Oncology, 2nd edition. By M. Bower and J. Waxman. Published 2010 by Blackwell Publishing Ltd.

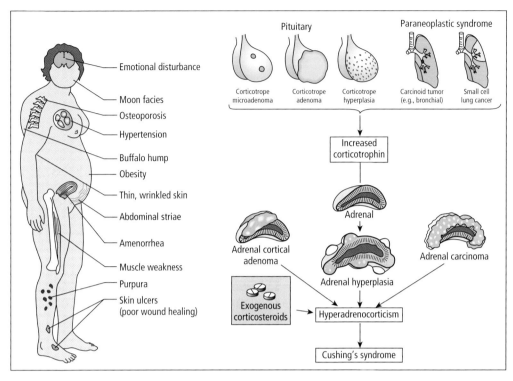

Figure 45.1 Causes and clinical features of Cushing's syndrome.

Table 45.1 Aetiology of Cushing's syndrome.

Type	Example
ACTH dependent	Pituitary adenoma (Cushing's disease)
	Ectopic ACTH secretion
	Ectopic CRH secretion (very rare)
ACTH independent	Exogenous glucocorticoid administration
	Adrenal adenoma
	Adrenal carcinoma
	Nodular adrenal hyperplasia

ACTH, adrenocorticotrophic hormone; CRH, corticotrophin-releasing hormone.

cortisol suppression in the low-dose dexamethasone (2 mg) test. After establishing the diagnosis, an elevated plasma ACTH supports the diagnosis of pituitary adenoma or ectopic ACTH syndrome. Failure of cortisol suppression following high-dose dexamethasone (2 mg four times daily for two days, or 8 mg overnight) and very high levels of ACTH (>200 pg/ml) suggest an ectopic source of ACTH. In difficult cases, a corticotrophin-releasing hormone (CRH) stimulation test, selective venous catheterization of the inferior petrosal sinus with ACTH estimations, somatostatin analogue scintigaphy and technetium-99 methoxyisobutylisonitrile (MIBI) imaging may be necessary to determine the source of ACTH.

The mainstay of palliative therapy for Cushing's syndrome due to ectopic ACTH production is inhibition of steroid synthesis, although inhibition of ACTH release and blocking glucocorticoid receptors have also been attempted. Several steroid synthesis inhibitors are available and successful use in these circumstances has been reported with aminoglutethamide, metyrapone, mitotane, ketoconazole and octreotide. On rare occasions laparoscopic bilateral adrenalectomy or adrenal artery embolization may be necessary to control symptoms.

Syndrome of inappropriate antidiuresis

Hyponatraemia is a common finding in association with advanced malignancy and many factors may contribute including cardiac and hepatic failure, hyperglycaemia and diuretics. However, the detection of concentrated urine in conjunction with hypo-osmolar plasma suggests abnormal renal free water excretion and the presence of the syndrome of inappropriate antidiuresis (SIAD). This acronym is better than the previous term 'SIADH' (syndrome of inappropriate antidiuretic hormone) since there is no vasopressin (ADH) secretion in approximately 15% of cases. In malignancy-related SIAD, tumours secrete ectopic arginine vasopressin or vasopressin-like peptides. In many respects SIAD is the opposite of diabetes insipidus; patients with SIAD are waterlogged with low plasma osmolality and sodium and high urine osmolality, whilst patients with diabetes insipidus are dehydrated with high plasma osmolality and sodium and low urine osmolality. SIAD is most frequently associated with small cell lung cancer or carcinoid tumours but has also been described in pancreatic, oesophageal, prostatic and haematological malignancies. Nonetheless many factors may contribute to SIAD (Table 45.2).

Significant symptoms of hyponatraemia appear at plasma sodium levels below 125 mmol/l, with confusion progressing to stupor, coma and seizures as levels fall. Nausea, vomiting and focal neurological deficits may also occur. The clinical features depend on both the levels of plasma sodium and the rate of decline. With gradual falls in sodium, the brain cells are able to compensate against cerebral oedema by secreting potassium and other intracellular solutes. Asymptomatic hyponatraemia therefore suggests chronic SIAD rather than acute SIAD. The division into chronic and acute SIAD is of therapeutic importance as their management differs. The diagnosis of SIAD requires the demonstration of plasma hyponatraemia and hypo-osmolality in the presence of concentrated urine and normal extracellular fluid volume (Table 45.3).

The management of SIAD depends upon the rate of onset of hyponatraemia and the presence of neu-

Table 45.2 Causes of the syndrome of inappropriate diuresis (SIAD).

Source of ADH	Examples
Ectopic ADH production	
Malignancy	Small cell lung cancer
Inappropriate pituitary secretion of ADH	
Malignancy	Lung cancer
	Lymphoma
Inflammatory lung disease	Pneumonia
	Lung abscess
Neurological disease	Meningitis
	Head injury
	Subdural haematoma
	Surgery
Drugs	Antidepressants
	(tricyclics, SSRIs)
	Carbamazepine
	Chlorpropamide
	Phenothiazines
	Vincristine
	Cyclophosphamide
	Ecstasy*
Postoperative	
Others	Hypothyroidism
	Porphyria
	Addison's disease

*Excessive water consumption may contribute to the development of hyponatraemia with ecstasy.
ADH, antidiuretic hormone; SSRI, selective serotonin reuptake inhibitor.

rological complications. Acute SIAD with an onset over two to three days and falls in serum sodium in excess of 0.5 mmol/l per day are associated with neurological sequelae and require prompt correction by intravenous hypertonic saline. In contrast, the mainstay of therapy for chronic asymptomatic SIAD is fluid restriction and inhibition of tubular reabsorption of water with drugs including the tetracycline antibiotic demeclocycline, which causes nephrogenic diabetes insipidus.

Non-islet cell tumour hypoglycaemia

Tumour-related hypoglycaemia is a frequent complication of β-islet cell tumours of the pancreas which secrete insulin (insulinomas), but occurs

Table 45.3 Diagnosis of the syndrome of inappropriate diuresis (SIAD).

Essential criteria to establish diagnosis
Plasma hypo-osmolality (plasma osmolality <275 mosmol/kg water and plasma sodium <135 mmol/l)
Concentrated urine (plasma osmolality >100 mosmol/kg water)
Normal plasma/extracellular fluid volume
High urinary sodium on a normal salt and water intake (urine sodium>20 mmol/l)
Exclude (i) hypothyroidism, (ii) hypoadrenalism and (iii) diuretics
Supportive criteria for diagnosis
Abnormal water load test (unable to excrete >90% of a 20 ml/kg water load in 4 hours and/or failure to dilute urine to osmolality <100 mosmol/kg water)
Elevated plasma arginine vasopressin levels

uncommonly with non-islet cell tumours. Most non-islet cell tumours produce hypoglycaemia through increased glucose use or by secreting insulin-like growth factors (IGF1 and IGF2). Non-islet cell tumours associated with hypoglycaemia are usually large retroperitoneal or intrathoracic sarcomas. Unlike other endocrine complications of malignancy, hypoglycaemia is very rarely associated with lung cancer. The clinical manifestations are due to cerebral hypoglycaemia and secondary secretion of catecholamines; they include agitation, stupor, coma and seizures that may follow exercise or fasting. Tumour-related hypoglycaemia should be differentiated from other causes of hypoglycaemia including drugs (e.g. sulphonylureas), hypoadrenalism, hypopituitarism and liver failure. In advanced malignancy the most common cause of hypoglycaemia is continued oral hypoglycaemic medication in long-standing diabetics.

Enteropancreatic hormone syndromes

Enteropancreatic hormone production is relatively uncommon in malignant disease. A variety of clinical syndromes occur associated with hormone secretion by endocrine tumours of the pancreas and less frequently tumours arising in other organs

(Table 45.4). The majority of pancreatic islet cell tumours are malignant (with the exception of most insulinomas) and metastases are frequently present at diagnosis. For many patients the distressing clinical manifestations arising from excessive secretion of gastrointestinal peptides require palliation and this may be difficult to achieve. These tumours often secrete more than one polypeptide hormone and may switch their hormone production during follow-up.

Carcinoid syndrome

Carcinoid tumours arise from enterochromaffin cells principally in the gastrointestinal tract, pancreas and lungs but occasionally in the thymus and gonads (Table 45.5). One in ten patients with carcinoid tumours develop the carcinoid syndrome after the development of hepatic metastases. This avoids the first pass metabolism of 5-hydroxytryptamine (serotonin, 5HT) and kinins in the liver so that the systemic symptoms occur. The acute symptoms are vasomotor flushing (typically of upper body lasting up to 30 minutes), fever, pruritic wheals, diarrhoea, asthma/wheezing, borborygmi and abdominal pain. Chronic complications include tricuspid regurgitation, arthropathy, pulmonary stenosis, mesenteric fibrosis, cirrhosis, pellagra (due to secondary deficiency of trytophan) and telangiectasia. The diagnostic investigation is 24-hour urinary collection of 5-hydroxyindoleacetic acid (5HIAA), a metabolite of 5HT. Somatostatin analogues are considered by most physicians to be the first-line treatment of choice for patients with carcinoid syndrome and indeed most enteropancreatic hormone syndromes. Palliation of the clinical manifestations of carcinoid syndrome includes symptomatic therapy of diarrhoea (codeine phosphate, loperamide or diphenoxylate), β₂-adrenergic agonists for wheezing, and avoiding precipitating factors to reduce flushing (including alcohol and some foods).

Phaeochromocytoma

Phaeochromocytomas arise from the chromaffin cells of the sympathetic nervous system, most

Table 45.4 Clinical manifestations of secretory endocrine tumours.

Tumour	Major feature	Minor feature	Common site	Percentage that are malignant	Percentage that are associated with MEN	Palliative treatments
Insulinoma	Neuroglycopenia (confusion, fits)	Permanent neurological deficits	Pancreas (β cells) >99%	10%	4–5%	Frequent feeding Glucose Glucagon Diazoxide Octreotide
Gastrinoma (Zollinger–Ellison syndrome)	Peptic ulceration	Diarrhoea Weight loss Malabsorption Dumping	Pancreas (D cells) 25% Duodenum 70%	>50%	20–25%	Gastrectomy Proton pump inhibitor H2 receptor antagonists Octreotide
VIPoma (Werner–Morrison syndrome)	Watery diarrhoea Hypokalaemia Achlorhydria	Hypercalcaemia Hyperglycaemia Hypomagnesaemia	Pancreas (A–D cells) 90% Neuroblastoma SCLC Phaeochromocytoma	>50%	6%	Octreotide Glucocorticoids
Glucagonoma	Migratory necrolyic erythema Mild diabetes mellitus Muscle wasting Anaemia	Diarrhoea Thromboembolism Stomatitis Hypoaminoacidaemia Encephalitis	Pancreas (α cells) 99%	>70%	1–20%	Octreotide Oral hypoglycaemics
Somatostatinoma	Diabetes mellitus Cholelithiasis Steatorrhoea Malabsorption	Anaemia Diarrhoea Weight loss Hypoglycaemia	Pancreas (β cells) 55% Duodenum and jejunum 45%	>60%	Case reports only	

H2, histamine type 2; MEN, multiple endocrine neoplasia; SCLC, small cell lung cancer; VIP, vasoactive intestinal polypeptide.

Table 45.5 Comparison of carcinoid tumours by site of origin.

Features	Foregut	Midgut	Hindgut
Frequency of occurrence	2–33% carcinoid tumours	75–87% carcinoid tumours	1–8% carcinoid tumours
Site	Respiratory tract, pancreas, stomach, proximal duodenum	Jejunum, ileum, appendix, Meckle's diverticulum, ascending colon	Transverse and descending colon, rectum
Tumour products	Low 5HTP, multihormones*	High 5HTP, multihormones*	Rarely 5HTP, multihormones*
Blood	5HTP, histamine, multihormones*, occasionally ACTH	5HT, multihormones*, rarely ACTH	Rarely 5HT or ACTH
Urine	5HTP, 5HT, 5HIAA, histamine	5HT, 5HIAA	Negative
Carcinoid syndrome	Occurs but is atypical	Occurs frequently with metastases	Rarely occurs
Metastasizes to bone	Common	Rare	Common

*Multihormones include tachykinins (substance P, substance K, neuropeptide K), neurotensin, PYY, enkephalin, insulin, glucagon, glicentin, vasoactive intestinal polypeptide, somatostatin, pancreatic polypeptide, ACTH and α-subunit of human chorionic gonadotrophin.
ACTH, adrenocorticotrophic hormone; 5HIAA, 5-hydroxyindole-acetic acid; 5HT, 5-hydroxytryptamine (serotonin); 5HTP, 5-hydroxytryptophan.

frequently in the adrenal medulla but occasionally from sympathetic ganglia. Phaeochromocytomas commonly secrete norepinephrine (noradrenaline) and epinephrine (adrenaline) but in some cases significant quantities of dopamine are also produced. Phaeochromocytomas are associated with a number of familial inherited cancer syndromes including multiple endocrine neoplasia (MEN) 2a, MEN 2b, von Hippel–Lindau syndrome and neurofibromatosis. The catecholamines cause intermittent, episodic or sustained hypertension and other clinical manifestations including anxiety, tremor, palpitations, sweating, flushing, headaches, gastrointestinal disturbances and polyuria. These symptoms are all attributable to excessive adrenergic stimulation.

24-hour urinary collection for urinary free catecholamines (epinephrine, norepinephrine and dopamine) is now the most widely employed diagnostic test although some centres also measure catecholamine metabolites such as metanephrines and vanillylmandelic acid (VMA). The tumour may be localized by radiolabelled meta-iodobenzyl guanidine (MIBG) scintography.

Initial treatment should be α-blockade to control hypertension followed by β-blockade to control tachycardia. This combination will control symptoms in most patients with malignant phaeochromocytoma. If palliation is not achieved, high-dose ^{131}I-MIBG may be used as therapy for phaeochromocytoma and neuroblastoma as it reduces catecholamine synthesis. This may only have a chance of success if the patient has small volume metastases, because ^{131}I-MIBG is β-emitting and β-particles have poor tissue penetration.

Gynaecomastia

Gynaecomastia results from elevation in the oestrogen : androgen ratio, which may be either a consequence of decreased androgen production or activity or increased oestrogen formation (usually by peripheral aromatization of circulating androgens to oestrogens). In men with advanced cancer, gynaecomastia is most often a consequence of drug therapy, either chemotherapy (alkylating agents, vinca alkaloids, nitrosoureas), anti-emetics (metoclopramide, phenothiazines), anti-androgens

Box 45.1: Oncological mnemonics

Causes of hypercalcaemia: GRIM FED

Granulomas (TB, sarcoid)
Renal failure
Immobility
Malignancy
Familial (familial hypocalciuric hypercalcaemia)
Endocrine **PATH** (**p**haeochromocytoma, **A**ddison's, **t**hyrotixicosis, **h**yperparathyroidism)
Drugs (thiazides, lithium, vitamins A and D, milk alkali syndrome)

Causes of SIADH: SIADH

Surgery
Intracranial (infection, head injury, cerebrovascular accident)
Alveolar (pus, cancer)
Drugs **ABCD** (**a**nalgesics: opiates, non-steriodal anti-inflammatory drugs, **b**arbiturates, **c**yclophosphamide/**c**arbamazepine/**c**hlorpromazine, **d**iuretic: thiazides))
Hormonal (hypothyroid, Addison's)

Causes of Cushingoid features: CUSHINGOID

Cataracts
Ulcers
Striae
Hypertension, hirsutism
Infections
Necrosis (avascular necrosis of femoral head)
Glycouria, glycaemia
Osteoporosis, obesity
Immunosuppression
Diabetes

Phaeochromocytoma: rule of 10s

This mnemonic applies to *adults* with phaeochromocytomas.
10% are extra-adrenal
10% are bilateral or multiple
10% are malignant
10% are familial

Phaeochromocytoma symptoms: 5 Hs

Headache
Hypertension
Hypotension (postural)
Heartbeat (palpitations)
Hyperhidrosis (sweating)

Causes of gynaecomastia: GYNAECOMASTIA

Genetic (Kleinfelter's, Kallman's)
Youth (puberty)*
Neonate*
Antifungals (ketoconazole)
Estrogen
Cirrhosis/cimetidine
Old age*
Marijuana
Alcoholism
Spirolonactone/stilboestrol
Tumours (testicular, adrenal)
Isoniazid
Alkylating agents

Causes of clubbing: CLUBBING

Cyanotic congenital heart disease
Lung disease (abscess, bronchiectasis, cystic fibrosis, empyema, fibrosing alveolitis)
Ulcerative colitis/Crohn's disease
Biliary cirrhosis
Birth defect (hereditary pachydermoperiostosis)
Infective endocarditis
Neoplasia (non-small cell lung cancer, mesothelioma, gastrointestinal lymphoma)
Goitre (thyrotoxicosis)

Features of MEN

MEN 1: 3Ps
Pituitary adenoma
Pancreatic islet cell tumours
Parathyroid

MEN 2: 2Cs
Catecholamines (phaeochromocytoma)
Cell carcinoma (medullary) of thyroid
Plus:
MEN 2a: parathyroid tumours
MEN 2b (also known as MEN 3): mucocutaneous neuromas

* Physiological causes.

(cyproterone acetate, flutamide, bicalutamide) or gonadotrophin-releasing hormone analogues (goserelin, leuprorelin). Occasionally other tumour secretion of oestrogens or gonadotrophins may be responsible. Tumours may either secrete oestrogens (Leydig cell testicular tumours and feminizing adrenocortical tumours), promote the conversion of androgens to oestrogens (Sertoli cell testicular tumours and hepatoma) or secrete human chorionic gonadotrophin (HCG) stimulating oestradiol production in the testes (testicular tumours, non-small cell lung cancers, hepatoma and islet cell tumours of the pancreas).

Paraneoplastic neurological conditions

In contrast to the metabolic and endocrine paraneoplastic conditions where products secreted by the tumours are responsible, most neurological paraneoplastic syndromes are immune mediated. Moreover with neurological paraneoplastic syndromes, the tumour may be asymptomatic or occult. It is thought that antibodies reacting to antigens on the surface of cancer cells cross-react with neural antigens and are the basis of these syndromes. The antibodies may be directed at ion channels, for example the presynaptic P-type voltage-gated calcium channel in the case of Lambert–Eaton myasthenic syndrome and the nictonic acetyl choline receptor in myasthenia gravis. Alternatively, antibodies may bind intracellular proteins such as Hu, a neuronal nuclear RNA-binding protein, and Yo, a cytoplasmic protein in Purkinje cells of the cerebellum. The most common paraneoplastic neurological manifestations are described in association with small cell lung cancer (Table 45.6).

Paraneoplastic dermatological conditions

A number of paraneoplastic dermatological manifestations have been described, and some are listed in Table 45.7. Amongst the most common paraneoplastic dermatological manifestation is clubbing

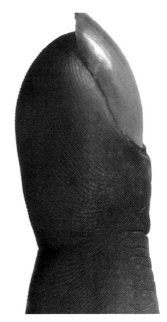

Figure 45.2 Finger nail clubbing is characterized by increased longitudinal curving of the nail, loss of the angle between the nail and its bed and bogginess of the nail fold.

(see Figure 45.2), a clinical sign beloved of physicians and first described by Hippocrates over 2400 years ago. It is characterized by softening of the nail bed and periungual erythema with loss of the normal 15 degree angle at the hyponychium. As this advances, bulging of the distal phalynx and curvature of the nail lead to a drumstick end appearance. Clubbing may be associated with hypertrophic osteoarthropathy with new subperiosteal cancellous bone formation at the distal ends of long bones, particularly the radius and ulna or tibia and fibula (Figure 45.3). A hereditary form of clubbing with hypertrophic osteo-arthropathy, Touraine–Solente–Golé syndrome, has recently been shown to be due to germline mutations of the 15-hydroxyprostaglandin dehydrogenase gene that catabolizes prostaglandin E2. Whether paraneoplastic clubbing is due to elevated levels of prostaglandin E2 or tumour-related secretion of growth factors, including PDGF (platelet-derived growth factor) and HGF (hepatocyte growth factor), remains unclear.

Table 45.6 Paraneoplastic neurological manifestations.

Condition	Clinical features	Antibodies	Percentage that are paraneoplastic	Underlying malignancy
Dermatomyositis	Erythematous rash, arthralgia	Anti-Jo-1	20%	NSCLC, SCLC, lymphoma
Encephalomyelitis	Fluctuating confusion, anxiety, depression, impaired short term memory	Anti-Hu, anti-CV2	10%	SCLC, thymoma
Lambert–Eaton syndrome	Proximal muscle weakness sparing eyes; power increases with repetition	Anti-VGCC	60%	SCLC
Myasthenia gravis	Muscle fatigability, ptosis, ophthalmoplegia	Anti-AChR	5%	Thymoma
Opsoclonus–myoclonus syndrome	Opsoclonus (irregular, rapid, horizontal and vertical eye movements) and myoclonus (brief, shock-like muscle spasms), intention tremor, unsteady gait	Anti-Hu, anti-Ri	20–50%	Neuroblastoma, breast
Polymyositis	Proximal muscle weakness, rash	Anti-Jo-1	10%	NSCLC, SCLC, lymphoma
Retinopathy	Night blindness, ring scotomas, photosensitivity	Anti-recoverin		SCLC, melanoma
Sensory neuropathy	Rapid progressive loss of all sensory modalities especially proprioception	Anti-Hu	10–20%	SCLC
Subacute cerebellar degeneration	Ataxia, nystagmus, dysarthria	Anti-Yo, anti-Hu, anti-VGCC, anti-Tr	50%	SCLC, ovary, Hodgkin's

NSCLC, non-small cell lung cancer; SCLC, small cell lung cancer.

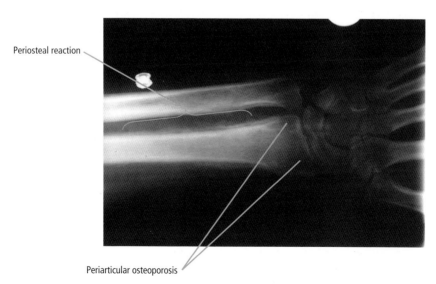

Figure 45.3 Forearm radiograph showing a periosteal reaction in the metaphysis and diaphysis of the radius and ulnar and periarticular osteoporosis due to hypertrophic osteoarthropathy secondary to non-small cell lung cancer (squamous cell).

Table 45.7 Paraneoplastic dermatological conditions.

Condition	Clinical features	Underlying malignancy
Acanthosis nigricans	Grey-brown, symmetrical, velvety plaques on neck, axillae and flexor areas	Adenocarcinoma, predominantly gastric
Acquired ichthyosis	Generalized dry, cracking skin; hyperkeratotic palms and soles	Hodgkin's disease, lymphomas, myeloma
Acrokeratosis paraneoplastica (Bazex syndrome)	Symmetrical psoriasiform hyperkeratosis with scales and pruritis on toes, ears and nose; nail dystrophy	Squamous carcinoma of oesophagus, head and neck, and lungs
Bullous pemphigoid	Large tense blisters; antibodies to desmoplakin	Lymphomas and others
Cushing's syndrome	Broad purple striae; plethora; telangiectasia; mild hirsutism	Small cell lung cancer, thyroid, testis, ovary and adrenal tumours, pancreatic islet cell tumours, pituitary tumours
Dermatitis herpetiformis	Pleomorphic, symmetrical, subepidermal bullae	Lymphoma and others
Dermatomyositis	Erythema or telangiectasia of knuckles and periorbital regions	Miscellaneous tumours
Erythema annulare centrifugum	Slowly migrating annular red lesions	Prostate tumours, myeloma and others
Erythema gyratum repens	Progressive scaling erythema with pruritis	Lung, breast, uterus and gastrointestinal tumours
Exfoliative dermatitis	Progressive erythema followed by scaling	Cutaneous T-cell lymphoma, Hodgkin's disease and other lymphomas
Flushing	Episodic reddening of face and neck	Carcinoid syndrome, medullary cell carcinoma of the thyroid
Generalized melanosis	Diffuse grey-brown skin pigmentation	Melanoma, ACTH-producing tumours
Hirsutism	Increased hair in male distribution	Adrenal tumours, ovarian tumours
Hypertrichosis lanuginosa	Rapid development of fine, long, silky hair	Lung, colon, bladder, uterus and gallbladder tumours
Muir–Torre syndrome	Sebaceous gland neoplasm	Colon cancer, lymphoma
Necrolytic migratory erythema	Circinate area of blistering and erythema on face, abdomen and limbs	Islet cell tumour of the pancreas (glucagonoma)
Pachydermoperiostosis	Thickening of skin folds, lips and ears; macroglossia; clubbing; excessive sweating	Lung cancer
Paget's disease of the nipple	Red keratotic patch over areola, nipple or accessory breast tissue	Breast cancer
Pemphigus vulgaris	Bullae of skin and oral blisters	Lymphomas, breast cancer
Pruritis	Generalized itching	Lymphoma, leukaemia, myeloma, central nervous system tumours, abdominal tumours
Sign of Leser–Trelat	Sudden onset of large number of seborrhoeic keratoses	Adenocarcinoma of the stomach, lymphoma, breast cancer
Sweet's syndrome	Painful, raised, red plaques; fever; neutrophilia	Leukaemias
Systemic nodular panniculitis (Weber–Christian disease)	Recurrent crops of tender, violaceous, subcutaneous nodules, which may be accompanied by abdominal pain and fat necrosis in bone marrow and lungs	Adenocarcinoma of the pancreas
Tripe palms	Hyperpigmented, velvety, thickened palms with exaggerated ridges	Gastric and lung cancer

ACTH, adrenocorticotrophic hormone.

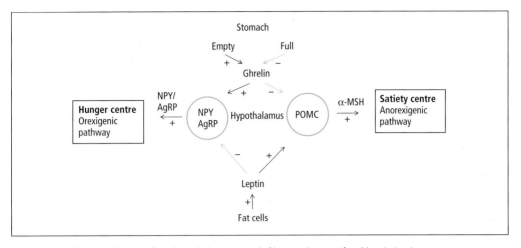

Figure 45.4 Schematic diagram of the hypothalamic control of hunger (see text for abbreviations).

Cachexia

Cachexia or severe protein-calorie malnutrition is one of the most debilitating and life-threatening aspects of cancer. This highly distressing symptom severely impairs the quality of life of many patients with cancer but is the focus of relatively little research. The normal balance between hunger and satiety, anorexia and obesity in humans is maintained by equilibrium between adipose-derived hormones including leptin and gut-derived hormones including ghrelin. An empty stomach stimulates ghrelin release which acts to promote neuropeptide Y (NPY) and Agouti-related peptide (AgRP) secretion in the hypothalamus, resulting in stimulation of the hunger centre. At the same time, ghrelin inhibits the release of pro-opiomelanocortin (POMC) hormones including α-MSH (melanocyte-stimulating hormone) from the hypothalamus, thus inhibiting the satiety centre and blocking anorexigenic pathways. Leptin, which is produced by fat cells, antagonizes ghrelin's actions on the hypothalamus by inhibiting NPY and AgRP release and stimulating α-MSH secretion (Figure 45.4). Amongst the mechanisms invoked in cancer cachexia is disruption of this delicate homoeostatic mechanism. In addition, tumour-related secretion of pro-inflammatory cytokines including interleukin-1 (IL-1) and interleukin-6 (IL-6), interferon gamma (IFN-γ) and tumour necrosis factor alpha (TNF-α) are thought to play a role in the pathogenesis of cancer cachexia. These effects may be mediated partly via the hypothalamic leptin/gherlin axis. Another clue to cancer cachexia has been found with the identification of proteolysis-inducing factor (PIF) and lipid-mobilizing factor (LMF). PIF causes breakdown of muscle proteins in skeletal muscle by activating the ubiquitin proteosome pathway and levels of PIF are raised in cancer patients with wasting. LMF, which is produced by tumour cells, causes lipolysis by raising the levels of the mitochondrial uncoupling proteins that turn brown fat into heat in hibernating animals.

The severe weight loss shortens survival and decreases quality of life substantially, indeed for many malignancies weight loss of >10% body weight is an independent adverse prognostic factor. The two major options for pharmacological therapy that aim to enhance appetite are progestogens, such as megestrol acetate, and corticosteroids. Neither these drugs nor enteral or parenteral nutrition has proved universally beneficial and both approaches are associated with appreciable toxicity. This is particularly so for corticosteroids, which, although they stimulate appetite, are catabolic in effect, leading to muscle loss. As the molecular aetiology of cancer cachexia is unveiled, novel therapeutic strategies are emerging.

Chapter 46

Oncological emergencies

Hypercalcaemia

One in ten cancer patients develop hypercalcaemia and malignancy accounts for about half the cases of hypercalcaemia amongst hospital inpatients. Hypercalcaemia occurs most frequently with myeloma, breast, lung and renal cancers, and 20% of cases occur in the absence of bone metastases. Most patients with hypercalcaemia of malignancy have disseminated disease and 80% die within one year. Thus hypercalcaemia is usually a complication of advanced disease and its treatment should be directed at palliation as it may produce a number of distressing symptoms (Table 46.1). The treatment of hypercalcaemia of malignancy frequently ameliorates these symptoms, and for this reason the diagnosis should always be sought.

In recent years there have been significant advances in our understanding of the biochemical processes that cause hypercalcaemia in malignancy, such that the factors involved in local osteolysis and in the evolution of humoral hypercalcaemia have now been delineated. A number of different cytokines have been implicated in the development of hypercalcaemia as a result of local osteolysis. These osteoclast-activating factors, which are released locally by metastatic tumour and stimulate osteoclastic resorption of

bone, include prostaglandin E2, tumour necrosis factors alpha (TNF-α) and beta (TNF-β), epidermal growth factor and transforming growth factor beta (TGF-β). It is probable that interleukin 1, epidermal growth factor and the tumour necrosis factors are the most important of these aetiological agents as the release of macrophage colony-stimulating factor by osteoblasts is enhanced by these factors. Since osteoclasts are derived from a haematopoietic stem cell progenitor, this release of macrophage colony-stimulating factor may be fundamental to oestoclastic bone resorption.

Humoral hypercalcaemia was described in 1941 by Albright but it was only in the late 1980s that the humoral factor causing hypercalcaemia was characterized. In the 1970s hypercalcaemia was thought to result from the ectopic production of parathyroid hormone (PTH) but this hypothesis remained unproven because the use of PTH antisera failed to demonstrate excessive secretion of PTH in patients with humoral hypercalcaemia. In addition, low serum concentrations of 1,25-vitamin D3 and urinary cyclic adenosine monophosphate (AMP) levels failed to reflect excess PTH activity and no PTH mRNA was found in the tumours of patients with humoral hypercalcaemia.

In the late 1980s polyadenylated RNA from a renal carcinoma from a patient with this syndrome was used to construct a cDNA library which was screened with a codon-preference oligonucleotide, synthesized on the basis of a partial N-terminal

Lecture Notes: Oncology, 2nd edition. By M. Bower and J. Waxman. Published 2010 by Blackwell Publishing Ltd.

Table 46.1 Clinical features of hypercalcaemia of malignancy.

General	Gastrointestinal	Neurological	Cardiological
Dehydration	Anorexia	Fatigue	Bradycardia
Polydipsia	Weight loss	Lethargy	Atrial arrhythmias
Polyuria	Nausea	Confusion	Ventricular arrhythmias
Pruritis	Vomiting	Myopathy	Prolonged P-R interval
	Constipation	Hyporeflexia	Reduced Q-T interval
	Ileus	Seizures	Wide T waves
		Psychosis	
		Coma	

amino acid sequence from a human tumour-derived peptide and a 2.0 kilobase cDNA was identified. The cDNA encoded a 177 amino acid prohormone, which consisted of a 36 amino acid leader sequence that is cleaved to produce a 141 amino acid, mature peptide and PTH-related peptide. The first 13 amino acids of the mature peptide have a sequence homology with PTH, and the *N*-terminal sequence is thought to be the PTH receptor-binding region. PTH-related peptide was found to be expressed in most normal human tissue, where its role is undetermined. The gene for PTH-related peptide has been mapped to the short arm of chromosome 12 and this is in contrast to the PTH gene which has been mapped to the short arm of chromosome 11. The gene for PTH-related peptide is complex and contains a six exon, 12 kilobase, single copy sequence, encoding up to five mRNA species. Exons 2, 3 and 4 are similar to the PTH gene.

A radioimmunoassay for PTH-related peptide was used to screen patients with hypercalcaemia-associated malignancy and the results contrasted with patients who were normocalcaemic and had malignant disease, patients with primary hyperparathyroidism and normal controls. PTH-related peptide was elevated in 19 of 39 (49%) patients with malignant hypercalcaemia, 12 of 74 (16%) normocalcaemic patients with malignancy, and four of 20 patients (20%) with hyperparathyroidism, but in none of 22 normal controls.

The clinical manifestations of hypercalcaemia are varied (Table 46.1) and many symptoms may be wrongly attributed to the underlying malignancy. A diagnosis of hypercalcaemia can only be made by biochemical investigation so all symptomatic patients with malignancy should have their corrected serum calcium measured if treatment is likely to be appropriate:

$$\text{Corrected calcium} = \text{measured calcium} + [(40 - \text{serum albumin (g/l)}) \times 0.02]$$

The mainstay of therapy is rehydration with large volumes of intravenous fluids followed by the administration of calcium-lowering agents, most commonly bisphosphonates. Low calcium diets are unpalatable, exacerbate malnutrition and have no place in palliative therapy. Drugs promoting hypercalcaemia (e.g. thiazide diuretics, vitamins A and D) should be withdrawn. The cornerstone of the re-establishment of normocalcaemia is treatment with a bisphosphonate. Bisphosphonates have multiple functions in hypercalcaemia. They reduce serum calcium levels by a direct effect on the osteoclast, by stabilizing hydroxyapatite crystals. There are two classes of effect of bisphosphonates. One group of bisphosphonates, which include clodronate and etidronate, acts through their incorporation into non-hydrolyzable analogues of adenosine triphosphate (ATP) that accumulate in osteoclasts and induce apoptosis. Alternately, agents such as pamidronate and zoledronate inhibit an enzyme called FPP synthase which functions in the mevalonate pathway. This leads to inhibition of protein prenylation. The bisphosphonates of choice are currently pamidronate, zoledronate and ibandronate. Approximately 80% of patients respond to hydration and bisphosphonate treatment by normalization of serum calcium levels. Calcium levels start to normalize within the first 24 hours of treatment with bisphosphonates and reach normal levels usually within three days. It is a dogma that treatment with bisphosphonates has to be repeated, usually on a three to four-weekly cycle. However, there is some information that suggests that a single treatment may be sufficient with re-setting of the calcium-stabilizing mechanisms. As well as these actions, bisphosphonates have valuable analgesic activity in patients with metastatic bone pain and reduce skeletal morbidity in patients with breast cancer and myeloma. In 20% of patients with hypercalcaemia, bisphosphonates do not work. Alternative treatments include the use of a somatostatin analogue such as octreotide which acts to reduce serum levels of PTHr-related peptide. Other more old fashioned treatments include calcitonin and mithramycin.

Superior vena cava obstruction

Superior vena cava obstruction (SVCO) restricts the venous return from the upper body resulting in oedema of the arms and face, distension of the neck and arm veins, headaches and a dusky blue skin discoloration over the upper chest, arms and face. SVCO is caused by a mediastinal mass compressing the vessel with or without intraluminal thrombus. Collateral circulation via the azygous vein may provide some drainage and over a period of weeks collaterals may form over the chest wall. In this case the flow of blood in these collateral veins will be from above downwards into the inferior vena cava circulation and this may be demonstrated clinically as an aid to confirm the diagnosis.

The presenting symptoms of SVCO include dyspnoea, swelling of the face and arms, headaches, a choking sensation, cough and chest pain (see Plate 46.1). The most important clinical sign is loss of venous pulsations in the distended neck veins. This is usually accompanied by facial oedema, plethora and cyanosis, and tachypnoea. The severity of the symptoms is determined by the rate of obstruction and the development of a compensatory collateral circulation. The symptoms may deteriorate when lying flat or bending, which further compromises the obstructed venous return. Careful assessment of the patient's history is frequently suggestive of a long period with minor symptoms of SVCO. In 9 out of 10 cases, the cause of SVCO is a malignancy, most often lung cancer (disproportionately more often small cell lung cancer) (Figure 46.1), lymphoma or metastatic breast or germ cell cancer. Rare non-malignant causes are listed in Table 46.2.

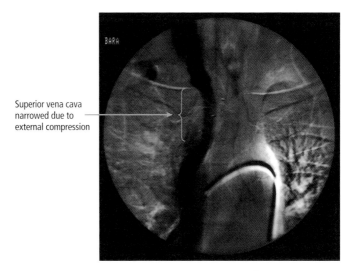

Superior vena cava narrowed due to external compression

Figure 46.1 Angiogram showing superior vena cava compression at the level of the carina due to small cell lung cancer.

Table 46.2 Non-maligant causes of superior vena cava obstruction (SVCO).

Mediastinal fibrosis	Idiopathic
	Histoplasmosis
	Actinomycosis
	Tuberculosis
Vena cava thrombosis	Idiopathic
	Behcet's syndrome
	Polycythemia vera
	Paroxysmal nocturnal haemoglobinuria
	Long-term venous catheters, shunts or pacemakers
Benign mediastinal tumours	Aortic aneurysm
	Dermoid tumour
	Retrosternal goitre
	Sarcoidosis
	Cystic hygroma

The management of SVCO depends upon the cause and severity, along with the patient's prognosis, and includes relieving symptoms as well as treating the underlying cause. SVCO is an oncological emergency in the presence of airway compromise and delays whilst histological findings are confirmed may adversely affect the outcome. In such circumstances patients are treated empirically with steroids and radiotherapy. However, when it is safe to do so, it is important to establish the diagnosis as this will determine the optimum treatment and a delay of one to two days to obtain a histological diagnosis is often appropriate, particularly in the context of a patient with minor symptoms and a long clinical history. Diagnostic procedures should include a plain chest X-ray (CXR), sputum cytology, bronchoscopy, thoracoscopy or mediastinoscopy, computed tomography (CT) scans or magnetic resonance imaging (MRI) and venography. A palpable lymph node may be amenable to biopsy, thereby providing a diagnosis.

Patients may respond to being sat upright with oxygen therapy and intravenous corticosteroids should be administered. In the majority of cases radiotherapy is the most appropriate treatment modality and relieves symptoms in up to 90% of patients within a fortnight. Where a diagnosis of lymphoma, small cell lung cancer or germ cell tumour has been obtained chemotherapy may be the optimal initial treatment.

For patients with recurrent SVCO, or in those where other therapeutic modalities are unsuitable, insertion of expandable wire stents under radiological guidance can be effective (Figure 46.2). Studies report instantaneous symptomatic relief with an excellent response rate. Although bypass of the obstruction has been performed surgically, this is usually reserved for patients with benign disorders. For central venous access catheter-associated thrombosis, removal of the line and anticoagulation should be commenced. The administration of low-dose warfarin has been reported to reduce the incidence of thrombosis associated with central venous access catheters.

Spinal cord compression

Spinal cord compression is a relatively common complication of disseminated cancer and affects 5% of patients with cancer. Spinal cord compression occurs with many tumour types but is particularly frequent in myeloma and prostate cancer. Up to 30% of these patients will survive for one year, so it is essential to be spared paraplegia for this remaining time by making the diagnosis swiftly and instituting treatment quickly. In general, the residual neurological deficit reflects the extent of deficit at the start of treatment, so early treatment leaves less damage. Neoplastic cord compression is nearly always due to extramedullary, extradural metastases usually from breast, lung, prostate, lymphoma or renal cancers. Commonly compression occurs by posterior expansion of vertebral metastases or extension of paraspinal metastases through the intervertebral foramina. These result in demyelination, arterial compromise, venous occlusion and vasogenic oedema of the spinal cord, all contributing to myelopathy; 70% occur in the thoracic spine, 20% in the lumbar spine and 10% in the cervical spine.

The earliest symptom of cord compression is vertebral pain, especially on coughing and lying flat. Subsequent signs include sensory changes one or two dermatomes below the level of compression. A complaint of back pain with focal weakness and

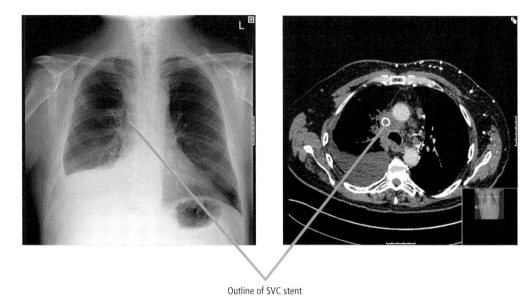

Outline of SVC stent

Figure 46.2 Chest X-ray and CT scan showing a superior vena cava (SVC) stent *in situ*.

bladder or bowel dysfunction with a sensory level requires urgent investigation in a patient with cancer. This will progress to motor weakness distal to the block and finally sphincter disturbance. If spinal cord compression is missed, or left untreated, patients can develop severe neurological deficits and double incontinence.

Spinal cord compression should be treated as a medical emergency. High-dose intravenous corticosteroids should be initiated on clinical suspicion alone to prevent further evolution of neurological deficit. Plain X-rays of the spine looking for vertebral collapse and MRI of the spinal axis to define the presence and level(s) of spinal cord compression should then be performed (Figures 46.3–46.5). 20 to 30% of patients have multiple levels of cord compression and imaging of the whole cord is therefore essential. If appropriate, a neurosurgical opinion should be obtained regarding the potential of surgical decompression, especially if there is vertebral instability or if the level of the compression has been previously irradiated. Otherwise, the definitive treatment is urgent local radiotherapy. It is important to provide adequate analgesia. Pretreatment ambulatory function is the main determinant of post-treatment gait function, thus prompt diagnosis and treatment is the key to gait and continence preservation.

Malignant effusions

Pleural effusions

Although not strictly an emergency, approximately 40% of all pleural effusions are due to malignancy (Table 46.3) and it frequently indicates advanced and incurable disease. The pleural space is normally filled with 10-40 ml of hypoproteinaceous plasma that originates from the capillary bed of the parietal pleura and is drained through the parietal pleura lymphatics. A pleural effusion is often the first manifestation of malignancy, and lung cancer and breast cancer account for almost two-thirds of cases. Malignant pleural effusions may be asymptomatic or cause progressive dyspnoea, cough and chest pain which may be pleuritic in nature. Malignant pleural effusions are usually exudates and this may be confirmed by a fluid lactate dehydrogenase (LDH) of >200 U/ml, a fluid : serum LDH ratio >0.6, a fluid : serum protein

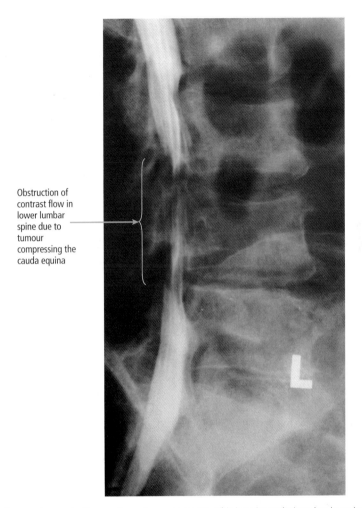

Obstruction of contrast flow in lower lumbar spine due to tumour compressing the cauda equina

Figure 46.3 Myelogram demonstrating cauda equine compression. This invasive technique has been largely replaced by CT and MRI.

ratio >0.5 and a fluid:serum glucose ratio of <0.5. The fluid may be blood stained and is typically hypercellular, containing lymphocytes, monocytes and reactive mesothelial cells; exfoliated tumour cells may be present also.

The management of malignant effusions should be tailored to the patient's symptoms as only half the patients will be alive at 3 months and over 90% of effusions will recur within 30 days of thoracocentesis. Reaccumulation of pleural effusions may be delayed by chemical pleurodesis (usually using talc or tetracycline) or video-assisted thoracic surgery (VATS) with pleurectomy and/or talc insufflation. Pleuroperitoneal shunts or chronic indwelling catheters may be considered for patients who fail pleurodesis, but this is rarely appropriate.

Pericardial effusions

The accumulation of fluid in the pericardial space around the heart may adversely affect cardiac function and like all effusions may be transudate, exudate or haemorrhage. Cardiac tamponade occurs when the pressure on the ventricles in

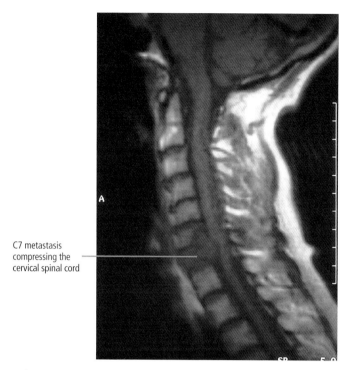

C7 metastasis compressing the cervical spinal cord

Figure 46.4 MRI scan demonstrating metastasis in a cervical C7 vertebral body with soft tissue extension posteriorly to cause compression of the cervical spinal cord.

diastole prevents them from filling, thus reducing the stroke volume and cardiac output. The classic sign of cardiac tamponade is Beck's triad of hypotension because of decreased stroke volume, jugular–venous distension due to impaired venous return to the heart, and muffled heart sounds due to fluid inside the pericardium (Figure 46.6).

Ascites

The most frequent malignancies causing ascites are primary tumours of the ovaries, pancreas, stomach and colon, breast and lungs. The distressing symptoms of ascites include abdominal distension or pain, dyspnoea due to diaphragmatic splinting, oedema of the legs, perineum and lower trunk, and a 'squashed stomach syndrome' leading to anorexia. If these symptoms are distressing, paracentesis is indicated – it offers rapid symptom relief but poor long-term control. Whilst anticancer therapy may reduce the subsequent reaccumulation of ascites, if this is not an option or is unsuccessful, diuretics may be helpful. Rarely a peritoneovenous shunt may be surgically placed under general anaesthetic if the ascites cannot be controlled.

Tumour lysis syndrome

The acute destruction of a large number of cells is associated with metabolic sequelae, and is termed the 'tumour lysis syndrome'. Cell destruction results in the release of different chemicals into the circulation, some of which may cause profound complications. Electrolyte release may cause transient hypercalcaemia, hyperphosphataemia and hyperkalaemia. The release of calcium and phosphate into the blood stream rarely causes any significant consequences. However, the calcium and phosphate may co-precipitate and cause some impairment of renal function. Hyperkalaemia can be a much more significant problem and may manifest as minor electrocardiograph (ECG) abnormal-

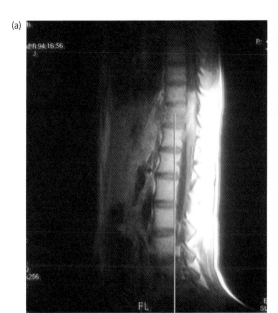

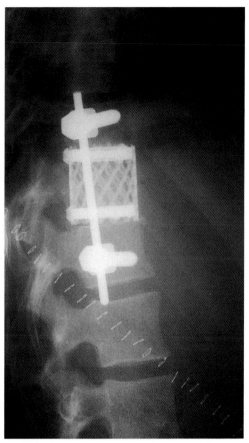

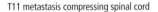

T11 metastasis compressing spinal cord

Figure 46.5 (a) MRI showing spine bone metastasis and cord compression at T11 due to vertebral metastasis with soft tissue extension. (b) A matched plain X-ray following surgical decompression and stabilization of the metastasis.

ities which, of course, all students reading this book can describe in intimate and complex detail (Table 46.4). Even more significant, however, are the cardiac arrhythmias, which may include ventricular tachycardia or ventricular fibrillation, and which may lead to the demise of the patient. Nucleic acid breakdown leads to hyperuricaemia and this, unless treated appropriately, can be complicated by renal failure due to the precipitation of uric acid crystals in the renal tubular system. So, of course, it is best that these things do not happen because we do not like our patients dying, least of all because of the complications of the treatment that we give them.

There are certain malignancies whose treatment is associated with a higher than usual risk of tumour lysis syndrome and these include acute promyelocytic leukaemia and high-grade lymphomas. Patients with acute promyelocytic leukaemia can develop the tumour lysis syndrome, with minor trauma to the patient, or even infection. In this instance there is a release of pro-coagulants from blast cells with the risk of a devastating coagulopathy. Patients with high-grade T-cell lymphomas may also be at risk from circumstances where one would not normally expect there to be a problem. For example, if these patients are started on steroids, they may develop tumour lysis because steroids have cytotoxic qualities in lymphoma. In these malignancies the risk of tumour lysis syndrome is pre-empted by a cunning pretreatment plan. Patients are started two days prior to

Table 46.3 Causes of pleural effusion.

Transudate	Cardiac failure
	Nephrotic syndrome
	Cirrhosis
	Protein-losing enteropathy
	Constrictive pericarditis
	Hypothyroidism
	Peritoneal dialysis
	Meig's syndrome (pleural effusion associated with ovarian fibroma)
Exudate	
Tumour	Primary: lung cancer, mesothelioma
	Secondary: breast or ovary cancer, lymphoma
Infection	Pneumonia
	Tuberculosis
	Subphrenic abscess
Infarction	Pulmonary embolus
Connective tissue disease	Rheumatoid arthritis
	Systemic lupus erythematosus
Others	Pancreatitis (usually left-sided pleural effusion)
	Dressler's syndrome (inflammatory pericarditis and pleurisy following myocardial infarction or heart surgery)
	Yellow nail syndrome (combination of discoloured hypoplastic nails, recurring pleural effusions and lymphedem; aetiology unknown)
	Asbestos exposure

chemotherapy or radiation therapy with allopurinol. The day before treatment intravenous hydration is started, and these efforts generally prevent the development of tumour lysis syndrome. Many clinicians advise alkalinization of the urine. However, in practice it is very difficult to achieve an alkaline urine and there are significant dangers inherent in the use of significant amounts of sodium bicarbonate. A proportion of patients will go on to develop tumour lysis syndrome despite these measures. For this reason patients who are treated require careful monitoring with two-hourly measurement of serum potassium levels for the

first 8–12 hours of treatment. Many clinicians will also advise ECG monitoring but it is our experience that these monitors are generally not observed to best effect. A new drug has become recently available for the treatment of this condition. Recombinant urate oxidase (rasburicase) converts uric acid, which is insoluble, into allantoin, which is. Clinical trials have shown that urate oxidase controls hyperuricaemia faster and more reliably than allopurinol, and its use is indicated in children and haematological malignancy.

Hyperviscosity syndrome

Blood hyperviscosity can be caused by too much protein or too many cells in the blood. The clinical features include spontaneous bleeding from mucous membranes, retinopathy, headache, vertigo, coma and seizures. The most frequent causes of excess proteins are monoclonal paraproteinaemias such as Waldenström's macroglobulinaemia (IgM) and myeloma (especially IgA and IgG3 myelomas). Hyperviscosity due to excess cell counts occurs in acute leukaemia blast crises. The retinopathy resembles retinal vein occlusion with dilated retinal veins and retinal haemorrhages. The serum viscosity may be measured (normal range: 0.14–0.18 cPa/s), but treatment of suspected hyperviscosity should be started before the results are available as they often take days to come back. Plasmapheresis should be used to decrease hyperviscosity related to excess proteins, whilst leukapheresis removes excess leukaemic blasts before definitive treatment can begin.

Myelosuppression

Neutropenia

We explain to our patients that chemotherapy puts them at risk of developing bone marrow suppression, as cancer treatments kill 'good' as well as 'bad' cells. In this case the 'good' cells are the haematological progenitor cells and patients are at risk of death if the effects of treatment upon the bone marrow are not recognized. Neutropenic sepsis is very common in cancer treatment and, if undiag-

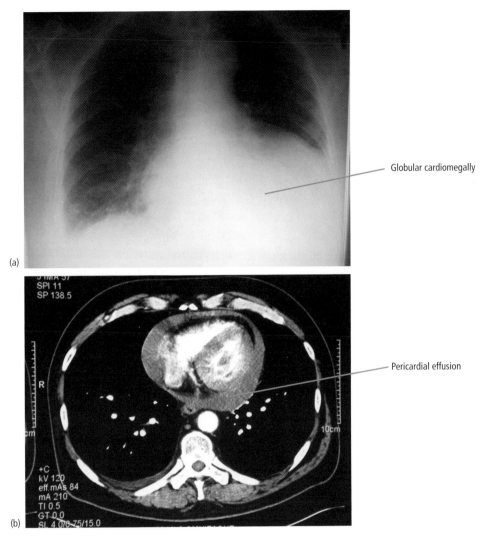

Globular cardiomegally

Pericardial effusion

Figure 46.6 (a) Chest X-ray showing a globular enlarged heart shadow and (b) CT scan confirming a malignant pericardial effusion due to metastatic non-small cell lung cancer. These effusions may present as a medical emergency with cardiac tamponade. The clinical symptoms include dyspnoea and cough and the signs are hypotension, tachycardia, pulsus paradoxus (fall of systolic blood pressure of >10 mmHg on inspiration), quiet muffled heart sounds and a raised jugular–venous pressure (JVP) with Kussmaul's sign (paradoxical rise in JVP on inspiration). The electrocardiograph may show pulsus alternans (alternating QRS voltages). The emergency treatment is by pericardiocentesis and a subsequent surgical formation of a pericardial window to prevent recurrence may be necessary.

nosed, leads to a mortality rate approaching 20–30%. Patients with neutropenic sepsis develop fevers and rigors with associated oral ulceration and candidiasis. It is standard practice for patients with neutropenic sepsis – which is defined by septic symptoms in the presence of a white count that is $<1.0 \times 10^9/l$ – to be admitted to hospital. The patient is resuscitated with intravenous fluids and blood cultures are taken. In the absence of any obvious focus of infection, such as the urinary tract, the advantage of culturing from sites other than blood is virtually zero. Cultures from other

Table 46.4 Electrocardiolgy for oncologists.

Oncological emergency	ECG features	Tracings
Hypercalcaemia	Short QT Broad-based, tall, peaked T waves wide QRS Low R wave Disappearance of P waves	
Pericardial effusion	Sinus tachycardia Low voltage complexes PR segment depression Alternation of the QRS complexes, usually in a 2 : 1 ratio (electrical alternans)	
Tumour lysis Hyperkalaemia	Peaked T waves Flattened P waves Prolonged PR interval Widened QRS complexes Deep S wave	
Hypocalcaemia	Long QT interval Narrow QRS Reduced PR interval Flat or inverted T waves Prominent U wave Ventricular arrhythmia	

sites merely act to swamp the microbiology lab with unnecessary requests for culture work without yielding any positive advantage. Just 20% of blood cultures from patients with neutropenic sepsis are positive for bacterial organisms. The cause for infection is generally not clear.

Antibiotic policies vary from hospital to hospital but there is good evidence that treatment with single-agent ceftazidime is as effective as treatment with combination antibiotic regimens. In the UK patients are generally admitted, though it is interesting to note that this conservative management policy is not strictly necessary. In one randomized study, treatment with oral ciprofloxacin in the community was compared with inpatient treatment with intravenous ceftazidime. The results were absolutely identical in terms of control of fever and patient outcome.

Over the last decade marrow growth factors have become available and granulocyte colony-stimulating factor (G-CSF), which stimulates the marrow to produce granulocytes, has entered wide use. There is no evidence that prophylactic use of G-CSF in any way prevents neutropenic sepsis or septic deaths. The evidence for its use in established infection is poor and the consensus view is that G-CSF is of value only in patients with established neutropenic sepsis who have a non-recovering marrow and in whom, additionally, an infective agent has been identified. G-CSF is of enormous value in transplantation programmes, where the mean period of time to engraftment has been reduced from 28 to 18 days by the use of these agents.

Anaemia

Anaemia is a very common complication of cancer and its treatment. It is estimated that up to 30% of all cancer patients will require a transfusion. In general, anaemia is cumulative and builds up over several cycles of chemotherapy. Recombinant erythropoietin is considered to be a valuable alternative to blood transfusion. The response of patients to erythropoietin is wide ranging and reported at between 20% and 60%. Haemoglobin levels increase after about six weeks of treatment with recombinant erythropoietin. The price of this agent used to be considered prohibitive, however it may become relatively more affordable as the cost of blood is widely predicted to increase significantly because of the increased costs of testing blood for infective agents such as Creutzfeldt–Jakob disease (CJD). The pharmaceutical industry markets erythropoietin for its effect upon the asthenia related to cancer treatment; claims are made for a far greater improvement in cancer fatigue than haemoglobin level.

Thrombocytopenia

Thrombocytopenia is not as significant a problem in the treatment of solid tumours as it is in the treatment of haematological malignancies. There is a significant risk of spontaneous major haemorrhage as the platelet count declines below 10–$20 \times 10^9/l$ and most oncologists advocate prophylactic platelet transfusions at this level or in the presence of bleeding. There are a number of regulatory molecules that stimulate early haematopoietic progenitors and these include the interleukins IL-1, IL-6 and IL-11. IL-1 and IL-6 have poor efficacy and significant toxicity, but IL-11 has been licensed for the prevention of chemotherapy-induced thrombocytopenia. The pharmaceutical industry continues to develop agents for the treatment of thrombocytopenia, and the focus recently has been on analogues of thrombopoietin, which appear to have more efficacy and less toxicity than the interleukins.

Cancer-related thromboses

Patients with cancer have an increased tendency to thrombosis, a problem that was first documented by Trousseau, who sadly went on to develop venous thromboses himself and died from cancer. Patients with cancer have an increased risk of developing thromboses for two major reasons. The first may be a pressure effect, where the primary tumour mass or secondary nodal masses impinge upon the vasculature, producing venous stasis and thrombosis. The second reason for the increased risk is the release from the tumour of pro-coagulants. A number of tissue pro-coagulants have been described, ranging from factors S and C to the current view that activated factor 10 is released by tumours, which sparks off the clotting cascade.

The incidence of venous thrombosis and thromboembolism in cancer patients is variably reported. One study looked at a group of patients presenting with deep venous thromboses (DVTs). Screening of these patients showed that almost 30% had a cancer that was most commonly a pelvic malignancy. As always in medicine, there is initial positive reporting, and later studies showed the true incidence of previously undetected cancer in patients presenting with venous thrombosis to be in the order of 5%. Once cancer has been diagnosed, thromboembolic events are remarkably common and described in about 10% of all patients. The incidence increases significantly

Thrombus in inferior vena cava

Metal filter in inferior vena cava

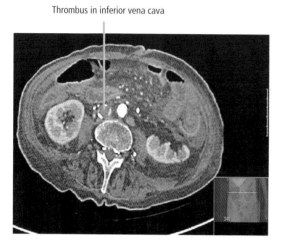 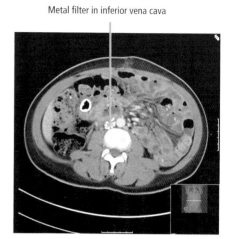

Figure 46.7 CT scan showing an inferior vena cava filter *in situ* in a woman with advanced ovarian cancer and recurrent thromboses.

Thrombus in left and right main pulmonary arteries suggesting saddle embolus

Ventilation scan

Perfusion scan

Large segmental perfusion defect

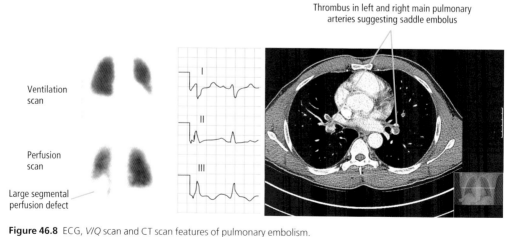

Figure 46.8 ECG, *V/Q* scan and CT scan features of pulmonary embolism.
V/Q scan showing large segmental perfusion defect in the left lower lung and normal ventilation.
ECG showing $Q_ιS_{III}T_{III}$ pattern (S wave in lead I, Q save in lead III and inverted T wave in lead III).
CT scan shows filling defects occluding the central pulmonary artery and extending into all the lobar branches due to saddle embolus.

when long lines are inserted in cancer patients for the purposes of chemotherapy or supportive care. In this group of patients the incidence of thromboembolism increases to 20%. For this reason prophylaxis with low-dose warfarin is recommended and this decreases the risk of subsequent thrombosis to between 2% and 5%. These statistics, however, are considered controversial and are debated endlessly. Because of the high risk of thrombosis in cancer patients it has been suggested that anticoagulation should be prophylactically prescribed. Logically, the best way of preventing thromboembolism would be with a heparin-like compound rather than with a coumarin. At the moment the evidence is that the low molecular weight heparins are probably more effective than warfarin in the prophylaxis of thromboembolism. There is an additional unexpected benefit to anticoagulation with low molecular weight heparins, and this is a modest survival advantage for patients, as demonstrated by randomized clinical trials. In some patients with pelvic tumours and recurrent thromboses, filters may be inserted into the inferior vena cava to reduce the risk of pulmonary embolism (Figures 46.7 and 46.8). The benefits of filters are transient.

Chapter 47

End of life care

Amongst the most important elements of oncological care is recognizing shifting goals as the cancer progresses. The balance of benefit and side effects of any intervention should be carefully weighed up. Whilst neurosurgical resection of solitary metastases from melanoma may be appropriate in some circumstances, venepuncture for measuring the serum electrolytes in a dying patient is rarely justifiable. These decisions should involve the patients wherever possible and require skilful use of communication. Throughout the cancer journey patients often enquire about their life expectancy and there is a temptation for clinicians to pluck some figure out of the air. An intelligent doctor will recognize the pitfalls of prognostication when applied to an individual and will appreciate that the median survival (the statistic most relevant in this circumstance) is the time when half the patients will still be alive. Stephen J. Gould, the evolutionary palaeontologist, explained this from a patient's perspective in the essay 'The median is not the message' published in the collection *Bully for Brontosaurus*. During the patient's journey with cancer a number of emotions are experienced and these may follow a stepwise succession originally described by the Swiss psychologist Elisabeth Kubler Ross. In her 1969 book

On Death and Dying she records the stages as denial, anger, bargaining, grieving and finally acceptance.

As the cancer progresses and the patient deteriorates, it is important that reviews are frequent and that problems are anticipated. This close follow-up is often best undertaken in the community by community palliative care services rather than bringing patients up to hospital or GP surgeries for regular appointments, but this approach requires excellent communication between all the health professionals involved. This may be facilitated by patient-held records similar to those used in shared care obstetrics. The anticipation of symptoms, including pain and diminishing mobility, should be addressed in advance so that analgesia is quickly available to patients.

Pain control

Nerve endings, or nociceptors, exist in all tissues and are stimulated by noxious agents including chemical, mechanical and thermal stimuli, giving rise to pain (Table 47.1). These stimuli are relayed by $A\beta$, $A\delta$ (fast transmitting fibres) and C (slow transmission of sensation) sensory nerve fibres to the dorsal horns of the spinal cord and different qualities of pain may use different sensory fibres.

Analgesic drugs form the mainstay of treating cancer pain and should be chosen based on the severity of the pain rather than the stage of the

Lecture Notes: Oncology, 2nd edition. By M. Bower and J. Waxman. Published 2010 by Blackwell Publishing Ltd.

Table 47.1 Definition of pain terms.

Term	Definition
Allodynia	Pain due to a stimulus that does not normally cause pain
Analgesia	Absence of pain in response to stimulation that would normally be painful
Dysesthesia	An unpleasant abnormal sensation, whether spontaneous or evoked
Hyperalgesia	Heightened response to a normally painful stimulus
Hyperpathia	An abnormally painful reaction to a stimulus, especially a repetitive stimulus, as well as an increased threshold
Hypoalgesia	Diminished pain in response to a normally painful stimulus
Neuralgia	Pain in the distribution of a nerve or nerves
Neuropathic pain	Pain initiated or caused by a primary lesion or dysfunction in the peripheral nervous system
Nociception	Nervous system activity resulting from potential or actual tissue-damaging stimuli
Paraesthesia	An abnormal sensation, whether spontaneous or evoked

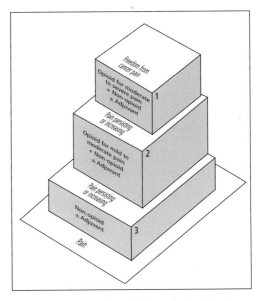

Figure 47.1 The World Health Organization's three step ladder to the use of analgesic drugs.

cancer. Drugs should be administered regularly to prevent pain using a stepwise escalation from non-opioid, to weak opioid and strong opioid analgesia (Figure 47.1). Adjuvant drugs may be added at any stage of the analgesic ladder as they may have additional analgesic effect in some painful conditions. Examples of adjuvant analgesics are corticosteroids, non-steroidal anti-inflammatory drugs, tricyclic antidepressants, anticonvulsants and some anti-arrythmic drugs. Morphine is the most commonly used strong opioid analgesic and whenever possible should be given by mouth. The dose of morphine needs to be tailored to each patient and be repeated at regular intervals so that the pain does not return between doses. There is no upper dose limit for morphine; however, a number of myths have arisen around opioid prescribing that may deter prescribers as well as patients. Firstly, opioid tolerance is rarely seen in patients with

cancer pain and neither psychological dependence nor addiction is a problem in this patient group. The toxicity of opioids may prove to be an obstacle for some patients (Table 47.2). Sedation is common at the start of opioid therapy but resolves in most patients within a few days. Similarly, nausea and vomiting may prove troublesome at the start of regular opioid dosing but usually dissipate within a few days and may be controlled with anti-emetics. Constipation develops in almost all patients on opioids and this toxicity persists and necessitates routine prophylactic laxatives for almost everyone receiving opioids. A careful explanation of these issues will result in the acceptance of opioid analgesia by almost all patients.

Care of the dying patient

The continuing attention to the needs and comfort of a dying patient is as important as the care given to any other patient and part of that care includes reducing the distress of relatives. Many issues may be raised by relatives that pose ethical dilemmas and these may make you question the therapy that has been or should be given. Amongst the most

269

Table 47.2 Side effects of opiates.

Side effect	Comments
Constipation	This affects almost all patients and all patients require prophylaxis with a stimulant laxative (e.g. senna, bisacodyl) and a softener (e.g. docusate sodium) or as a combined preparation (e.g. co-danthramer, co-danthrusate)
Drowsiness	Generally remits after a few days
Nausea	Affects one-third of opioid naïve patients but usually resolves within 1 week. Consider prophylaxis for 1 week
Hallucinations	An uncommon side effect that often features images in the peripheral vision
Nightmares	Vivid and unpleasant but rare
Myoclonic jerks	Occur usually with excess doses and may be mistaken for fits
Respiratory depression	Not a problem in patients with pain

frequent scenarios is the role of intravenous hydration, evaluating the balance between painful cannulation and restriction of mobility versus an uncomfortable dry mouth and thirst. To address these questions you should consider whether death from the cancer is now inevitable, whether interventions would relieve symptoms and whether treatment would cause harm. Careful explanation to the relatives is essential; in this circumstance, for example, they need to be reassured that the patient is not dying because of dehydration but rather because of progression of the cancer.

Symptom control in the dying patient often requires a different route of administration as swallowing may be difficult and agitation and restlessness are often prominent features as death approaches. A number of factors may contribute to terminal agitation including physical causes such as pain, sore mouth and full bladder or rectum, along with emotional factors including fear of dying and the distress of relatives. The physical causes should be addressed appropriately and unnecessary medications should be stopped. Often the best method of delivering analgesia, anti-emetics and sedation, if appropriate, is via a subcutaneous syringe driver. Similarly, oral secretions accumulating in a patient who is too weak to cough may be distressing to the patient and family alike. Drug treatment for terminal secretions includes hyoscine hydrobromide and glycopyrronium bromide, which is less sedating. It is important to recall that not all patients wish to be sedated and this should be discussed with them and their families.

The last hours and days

For many patients with cancer the last hours and days are heralded by a deterioration to semiconsciousness. At this time patients are usually unable to take oral medication and prescriptions need to be reconsidered. Many medicines may be stopped altogether and alternative routes of administration, including subcutaneous, rectal and transdermal routes, may be employed for other necessary medications including analgesia. Although patients may no longer be receiving medicines by mouth, oral hygiene remains an important part of overall care. It is particularly important to avoid unnecessary unpleasant interventions at this time and to adopt a practical problem-oriented approach to symptom control. A practical guide to the care of the dying patient in a hospital was developed at the Royal Liverpool Hospital in conjunction with Marie Curie Cancer Care to transfer best practice learnt from hospice care. The Liverpool Care of the Dying Pathway helps members of the multidisciplinary team in making a decision about which medical interventions should be stopped and which continued (including anticipatory prescribing) and what comfort measures should be started. It also promotes psychological support of the patients, family and carers as well as addressing spiritual needs and bereavement. There has been debate recently about the value of the Liverpool Pathway, with some critics suggesting that it is a one-way road that sanitizes and precipitates the process of dying without allowing thought or revison of decisions.

When death is inevitable, as it is for all of us, and is approaching rapidly it is the policy in many UK hospitals to discuss resuscitation policies with patients and their relatives. Under these circumstances resuscitation is rarely appropriate and, if deemed futile, the lead clinician may make a DNAR (do not attempt resuscitation) decision. These DNAR decisions should be discussed with patients who wish to engage in advanced care planning. However, prolonged discussions about DNAR policies with patients who do not wish to contemplate their future are, in the view of these authors, distressing and irrelevant. The reason for our autocratic view is that cardiac resuscitation cannot return the patient who has died from cancer from his journey across the River Styx, and it causes distress in the relatives and the arrest team.

Bereavement

Bereavement care and support includes recognizing the physical and emotional needs of families and carers and continues after the patient's death. A number of features have been identified that are associated with the risk of severe bereavement reactions (Table 47.3), and the recognition of these risks prior to death can allow planning of care for those left behind after the death. Health professionals are not immune to bereavement, or at least the good ones are not, and our need for support should not be ignored.

The culture of death and dying

Just as different cultures, regardless of the scientific evidence, have developed distinct explanations for

the origins of life ranging from Big Bangs and evolution to creationist genesis, similar cultural variations affect attitudes to death. For example, Christians, Jews (Box 47.1) and Sufis believe in resurrection whilst Hindi, Buddhists (Box 47.2) and Sikhs believe in reincarnation. These cultural discrepancies must be recognized and respected, particularly where patients' and carers' views differ.

Box 47.1: Jewish mourners' Kaddish prayer

Glorified and sanctified be God's great name throughout the world which He has created according to His will. May He establish His kingdom in your lifetime and during your days, and within the life of the entire House of Israel, speedily and soon; and say, Amen.

May His great name be blessed forever and to all eternity. Blessed and praised, glorified and exalted, extolled and honoured, adored and lauded be the name of the Holy One, blessed be He, beyond all the blessings and hymns, praises and consolations that are ever spoken in the world; and say, Amen.

May there be abundant peace from heaven, and life, for us and for all Israel; and say, Amen.

He who creates peace in His celestial heights, may He create peace for us and for all Israel; and say, Amen.

With a strong belief in an afterlife, mourning practices in Judaism are extensive, but are not an expression of fear of death. Instead they aim to show respect for the dead and to comfort the living. As an expression of respect, following death the body is never left alone and on hearing of the death, friends and relatives tear a portion of their clothes. Burial is prompt, within 2 days, and is followed by 7 days of mourning (shiva). Mourners sit on low stools or the floor instead of chairs, do not wear leather shoes, do not shave or cut their hair, do not wear cosmetics, do not work and do not do things for comfort or pleasure, such as bathe, have sex or put on fresh clothing. Mourners wear the clothes that they tore at the time of learning of the death and mirrors in the house are covered. The Jewish Kaddish prayer is recited for the first 11 months following a death by identified mourners and on each anniversary of the death (Yahrzeit). It is remarkable that there is no reference to death in the prayer but rather it focuses on the greatness of God and on a call for peace.

Table 47.3 Risk factors for bereavement.

Patient	Young
Cancer	Short illness, disfiguring
Death	Sudden, traumatic (haemorrhage)
Relationship to patient	Dependent or hostile
Main carer	Young, other dependents, physical or mental illness, unsupported

Box 47.2: The *Tibetan Book of the Dead* (bardo thodol)

A fundamental tenet of Buddhism is that death is not something that awaits us in some distant future, but something that we bring with us into the world and that accompanies us throughout our lives. Rather than a finality, death offers a unique opportunity for spiritual growth with the ultimate prospect of transformation into an immortal state of benefit to others. Among Tibet's many and varied religious traditions are esoteric teachings that address compassionate death including the *Tibetan Books of the Dead*. These popular texts are manuals of practical instructions for the dying, who are immediately facing death; for those who have died, who are wandering in the intermediate state between lives; and for the living, who are left behind to continue without their loved ones.

Before death, friends and relatives are encouraged to bid farewell without excess drama so that neither regret nor longing is experienced by the dying as their state of mind at death must be positive. This may be facilitated by a spiritual master (lama) whispering guiding instructions from *Liberation Through Hearing during the Intermediate State* commonly known as the *Tibetan Book of the Dead* into the dying person's ear.

Tibetan Buddhism recognizes that spiritual growth may be derived from acknowledging death and proposes detailed meditation strategies that relate to the acceptance of death in order to comprehend the nature of human existence. Four human life cycle stages are recognized: birth, the period between birth and death, death, and the interval between death and rebirth (the bardo). This post-mortem bardo lasts seven weeks and is followed by rebirth into a worldly state that is influenced by past actions or karma. The cycle of rebirth (samsara) may be broken by enlightenment, culminating in the final liberation of buddhahood.

Self-assessment MCQs

1. In a woman, what carries the greatest risk for breast cancer?
   a. family history of breast cancer
   b. previous contralateral breast cancer
   c. benign breast disease
   d. oral contraceptive usage
   e. nulliparity

2. A 30-year-old man receives BEP chemotherapy for a metastatic germ cell tumour. He develops interstitial lung disease. Which drug is most likely to be responsible?
   a. bleomycin
   b. etoposide
   c. cisplatin
   d. ondansetron
   e. filgrastim (G-CSF)

3. A 55-year-old woman had surgery, radiotherapy and adjuvant chemotherapy for breast cancer three years previously. She presents with lower back pain and mild leg weakness. An MRI scan reveals vertebral bone metastases and cord compression at L1. What is the most appropriate treatment?
   a. physiotherapy and mobilization
   b. surgical decompression and radiotherapy
   c. chemotherapy
   d. endocrine therapy
   e. non-steroidal anti-inflammatory drugs and bed rest

4. A 79-year-old smoker presented with dyspnoea. Investigations reveal a 10 cm lung mass and a serum sodium of 112 mmol/l. What histological subtype of lung cancer is most likely?
   a. small cell carcinoma
   b. adenocarcinoma
   c. squamous cell carcinoma
   d. large cell carcinoma
   e. carcinoid

5. A woman received extended field mantle radiotherapy for stage 2A Hodgkin's lymphoma; 10 years later, what malignancy is the most likely sequelae?
   a. thyroid carcinoma
   b. acute myeloid leukaemia
   c. non-Hodgkin's lymphoma
   d. breast cancer
   e. ovarian germ cell tumour

6. A 26-year-old man is treated with the CODOX-M/IVAC chemotherapy regimen for sporadic Burkitt lkymphoma. Which cytotoxic drug causes the least bone marrow suppression?
   a. cyclophosphamide
   b. doxorubicin
   c. ifosfamide
   d. etoposide
   e. vincristine

7. What is the most common site of spread of epithelial ovarian tumours?
   a. inguinal lymph nodes
   b. adnexae
   c. bone
   d. lungs
   e. liver

8. A 28-year-old woman presents with amenorrhoea, a large uterus and multiple rounded opacities on her chest X-ray. Which serum tumour marker is most helpful in establishing a diagnosis of choriocarcinoma?
   a. carcinoembryonic antigen
   b. human chorionic gonadotropin
   c. α-fetoprotein
   d. CA-125
   e. Ca199

9. A 60-year-old woman undergoing chemotherapy for acute myeloid leukaemia develops chemotherapy refractory disease. Which of the following is most likely to be overexpressed by the leukaemia cells and account for the chemotherapy resistance?
   a. P glycoprotein
   b. p53
   c. Bcl-2
   d. P450
   e. myc

10. Which cancer is most likely to produce bone metastases that are osteoblastic rather than osteolytic?
   a. choriocarcinoma
   b. endometrial cancer
   c. colorectal cancer
   d. ovarian cancer
   e. prostate cancer

11. What is the most common site of tumours in adults who present with myasthenia gravis?
   a. skeletal muscle
   b. stomach
   c. lung
   d. thymus
   e. thyroid

12. Red cell aplasia due to failure to produce erythrocytes is a paraneoplastic syndrome. What tumour type is most frequently associated with it?
   a. carcinoid
   b. glucagonoma
   c. insulinoma
   d. neuroblastoma
   e. thymoma

13. Which secretory endocrine islet cell tumour produces a distinctive, severe rash?
   a. gastrinoma
   b. glucagonoma
   c. insulinoma
   d. somatostatinoma
   e. VIPoma

14. Which of the following facts concerning the risk of mesothelioma is true?
   a. mesothelioma is more common in women than men
   b. the wives of asbestos workers have an increased risk of mesothelioma
   c. since the banning of asbestos in the 1980s the incidence of mesothelioma is falling
   d. the risk of mesothelioma decreases with age
   e. asbestos exposure is not a risk for peritoneal mesothelioma

15. The high incidence of hepatitis B infection in Africa and parts of Asia is thought to be causally associated with increased incidence of which malignancy?
   a. hepatocellular carcinoma
   b. oesophageal cancer
   c. Burkitt lymphoma
   d. gastric carcinoma
   e. Kaposi's sarcoma

16. Brachytherapy involves the delivery of radiation therapy locally by direct apposition to the treated tissue. What is the most common radioisotope used in this application?
   a. iodine-125
   b. carbon-14

c. hydrogen-3

d. phosphorus-34

e. fluorine-18

17. DNA viruses have been implicated in several human tumours. Evidence for a causative role exists for which of the following neoplasms?

a. Burkitt lymphoma

b. testicular germ cell tumour

c. mesothelioma

d. osteogenic sarcoma

e. oesophageal carcinoma

18. A woman of 63 years has advanced metastatic breast cancer and is confined to bed due to painful bone metastases. What is her ECOG (Eastern Co-operative Oncology Group) performance status?

a. 0

b. 1

c. 2

d. 3

e. 4

19. Childhood retinoblastoma occurs in both sporadic and familial forms. What feature occurs more often in the sporadic form?

a. bilateral retinoblastoma

b. later age at retinoblastoma onset

c. family history of retinoblastoma

d. germline mutation of the Rb gene

e. development of osteosracoma

20. A 45-year-old man with long-standing gastro-esophageal reflux undergoes upper endoscopy that reveals patchy areas of epithelium resembling gastric mucosa extending 5 cm proximal to the oesophagogastric junction. Biopsies are obtained. The pathological report describes 'Barrett's epithelium'. Which of the following processes does this finding represent?

a. cellular hyperplasia

b. cellular hypertrophy

c. metaplasia

d. carcinoma *in situ*

e. cellular atrophy

21. What are the chances that you will die of cancer?

a. 1 in 4

b. 1 in 8

c. 1 in 9

d. 1 in 20

e. 1 in 40

22. Which skin condition is premalignant?

a. seborrhoeic keratosis

b. actinic keratosis

c. blue naevus

d. strawberry naevus

e. haemangioma

23. How much does it cost to develop a new cancer drug?

a. £1 billion

b. £750 million

c. £100 million

d. £10 million

e. £1 million

24. What is the current UK NHS budget?

a. £100 million

b. £200 million

c. £10 billion

d. £100 billion

e. Not enough

25. What proportion of the European average does the UK spend on cancer drugs?

a. 60%

b. 100%

c. 150%

d. 10%

e. 200%

26. What percentage of patients with humeral hypercalcaemia of malignancy respond to bisphosphonates?

a. 80%

b. 96%

c. 42%

d. 50%

e. 10%

27. What is the main obstacle to cancer cure?
    a. money
    b. love
    c. lifestyle
    d. big pharma
    e. doctors

28. What is the source of at least 95% of the drugs that we use for cancer treatment?
    a. big pharma
    b. universities
    c. crackpot researchers
    d. government
    e. World Health Organization

29. What is the androgen receptor?
    a. an oncogene
    b. something that you take with a sip of water
    c. a transcription factor
    d. a source of embarrassment
    e. cytoplasmic and nuclear protein that trimerizes when activated

Answers to MCQs

1. b
2. a
3. b
4. a
5. d
6. e
7. b
8. b
9. a
10. e
11. d
12. e
13. b
14. b
15. a

16. a
17. a
18. e
19. b
20. c
21. a
22. b
23. b
24. d
25. a
26. a
27. c
28. a
29. d

Index

Page numbers in italic, e.g. *214*, refer to boxes, figures or tables.